A CON
GUI
OVER THE COUNTER
MEDICINES

A CONSUMER'S GUIDE TO OVER THE COUNTER MEDICINES

Dr Barrington Cooper, Dr Laurence Gerlis,
and Elizabeth Jeannet

Pharmaceutical Consultant: Dawn Hurrell

● Fully revised and reorganized to take account of the latest developments ●
● Over 1600 over-the-counter medicines and remedies listed ●
● All widely available herbal remedies included ●
● All widely available homeopathic preparations included ●
● Completely new sections to include fluoride supplements, sleeping
problems and stress, anti-smoking treatments, contraceptives, and more ●
● Key medical terms explained ●
● Now with a Glossary of Herbal Remedies ●

HAMLYN

Edited and typeset by Neil Curtis, Publishing Services
Designed by Richard Garratt

This edition first published 1996
Hamlyn is an imprint of Reed International Books
Michelin House, 81 Fulham Road, London SW3 6RB
and Auckland, Melbourne, Singapore and Toronto

A catalogue record for this book is available from the British Library.

ISBN 0 600 58898 X

Printed in Great Britain

IMPORTANT

As the introduction explains, *A Consumer's Guide to Over
the Counter Medicines* is designed to be a self-treatment book
only for minor conditions. It would be used, therefore,
before consulting a physician to gain information about
medicines which are available, without a prescription, from
pharmacies, health food shops, and so on. On the other
hand, the *Guide* is **not intended** to be a substitute for the
advice of a prescribing physician nor for the instructions on
the medicine's package. Similarly, it is advisable to consult a
herbal or homoeopathic practitioner if you intend to use
alternative therapies.

Every effort has been made to ensure that the information
contained in the book is as accurate and up-to-date as possible at the time of going to press but medical and pharmaceutical knowledge continues to progress, and the use of a
particular medicine may be different for every patient.
Always consult your medical practitioner if any symptoms
from which you are suffering persist or worsen.

The authors, editors, consultants, and publishers of this book
can not be held liable for any errors or omissions, nor for
any consequences of using it.

CONTENTS

Introduction

This is the second edition of *A Consumer's Guide to Over the Counter Medicines*. It is a companion to our other books *A Consumer's Guide to Prescription Medicines* and *Your Symptoms Diagnosed*.

More people are turning to self-medication, and society is also turning towards it. This book arms them with the information to self-treat with acceptable safety margins. There is no such thing as 100 per cent safety in medicines, and readers of this book are encouraged to seek medical advice if they suffer serious side effects or if their symptoms worsen or persist.

Since the last edition of this book was published, a number of former prescription-only medicines have moved to over-the-counter status. These include powerful anti-ulcer remedies, such as Zantac and Tagamet, as well as the anti-viral cream Zovirax. This trend is to be encouraged, because it will allow those patients who are interested in self-treatment to treat themselves under the supervision of an experienced pharmacist. With healthcare costs increasing, this will relieve the burden on the health service and allow more serious conditions more time and resources. We do not, however, wish to promote excessive self-medication nor drive ill patients away from doctors' surgeries. We do believe in a partnership between doctors, patients, and pharmacists in caring for patients rather than the professions being simply distant, advisory, and sometimes adversarial. This book contains homeopathic and herbal remedies as well as more orthodox treatments. We do not endorse any product, however, since effects vary from person to person.

In general terms, this book is intended for the treatment of minor conditions. Potentially serious conditions, such as headache, chest pain, abdominal pain, painful eye, or ear ache, should be referred to a medical practitioner, particularly if they occur as a result of injury. Where possible, a diagnosis should be made before treatment begins. Our intention is to help you make informed choices.

Dr Barrington Cooper
Dr Laurence Gerlis
21 Devonshire Place
London
W1
1996

Alternative therapies

As orthodox practitioners, we rarely recommend or prescribe alternative or natural remedies. Having said this, we often use multivitamin preparations in recovery from viral infections such as ME (myalgic encephalomyelitis). Until recently, we used tryptophan in high doses to treat depression but this has now fallen into disrepute because one source of this amino acid caused a side effect known as EMS (eosinophilic myalgic syndrome). This is a reminder to us that alternative remedies, which use small quantities of proteins, minerals, vitamins, and herbs, may still cause allergic reactions, and some suppliers have better quality control than others.

Because increasing numbers of people are turning to alternative therapies, we have included alternative preparations in the relevant sections of this book, (and homeopathic remedies are listed separately). We are not in a position to recommend any particular treatment, and readers are advised to consult an alternative medicine practitioner or to discuss their treatment with their supplier. We can, however, give a few points of guidance.

Although most alternative remedies have not undergone formal clinical trials, there are some areas where specific products have achieved generally accepted success. Herbs have a longer history of use than any other form of medicine, and more than 25 per cent of existing medicinal drugs are extracted or have originated from plant materials. Many herbal remedies, therefore, are well known for their effects. Garlic is felt to be responsible for the low incidence of heart disease among French people. Peppermint oil is used to treat irritable bowel, and bran to treat bowel disorders. Herbal extracts such as kelp (seaweed), may often be rich in minerals.

Live yoghurt extracts may treat candida (thrush). In France, doctors routinely prescribe acidophilus (a bacterial extract) with antibiotics to prevent thrush but, in the United Kingdom, the only such preparation available is an alternative therapy (*see* 'Miscellaneous' section). Many rheumatologists see patients who claim to have benefited from either mussel extracts or cod liver oil. Similarly, many women take evening primrose oil or vitamin B6 for premenstrual symptoms.

Many of the alternative remedies are amino acid or protein extracts. Amino acids are the building blocks of proteins, and they cannot be stored in the body. True deficiency is rare, but many people believe that one can build up muscle and lose fat by taking high-protein supplements. These proteins may have an antidepressant effect.

Many of the preparations listed here are licensed under the Medicines Act of 1968. (Those not so licensed are marked * to denote unlicensed status). The granting of a product licence means that they are entitled to be called medicines, and that there are specific controls over what the product contains, where it may be sold, in what form, and with what recommendations for use. Manufacture is subject to Department of Health inspection, and the licence ensures that the product has been screened for safety, quality, and efficacy. The PL number that you will see on the product packet indicates that the medicine holds a full product licence. A PLR number denotes a product licence of right, and the product has not been so completely screened, because it was on the market before the introduction of the licensing scheme. An HR number relates to homeopathic remedies (*see* 'Homeopathic preparations' section), and indicates that the product has been screened for safety and quality.

There are many unlicensed alternative remedies to be found in health food shops and pharmacies. If they do not hold a licence, however, they may only describe themselves as food supplements and not as medicines. The licensing procedure is costly and so, for financial reasons, many smaller companies may choose not to apply for licences. Many of these unlicensed supplements may be excellent and may be closely comparable to their licensed counterparts.

It is important not to treat alternative remedies lightly, simply because they are not classified as medicines. Remember that there is always the possibility of allergic reaction, and many of them may be toxic in high doses. The manufacturer's directions must always be followed accurately. It is worth remembering that side effects can occur with all treatments, whether orthodox or alternative. If you are already taking medication, you should consult your doctor, pharmacist, or alternative practitioner about the advisability of taking an alternative medicine. Advice should always be sought before taking alternative medicines during pregnancy or breastfeeding, or before giving alternative medicines to young children.

How to use this book

A Consumer's Guide to Over-the-Counter Medicines is divided into a series of sections. Each section is concerned with the various disorders of one part of the body. Thus, anyone with an eye or ear condition should consult the relevant section. (Treatments on skin infections should be sought under the section on skin disorders, as well as among the antiseptics and antifungals.) Each product is listed with information such as side effects, contra-indications (when the drug should not be used), and interactions (what the drug should not be mixed with).

We have grouped preparations according to their general use, and have tried to include as many preparations as possible. If you cannot find any particular preparation, the other products used for that condition will give general guidance for use, provided the ingredients are the same. For example, many iron supplements may cause stomach upset, and should not be used with some antibiotics. The entry for ferrous sulphate is typical of medications in this category, and, if you cannot find your iron supplement listed, ferrous sulphate will give you some general information.

The paragraph headed 'not to be used with' includes other medicines, substances such as alcohol, or even foods that should not be taken at the same time as the drug prescribed. This is because the medicine may interact with one or more of the substances mentioned in an unpleasant, harmful, or potentially dangerous way. On the other hand, for an individual patient, there may be no serious interaction at all, but this cannot be predicted. It may be possible to take the medicines at different times of day to eliminate an adverse effect, but this is variable according to the nature of the interaction. Always consult your doctor or pharmacist before taking such a mixture.

All the preparations included in this book are also listed in the index so that you may check on a drug that has been recommended to you. Please remember that a drug that is suitable for one person may be totally inappropriate for another. The information contained in this guide will help you to use over-the-counter medicines safely, but ask for advice at a pharmacy if you require further assistance.

manufacturer's brand name or generic name

manufacturer

dose range, including variations for children or for the elderly (note: this is for guidance only and you always follow the instructions on the medicine's label

general description, including physical appearance, the type of drug, and the conditions it is used to treat

Actifed Compound
(Warner Wellcome Consumer Healthcare)

A linctus used as an antihistamine opiate cough suppressant and sympathomimetic decongestant to treat dry cough and nasal congestion.

Dose: adults 10 ml 4 times a day; (children 2-5 years ¼ adult dose, 6-12 years ½ adult dose).

Side effects: drowsiness, rapid or abnormal heart rate. dry mouth, anxiety, shaking hands.

Caution: pregnant women, asthmatics, and patients taking other medication should consult a doctor before taking this product.

Not to be used for: children under 2 years, or for patients with high blood pressure, thyroid disease, heart disease, or diabetes.

Not to be used with: alcohol, other sedating medicines, MAOIs, betablockers, antihypertensives, tricyclic antidepressants.

Contains: triprolidine hydrochloride, pseudoephedrine hydrochloride, dextromethorphan hydrobromide.

these are the most commonly noted side effects. In many cases, however, no side effects or only some will be experienced

circumstances where care should be exercised by certain groups of patients or those taking other medicines

any groups of patients who should not take this medication

these are substances, such as alcohol or foods, or other drugs, with which this medicine should not be taken

the active ingredients of the medicine

Eye conditions

The main eye disorders are infections, inflammations, cataract, and glaucoma. Because of the sensitive nature of the eyes, most of these should be treated by a doctor using a prescription medicine. A few eye preparations are available over the counter, and some of these can be used in the early stages of eye infections to irrigate and to disinfect the eye. Others contain lubricants for those people whose natural tear production is reduced. Contact lens solutions are also licensed medicinal products available without prescription.

Whatever the symptoms, self-treatment should not be prolonged beyond twenty-four hours unless there is definite improvement in the condition. Redness of the eye, pain in the eye, altered vision, painful reaction to light, and pus in the eye are all symptoms that require medical attention relatively quickly. Insertion of drops or ointments into the eye may cause temporary blurring of the vision, and you should not drive or operate machinery while the eyesight is affected.

Eye infections are most commonly due to bacteria, and may improve after twenty-four hours' use of one of the products listed here. If not, antibiotic treatment may be necessary after a consultation with a doctor. Some viruses affect the eye and can cause permanent damage. (A medical opinion and the use of antiviral drugs will be needed to resolve the virus).

Hayfever sufferers (and people with other allergies) can experience reddening, itching, and watering of the eyes. Specific anti-allergy drops are available to treat this type of condition (see 'Allergic disorders' section).

Red eyes may be due simply to irritation caused by cigarette smoke, dust, chlorine, etc., but prolonged

10/10
(CIBA Vision)

A cleaning and disinfection system (consisting of two different solutions) for all types of contact lenses.

Use: clean and rinse lens, soak for at least 10 minutes in the cleaning/disinfecting solution, then rinse in the rinsing/ neutralizing solution.

Aosept
(CIBA Vision)

A disinfecting, neutralizing, and storing solution (supplied with Aodisc neutralizing catalyst) for all types of contact lenses.

Use: soak for 6 hours (or overnight) in solution containing Aodisc neutralizing catalyst.

Artificial Tears Minims
(Chauvin)

Drops packed in single-use containers and used to treat dry eyes.

Dose: 1-2 drops in the eye 3 or 4 times a day.
Side effects:
Caution:
Not to be used for:
Not to be used with:
Contains: hydroxyethylcellulose, sodium chloride.

Bausch & Lomb
(Bausch & Lomb)

A care system consisting of a cleaner and wetting/soaking

solution for gas-permeable contact lenses.

Use: clean lens with cleaning solution, then soak in wetting/ soaking solution for 10 hours before rinsing and inserting into eye.

Boots Easiclens see Opti-free
(Boots)

Boots Effervescent Protein Remover Tablets see Hydrocare Fizzy
(Boots)

Boots Eye Drops
(Boots)

Soothing and antiseptic eye drops used to refresh tired and irritated eyes.

Dose: 1-2 drops in each eye when required.
Side effects:
Caution:
Not to be used for: patients who wear contact lenses.
Not to be used with:
Contains: witch hazel, cetrimide (in a solution buffered with borax and boric acid).

Boots Gas-permeable All-in-One Solution see Total
(Boots)

Boots Hard Lens Cleaning Solution see Contactaclean
(Boots)

Boots Hard Lens Soaking Solution see **Contactasoak**
(Boots)

Boots Hard Lens Wetting Solution see **Contactasol**
(Boots)

Boots Preservative Free Contact Lens System see **10/10**
(Boots)

Boots Preservative Free Cleaner see **LC65**
(Boots)

Boots Soft Lens Cleaning Solution see **Hydroclean**
(Boots)

Boots Soft Lens Comfort Solution see **Hydrosol**
(Boots)

Boots Soft Lens Soaking Solution see **Hydrosoak**
(Boots)

Boston
(Mid-Optic)

A care system consisting of a cleaner and wetting/soaking
solution for gas-permeable contact lenses.

Use: clean lens by rubbing for 20 seconds with cleaning
solution, then soak for at least 10 hours in soaking/wetting
solution, before rinsing with fresh soaking/wetting solution and
inserting into eye.

Brolene Eye Drops
(Rhone-Poulenc Rorer Family Health)

Drops supplied with or without autodrop device (to aid administration) and used to treat minor eye infections such as sticky eyes and conjunctivitis.

Dose: 1-2 drops up to four times a day.
Side effects: rash or itching around eyes.
Caution: pregnant women and nursing mothers should consult a doctor before using this product. Consult a doctor if no improvement after 2 days.
Not to be used for: patients who wear contact lenses.
Not to be used with:
Contains: propamidine isethionate.

Brolene eye ointment
(Rhone-Poulenc Rorer Family Health)

An ointment used to treat minor eye and eyelid infections, such as conjunctivitis, styes, and blepharitis.

Dose: apply once or twice a day.
Side effects: rash or itching around the eyes.
Caution: pregnant women and nursing mothers should consult a doctor before using this product. Consult a doctor if no improvement after 2 days.
Not to be used for:
Not to be used with:
Contains: dibromopropamidine isethionate.

Clean-n-Soak
(Allergan)

A cleaning and soaking solution for use with hard and gas-permeable contact lenses.

Use: rub lens with solution to clean, then soak in solution for 4 hours (or overnight) to disinfect.

Clen-zym
(Alcon)

Protein-removing tablets for use with soft contact lenses.

Use: dissolve tablet in saline. Clean lens, rinse then soak in prepared solution for 2-12 hours. Use weekly before disinfection.

Clerz
(CIBA Vision)

Comfort drops for use with all types of contact lenses.

Use: 1-2 drops applied to the eye when needed for extra comfort.

Complete
(Allergan)

A complete contact lens solution, to clean, rinse, and disinfect all soft contact lenses.

Use: clean lens for 15 to 20 seconds, then rinse and soak for at least 4 hours.

Contactaclean
(CIBA Vision)

A cleaning solution for use with hard and gas-permeable contact lenses.

Use: clean lens with this product before disinfecting with appropriate solution.

Contactasoak
(CIBA Vision)

A soaking solution for use with hard and gas-permeable contact lenses.

Use: soak in this product after cleaning, then wet (using appropriate wetting solution) before insertion.

Contactasol
(CIBA Vision)

A wetting solution for use with hard and gas-permeable contact lenses.

Use: wet lens with this solution after disinfection and before insertion into eye.

Eye Dew
(Crookes Healthcare)

Soothing and sympathomimetic drops used to give bright, sparkling, or white eyes.

Dose: 1-2 drops in each eye up to 4 times a day.
Side effects: temporary irritation.
Caution: patients with heart disease, high blood pressure, depression, glaucoma, diabetes or overactive thyroid should consult a doctor before using this product.
Not to be used for: prolonged use, or patients with eye pain or wearing soft contact lenses.
Not to be used with: MAOIs.

Contains: witch hazel, naphazoline hydrochloride.

Fizziclean
(Bausch & Lomb)

Protein-removing tablets for use with soft and hard contact lenses.

Use: Dissolve tablet in saline. Clean lens, then soak in prepared solution for 15 minutes-12 hours. Clean, rinse, and disinfect lens with appropriate solutions before insertion into eye. Use weekly.

Golden Eye see **Brolene**
(Typharm)

Hydrocare Fizzy
(Allergan)

Protein-removing tablets for use with soft or gas-permeable contact lenses.

Use: dissolve tablet in saline solution, soak lens for 15 mins-2 hours, then rinse and disinfect with appropriate solutions. Use weekly.

Hydrocare Preserved Saline with Calcium Deposit Preventer
(Allergan)

Preserved saline solution for use with soft contact lenses (for all procedures where the use of preserved saline is recommended).

Hydroclean
(CIBA Vision)

Cleaning solution for soft contact lenses.

Use: clean with this product, then rinse and disinfect with appropriate solutions before use.

Hydrosoak
(CIBA Vision)

A cleaning and soaking solution for soft contact lenses.

Use: Clean lens with Hydroclean, then soak overnight in this product. Lenses may be inserted straight from soaking solution, or add Hydrosol for extra comfort.

Hydrosol
(CIBA Vision)

A comfort solution for soft contact lenses.

Use: apply when needed for extra comfort, or when first inserting lens into eye.

Hypotears
(CIBA Vision Ophthalmics)

Drops used to moisten dry eyes.

Dose: 1-2 drops when needed.
Side effects:
Caution:
Not to be used for: patients who wear soft contact lenses.
Not to be used with:

Contains: polyvinyl alcohol.

---

hypromellose eye drops

Drops available in various strengths and used to treat tear deficiency.

Dose: 1-2 drops 3 times a day or as required.
Side effects:
Caution:
Not to be used for: patients who wear soft contact lenses.
Not to be used with:
Contains: hypromellose.

Isopto Alkaline see hypromellose eye drops
(Alcon)

Isopto Frin
(Alcon)

Drops to relieve redness of the eye caused by minor irritations.

Dose: 1-2 drops into the eye up to 4 times a day.
Side effects:
Caution: infants and patients who have had eye surgery or who are suffering from glaucoma, high blood pressure, or depression should be seen by a doctor before using this product.
Not to be used for: patients who wear soft contact lenses.
Not to be used with:
Contains: phenylephrine hydrochloride, hypromellose.

Isopto Plain see hypromellose eye drops
(Alcon)

Lacri-Lube
(Allergan)

A preservative-free ointment used for lubricating the eyes and protecting the cornea.

Dose: apply into the eye as needed.
Side effects:
Caution:
Not to be used for:
Not to be used with:
Contains: white soft paraffin, mineral oil, lanolin.

Larch Resin Comp. Lotion
(Weleda)

A lotion used as a herbal remedy to relieve the symptoms of tired, strained eyes.

Dose: apply sparingly around the eyes on the lids and temples as required.
Side effects: irritation.
Caution: keep out of the eyes.
Not to be used for: inflamed eyes.
Not to be used with:
Contains: ananassa fruit, lavender oil.

LC-65
(Allergan)

A non-abrasive daily cleaning solution for all types of contact lenses. (Compatible with all disinfection systems.)

Use: rub lens with solution for 15-20 seconds, then rinse and disinfect with appropriate solutions.

LensFresh
(Allergan)

Comfort drops for all contact lenses.

Use: apply when required to add comfort.

Lens Plus see **saline solution**
(Allergan)

Lensept
(CIBA Vision)

A cleaning and disinfecting solution for soft contact lenses.

Use: clean lens with solution, then soak for 10-20 minutes. Lenses must then be soaked in Lensrins before use.

Lensrins
(CIBA Vision)

A rinsing and storing solution for soft contact lenses.

Use: soak lens for at least 4 hours after cleaning and disinfecting with Lensept.

Liquifilm
(Allergan)

A wetting solution for use with hard or gas-permeable contact lenses.

Use: wet lens before insertion into the eye.

Liquifilm Tears
(Allergan)

Drops available as a multidose bottle or as preservative-free, single-use containers, and used to lubricate dry eyes.

Dose: 1 or 2 drops into the eye as needed.
Side effects:
Caution:
Not to be used for: patients who wear soft contact lenses.
Not to be used with:
Contains: polyvinyl alcohol; (preservative-free drops also contain povidone iodine).

Lubrifilm
(Cusi)

An eye ointment used to lubricate the eye.

Dose: apply when required.
Side effects:
Caution:
Not to be used for:
Not to be used with:
Contains: wool fat, yellow soft paraffin, liquid paraffin.

Miraflow
(CIBA Vision)

A daily cleaning solution for all types of contact lenses.

Use: clean lens before disinfecting with appropriate solution.

Murine see Optrex Clearine
(Abbott)

Normasol
(Seton Healthcare)

A sachet of sterile saline solution, used to wash out the eye, or to wash wounds and burns on the skin.

Dose: use to wash the eye.
Side effects:
Caution: for single use only – do not store the remaining contents of the sachet.
Not to be used for:
Not to be used with:
Contains: sodium chloride solution.

Opti-clean
(Alcon)

A cleaning solution for all types of contact lenses.

Use: apply 1-2 drops to the lens, rub for 20 seconds, then rinse with saline and disinfect with appropriate solution.

Opti-free
(Alcon)

A cleansing and disinfecting system for all soft contact lenses.

Use: clean lenses with Opti-clean, rinse with saline, then soak in Opti-free for at least 6 hours (or overnight) before inserting lenses.

Optrex
(Crookes Healthcare)

Drops and lotion used as an astringent and antiseptic to relieve tired or sore eyes and minor eye irritations.

Dose: 1-2 drops in each eye, or bathe the eye with lotion, when required.
Side effects: allergy.
Caution: children under 3 years should be seen by a doctor before using these products.
Not to be used for: patients who wear soft contact lenses.
Not to be used with:
Contains: witch hazel.

Optrex Clearine
(Crookes Healthcare)

Sympathomimetic and astringent eye drops used to reduce redness in the eye due to minor eye irritations, such as smoke, chlorine, and dust.

Dose: 1-2 drops in each eye up to 4 times a day.
Side effects: temporary irritation.
Caution: patients with eye disease, overactive thyroid, glaucoma, high blood pressure, heart disease, or diabetes should consult a doctor before using this product.
Not to be used for: children under 12 years, or for patients who wear contact lenses or who have pain in the eye.
Not to be used with:
Contains: witch hazel, naphazoline.

Optrex Sterile Emergency Eye Wash
(Optrex)

A bottle of eye wash for single use as a first aid measure in case of accidental injury to the eye (where chemicals, irritants or foreign bodies enter the eye).

Dose: apply to the eye to wash out.
Side effects:
Caution:

Not to be used for:
Not to be used with:
Contains: sodium chloride solution.

Oxysept
(Allergan)

Contact lens solutions available as no. 1 (disinfecting solution) and no. 2 (rinsing and neutralizing solution) for soft lenses.

Use: soak in solution no. 1 for at least 10 minutes (or overnight), then soak in solution no. 2 to neutralize (for 10 mins-12 hours).

Oxysept 1-Step
(Allergan)

Contact lens solutions and tablets used as a disinfecting and neutralizing system for soft contact lenses.

Use: Soak lens for 4 hours (or overnight) in solution containing tablet.

Pliagel
(Alcon)

A daily cleaning solution for use with soft or gas-permeable contact lenses.

Use: Rub solution on to lens, then rinse and disinfect with appropriate solutions before use.

Preflex
(Alcon)

A daily cleaning solution for soft contact lenses.

Use: clean lens for at least 30 seconds, then rinse with appropriate solution before insertion into eye.

Refresh see **Liquifilm Tears**
(Allergan)

Lubricating drops, packed in single-use containers, to treat dry eyes.

Refresh Night Time
(Allergan)

An ointment used as a lubricant to treat dry eyes.

Dose: apply at night.
Side effects:
Caution:
Not to be used for:
Not to be used with:
Contains: white soft paraffin, mineral oil, lanolin alcohols.

Renu Multipurpose Solution
(Bausch & Lomb)

A complete solution for rinsing, disinfecting, lubricating, and cleaning soft contact lenses.

Use: clean lens, rinse with fresh solution, soak for at least 4 hours (or overnight) to disinfect, then rinse with more solution prior to insertion. 1-2 drops may be inserted directly into the eye for lubrication.

Salette see **saline solution**
(Alcon)

saline solution
(Alcon, Allergan, Boots, CIBA Vision)

Sterile saline solution for use with contact lenses (e.g. rinsing, dissolving enzyme tablets, etc.).

---

simple eye ointment see **Lubrifilm**

Sno Tears see **Liquifilm Tears**
(Chauvin)

Soaclens
(Alcon)

A wetting and soaking solution for use with hard and gas-permeable contact lenses.

Use: Soak lens for at least 4 hours before insertion.

Sodium Chloride Minims
(Chauvin)

Drops packed in single-use containers, used to irrigate the eyes.

Softab
(Alcon)

Disinfecting tablets for use with soft contact lenses.

Use: dissolve tablet in non-preserved saline, clean lens, and rinse (using appropriate solutions), then soak in prepared solution for 4 hours or overnight.

Solar Saline Aerosol see **saline solution**
(CIBA Vision)

Sootheye
(Rhone-Poulenc Rorer Family Health)

Eye drops supplied with autodrop appliance for ease of administration, and used to treat minor eye irritations.

Dose: 1-2 drops up to 4 times a day.
Side effects: temporary mild stinging.
Caution:
Not to be used for: patients who wear soft contact lenses.
Not to be used with:
Contains: zinc sulphate.

Steripod Blue
(Seton Healthcare)

A plastic ampoule containing sterile saline solution, used to wash out the eye, or to wash wounds and burns on the skin.

Dose: use to wash the eye.
Side effects:
Caution: for single use only – do not store the remaining contents of the ampoule.
Not to be used for:
Not to be used with:
Contains: sodium chloride solution.

Tears Naturale
(Alcon)

Drops used to lubricate dry eyes.

Dose: 1-2 drops into the eye as needed.

Side effects:
Caution:
Not to be used for: patients who wear soft contact lenses.
Not to be used with:
Contains: dextran, hypromellose.

Total
(Allergan)

A complete solution for wetting, soaking, and cleaning hard and gas-permeable contact lenses.

Use: clean lens, soak overnight, then rinse and wet with fresh solution.

Total Care
(Allergan)

A care system consisting of a cleaning solution, protein-remover tablet, and disinfecting/wetting/storing solution for hard and gas-permeable contact lenses.

Use: clean lens with cleaning solution, rinse with disinfecting solution or saline, then store in disinfecting solution for 6 hours (or overnight). Rinse with fresh disinfecting solution if necessary, and insert into eye. Use the protein-remover tablets weekly by dissolving 1 tablet in disinfecting solution and soaking lens for 6-12 hours. (Rinse with fresh disinfecting solution before insertion into eye.)

Transclean
(Chauvin)

A cleaning solution for use with hard and gas-permeable contact lenses.

Use: clean lens before disinfecting with appropriate solution.

Transdrop
(Chauvin)

An in-use comfort solution for use with hard and gas-permeable contact lenses.

Use: add when required for comfort.

Transoak
(Chauvin)

A soaking solution for hard and gas-permeable contact lenses.

Use: soak after cleaning lens with cleaner, then wet using appropriate solution before insertion.

Transol
(Chauvin)

A wetting solution for hard and gas-permeable contact lenses.

Use: apply to lens before insertion.

Ultrazyme
(Allergan)

Protein-removing tablets for use with soft contact lenses.

Use: dissolve tablet in Oxysept-1 solution, then soak lens for 15 minutes (or overnight). Soak in Oxysept-2 solution for 10 minutes before inserting lens into eye.

Viscotears
(CIBA Vision Ophthalmics)

A liquid gel for treating dry eyes.

Dose: 1 drop in the eye 3-4 times a day.
Side effects: temporary irritation, sticky eyelid.
Caution: children, pregnant women, nursing mothers, and patients with any other eye disorder should consult a doctor before using this product.
Not to be used for: patients who wear contact lenses.
Not to be used with:
Contains: carbomer 940.

Ear conditions

The ear, like the eye, is a delicate organ. Infections in the outer and middle ear are common, and usually respond to prescribed antibiotics. Because infections may involve rupture of the eardrum, they are best seen by a doctor. Most of the preparations below are used for clearing ear wax, although Audax is also licensed for use in painful inflammatory conditions. When there is any pain in the ear, however, it should be examined by a doctor before inserting any drops at all.

Ear wax itself is a simple condition but, even so, patients with known (or suspected) perforated eardrums need to be careful when putting anything into the ears. For the same reason, syringeing the ears must be carried out under medical supervision.

Wax blocking the ears may cause deafness, and wax-removing drops may improve the situation. Deafness may be due to infections behind the eardrum, however, and in children a chronic state of glue ear may develop. Hearing does deteriorate with age and, in addition, many people complain of noises in the ear (tinnitus). This can be due to wax or infections, or to Ménière's disease, which should be treated by a doctor. Vertigo or dizziness is also a symptom of ear disease, because the balance mechanism is located near to the ear. Circulatory problems can also cause dizziness, and many drugs (such as aspirin) can cause buzzing in the ears. Certain antibiotics can affect the ears, particularly in patients with impaired kidney function.

Catarrh can accumulate behind the eardrum, (particularly following a cold), and can cause pain, dizziness, or reduced hearing. In this case, the use of decongestant medicines or nasal sprays (to help clear the catarrh) and steam inhalations (to open the internal passages leading to the ear) may ease the problem. (See 'Respiratory Conditions' section for products available.)

Audax
(Seton Healthcare)

Drops used as an analgesic to relieve pain associated with acute inflammation of the outer or middle ear, and to soften wax.
Dose: for pain, fill the ear with the liquid and plug it every 3-4 hours. To soften wax, use twice a day for 4 days.
Side effects:
Caution: painful or inflamed ears should be examined by a doctor as soon as possible.
Not to be used for: children under 1 year, patients allergic to aspirin or salicylates, or for anyone with a perforated eardrum.
Not to be used with:
Contains: choline salicylate, glycerol.

Boots Ear Wax Remover
(Boots)

A solution applied to the ear to remove hardened ear wax.

Dose: apply daily for up to 4 days.
Side effects: irritation of sensitive skin.
Caution: patients with a history of severe ear infection should consult a doctor before using this product.
Not to be used for: patients with a perforated eardrum.
Not to be used with:
Contains: docusate sodium.

Cerumol
(LAB)

Drops used as a wax softener to remove wax from the ears.

Dose: 5 drops into the ear 2-3 times a day for up to 3 days (leave the drops in for 20 minutes).

Side effects:
Caution: discard 6 months after opening.
Not to be used for: inflammation of the outer ear, dermatitis, eczema, perforated eardrum.
Not to be used with:
Contains: paradichlorobenzene, chlorbutol, arachis oil.

Dioctyl Ear Drops
(Schwarz Pharmaceuticals)

Drops used as a wax softener to remove wax from the ears.

Dose: 4 drops into the ear twice a day and plug with cotton wool (use for 2-3 days).
Side effects:
Caution:
Not to be used for: patients suffering from perforated eardrum.
Not to be used with:
Contains: sodium docusate.

Earex
(Seton Healthcare)

A solution applied to the ear to clear excess wax.

Dose: 4 drops to be used night and morning for up to 4 days.
Side effects:
Caution: discard 8 weeks after opening.
Not to be used for: patients with inflamed or infected ears, or damaged eardrum.
Not to be used with:
Contains: arachis oil, almond oil, camphor oil.

Exterol
(Dermal)

Drops used as a wax softener to remove hardened wax from the ears.

Dose: 5-10 drops in the ear 1-2 times a day for 3-4 days, or until symptoms clear.
Side effects: slight fizzing, irritation.
Caution:
Not to be used for: patients suffering from known or suspected perforated eardrum.
Not to be used with:
Contains: urea hydrogen peroxide.

Molcer
(Wallace)

Drops used as a wax softener to soften ear wax.

Dose: fill the ear with the drops and plug with cotton wool; leave for 2 nights and then clean out.
Side effects:
Caution:
Not to be used for: patients suffering from perforated eardrum.
Not to be used with:
Contains: dioctyl sodium sulphosuccinate.

Otex see **Exterol**.
(DDD)

Otovent*
(Inphormed)

A balloon device used to equalize pressure in the middle ear.

Dose: use 2-3 times a day for 2-3 weeks.
Side effects: initially discomfort in ear.
Caution: children should be supervised by an adult during use.

Not to be used for: children under 3 years, or for anyone with nasal congestion.
Not to be used with:
Contains:

Wax-Aid
(Seton Healthcare)

Ear drops used to soften hardened ear wax.

Dose: 3-4 drops in the ear twice a day.
Side effects:
Caution: see a doctor before using this product if there is any pain in the ear.
Not to be used for: infected or inflamed ears, or for patients with perforated eardrum.
Not to be used with:
Contains: paradichlorobenzene, chlorbutol, turpentine oil.

Waxsol
(Norgine)

Drops used as a wax softener to remove wax from the ears.

Dose: fill the ear with the solution for 2 nights before they are to be syringed.
Side effects: temporary irritation.
Caution:
Not to be used for: patients suffering from pain or inflammation in the ear or history of perforated eardrum.
Not to be used with:
Contains: docusate sodium.

Wax Wane
(Thornton & Ross)

Ear drops used to soften hard wax before syringing.

Dose: 4-5 drops in the ear 2-3 times a day for a few days.
Side effects:
Caution:
Not to be used for: patients with inflamed or infected ears, or damaged eardrum.
Not to be used with:
Contains: turpentine oil, chloroxylenol, terpineol.

Diseases of the mouth and throat

Many of the mouth conditions people complain of can be treated with antiseptic mouthwashes and lozenges. These comprise most of the preparations available over the counter, although there are some other interesting drugs that can be bought without a prescription.

Local anaesthetics are available to numb soreness in the mouth and throat; these include Merocaine, Tyrozets, and Ultra Chloraseptic Spray. (Hot drinks should be avoided after using anaesthetic products, because burns can result while sensation in the mouth and throat is diminished.) Aezodent is a dental anaesthetic, and Bonjela is useful for painful mouth conditions, including ulcers and teething.

Bioral is a formulation of an anti-ulcer drug that can be used for treating mouth ulcers. Blisteze lip salve is to be recommended for chapped or painful lips. (Unlicensed lip salves are also available in stick form – e.g. Lypsyl and Chapstick.) Artificial saliva products, such as Glandosane, are also available for anyone with reduced salivary gland actions. Persistent problems should be seen by a doctor or dentist.

Products for preventing dental decay are listed in a separate section (see 'Fluoride Supplements and Decay Prevention').

Vitamin deficiencies may cause soreness in or around the mouth, and dental conditions will often present as soreness or pain in the mouth. Thrush (fungal infections) are common in the mouth, particularly in patients taking powerful antibiotics or corticosteroid inhalers (see 'Antifungal Preparations' section). Ulcers that do not heal may need medical assessment. Bad breath can be caused by stomach or chest conditions or by sinusitis; similarly, loss of taste can be caused by sinus infections. A sensation of water in the mouth (waterbrash) is caused by stomach acidity (see 'Stomach Preparations' section). Many virus infections (including measles) can cause spots in the mouth. White patches in the mouth can be due to fungus or leukoplakia – the latter should be seen by a doctor. Cold sores are caused by a herpes infection on the mouth, and they usually respond to antiviral agents such as Zovirax. Stones in the mouth can result from salivary glands, and occasionally these stones can block the gland and cause swelling. Gum infections (gingivitis) may respond to antiseptic mouthwashes but, if persistent, such infections should be seen by a dentist. Spots on the tongue may be alarming, but often these are normal taste buds!

AAA Spray
(Rhone-Poulenc Rorer)

An aerosol used as a local anaesthetic to treat sore throat and minor infections of the mouth.

Dose: 2 sprays every 2-3 hours up to a maximum of 16 sprays in 24 hours; children over 6 years half adult dose.
Side effects:
Caution: avoid the eyes. Avoid inhaling the spray.
Not to be used for: children under 6 years.
Not to be used with:
Contains: benzocaine.

Adcortyl in Orabase
(Squibb)

A paste used as a corticosteroid treatment for common mouth ulcers.

Dose: apply up to 4 times a day (but especially at night) after meals, for up to 5 days only. (Do not rub in.)
Side effects: irritation.
Caution: pregnant women, nursing mothers, patients with a history of stomach ulcers or diabetes, and patients suffering from their first mouth ulcer or with recurrent mouth ulcers should consult a doctor before using this product. Patients using prescribed corticosteroid treatments should also consult a doctor or pharmacist.
Not to be used for: patients suffering from tuberculosis of the skin, cowpox, chickenpox, or mouth infections.
Not to be used with:
Contains: triamcinolone acetonide.

Aezodent
(Associated Dental)

An ointment used as an antiseptic and anaesthetic to treat discomfort due to dentures.

Dose: apply to gums and denture.
Side effects:
Caution:
Not to be used for:
Not to be used with:
Contains: chlorbutol, methyl salicylate, benzocaine, menthol, eugenol.

Anbesol
(Whitehall)

An antiseptic and anaesthetic liquid used to relieve pain from mouth ulcers, dentures, and babies' teething.

Dose: make 2 applications when required. (For teething babies make only 1 application). Do not repeat for at least half an hour.
Side effects:
Caution:
Not to be used for:
Not to be used with:
Contains: lignocaine hydrochloride, chlorocresol, cetylpyridinium chloride.

Anbesol Adult Strength
(Whitehall)

An anaesthetic and antiseptic gel used temporarily to relieve pain from mouth ulcers and irritation from dentures.

Dose: apply up to 4 times a day for a maximum of 7 days.
Side effects:
Caution:
Not to be used for: infants or small children.
Not to be used with:
Contains: lignocaine hydrochloride, chlorocresol, cetylpyridinium chloride.

Anbesol Teething Gel
(Whitehall)

An anaesthetic and antiseptic gel used to relieve pain from mouth ulcers, dentures, and babies' teething.

Dose: make 2 applications up to 4 times a day. (For teething babies make only 1 application).
Side effects:
Caution:
Not to be used for:
Not to be used with:
Contains: lignocaine hydrochloride, chlorocresol, cetylpyridinium chloride.

Bansor
(Thornton & Ross)

A liquid used as an antiseptic to treat sore gums.

Dose: apply to the affected gums. Suitable for adults, babies, and children.
Side effects:
Caution:
Not to be used for:
Not to be used with:
Contains: cetrimide.

Betadine Gargle and Mouthwash
(Seton Healthcare)

A solution used as an antiseptic to treat mouth and throat infections.
Dose: rinse or gargle with the solution up to 4 times a day for up to 14 days.
Side effects: rarely irritation and allergy.
Caution: do not swallow. Pregnant women and nursing mothers should use for a maximum of 3 days only.
Not to be used for: children under 6 years.
Not to be used with:
Contains: povidone-iodine.

Betasept Antiseptic Gargle and Mouthwash Concentrate
(Seton Healthcare)

An antiseptic liquid used as a mouthwash or gargle to treat viral, bacterial, and fungal throat and mouth infections.

Dose: use 10 ml liquid, undiluted or added to 10 ml warm water, and gargle or rinse the mouth for 30 seconds. Use 4 times a day for up to 14 days.
Side effects:
Caution: do not swallow. Pregnant women and nursing mothers should not use for more than 2-3 days. (Pregnant women should not repeat the treatment during the pregnancy).
Not to be used for: children under 6 years, or for patients with allergy to iodine, or thyroid disorders.
Not to be used with: lithium treatment.
Contains: povidone-iodine.

Bioral
(Sterling Health)

A gel used as a cell-surface protector to treat mouth ulcers.

Dose: apply after meals and at bed time.
Side effects:
Caution: not suitable for teething problems.
Not to be used for:
Not to be used with:
Contains: carbenoxolone sodium.

Bio-Strath Chamomile Formula
(Cedar Health)

A liquid used as a herbal remedy to relieve the symptoms of minor acute painful conditions of the mouth and throat.

Dose: 20 drops (0.6 ml) in a little water, 3 times a day before meals, or as directed by a doctor.
Side effects:
Caution: pregnant women should consult a doctor before using this product.
Not to be used for: children.
Not to be used with:
Contains: yeast, sage, camomile.

Blisteze
(Dendron)

A cream applied to relieve occasional cold sores, cracked lips, and chapped lips.

Dose: apply every hour.
Side effects:
Caution:
Not to be used for:
Not to be used with:
Contains: strong ammonia solution, aromatic ammonia solution, phenol.

Bocasan
(Oral-B)

A sachet of white granules used as an antiseptic and cleanser to aid treatment of gingivitis and other mouth infections.

Dose: use as a mouthwash 3 times a day after meals for a maximum of 7 days.
Side effects:
Caution: children under 12 years should be supervised while using this product. Do not swallow.
Not to be used for:
Not to be used with:
Contains: sodium perborate monohydrate, sodium hydrogen tartrate.

Bonjela
(Reckitt & Colman)

An antiseptic gel used to relieve the pain of teething in infants, and of mouth ulcers, cold sores, and irritation from dentures.

Dose: use every 3 hours (up to 6 times a day). Babies under 4 months should not be treated for more than 7 days.
Side effects:
Caution: do not apply directly to dentures. Apply only small quantities of gel, particularly in children.
Not to be used for: infants under 4 months.
Not to be used with:
Contains: choline salicylate, cetalkonium chloride.

Bonjela Pastilles
(Reckitt & Colman)

A pastille used as an antiseptic and pain-relieving treatment for mouth ulcers and soreness from dentures.

Dose: allow 1 pastille to dissolve near the sore area when required.
Side effects:
Caution:
Not to be used for: children under 6 years, or for more than 7 days.
Not to be used with:
Contains: lignocaine hydrochloride, aminacrine hydrochloride.

Boots Antiseptic Lozenges see Tyrozets.
(Boots)

Boots Antiseptic Throat Drops
(Boots)

An antiseptic lozenge used to treat sore throats.

Dose: 1 lozenge sucked slowly. (Maximum of 8 in 24 hours).
Side effects:
Caution:
Not to be used for: children under 5 years.
Not to be used with:
Contains: amylmetacresol.

Boots Children's Teething Gel
(Boots)

A sugar-free gel used as an antiseptic and pain-relieving gel to treat teething pain.

Dose: apply every 3 hours when required.
Side effects: allergy.
Caution:
Not to be used for:
Not to be used with:

Contains: cetylpyridinium chloride, lignocaine hydrochloride.

Boots Cold Sore and Lip Ointment
(Boots)

A healing ointment used to relieve pain and heal cold sores and dry, cracked, or chapped lips.

Dose: apply 5-6 times a day when required.
Side effects:
Caution:
Not to be used for: children under 12 years.
Not to be used with:
Contains: zinc oxide, allantoin, diperodon hydrochloride, camphor.

Boots Cold Sore Lotion
(Boots)

A lotion used to soothe and relieve cold sores.

Dose: dab on to sore and repeat frequently.
Side effects:
Caution:
Not to be used for:
Not to be used with:
Contains: dichlorobenzyl alcohol, levomenthol, camphor, benzyl alcohol.

Boots Glycerin of Thymol Pastilles
(Boots)

A pastille used as an antiseptic to treat sore throat and laryngitis.

Dose: 1 pastille sucked when required.
Side effects:

49

Caution:
Not to be used for: children under 12 years.
Not to be used with:
Contains: amylmetacresol.

Boots Oral Antiseptic
(Boots)

A mouthwash and gargle used to relieve mouth and throat infections.

Dose: use 15 ml to rinse mouth or gargle 2-3 times a day.
Side effects: allergy, nausea, vomiting.
Caution: pregnant women and nursing mothers should consult a doctor before using this product.
Not to be used for: children under 6 years.
Not to be used with:
Contains: cetylpyridinium chloride.

Boots Sore Mouth Gel
(Boots)

An anaesthetic and antiseptic gel used to relieve the pain of mouth ulcers.

Dose: adults and older children, apply every 3 hours; for babies teething apply to gums and repeat after 20 minutes if necessary. (Maximum of 6 doses in 24 hours.)
Side effects:
Caution:
Not to be used for:
Not to be used with:
Contains: lignocaine hydrochloride, cetylpyridinium chloride.

Boots Sore Mouth Pastilles
(Boots)

An antiseptic pastille used to relieve soreness in the mouth.

Dose: dissolve one pastille in the mouth (near the sore area) every 2-3 hours.
Side effects:
Caution:
Not to be used for: children under 3 years.
Not to be used with:
Contains: dichlorobenzyl alcohol.

Bradosol
(Zyma Healthcare)

A sugar-free lozenge used as an antibacterial treatment for infections of the throat, and to relieve soreness.

Dose: 1 lozenge to be sucked when required.
Side effects:
Caution:
Not to be used for: children under 5 years.
Not to be used with:
Contains: benzalkonium chloride.

Bradosol Plus
(Zyma Healthcare)

An anaesthetic, antibacterial, and soothing lozenge used to treat painful sore throats.

Dose: suck 1 lozenge slowly every 2-3 hours (maximum 8 in 24 hours), for up to 5 days.
Side effects:
Caution: do not eat or drink for 1 hour after sucking lozenge. Patients with severe sore throat, or also suffering from fever, headache, nausea, or vomiting should consult a doctor before using this product.

Not to be used for: children under 12 years.
Not to be used with:
Contains: domiphen bromide, lignocaine hydrochloride.

Brush Off
(Seton Healthcare)

An antiseptic, antiviral, and antibacterial solution used to treat and prevent cold sores.

Dose: apply twice a day.
Side effects: allergy.
Caution: pregnant women and nursing mothers should use on minor cold sores only. Patients with thyroid disorder should consult a doctor before using this product. Discard the solution 28 days after opening.
Not to be used for: patients allergic to iodine.
Not to be used with:
Contains: povidone-iodine.

Calgel
(Warner Wellcome Consumer Healthcare)

A sugar-free gel used as an antiseptic and local anaesthetic to treat teething pain.

Dose: apply up to 6 times a day. Leave at least 20 minutes between applications.
Side effects:
Caution:
Not to be used for: children under 3 months.
Not to be used with:
Contains: lignocaine hydrochloride, cetylpyridinium chloride.

---

clove oil BP

A liquid used as a temporary treatment for toothache.

Dose: apply to the affected tooth as required, but do not use continuously. (Seek dental treatment as soon as possible.)
Side effects:
Caution: consult a dentist as soon as possible.
Not to be used for: infants.
Not to be used with:
Contains: clove oil.

Colgate Chlorohex 2,000 see **Corsodyl Mouthwash**
(Colgate Oral Pharmaceuticals)

Colsor
(Pickles)

A cream and lotion used as an antiseptic to treat cold sores.

Dose: apply lotion sparingly 2-3 times a day, or apply cream when required.
Side effects:
Caution: avoid contact with the eyes.
Not to be used for:
Not to be used with:
Contains: tannic acid, phenol, menthol.

Corlan
(Evans)

A pellet used as a corticosteroid to treat recurrent mouth ulcers.

Dose: allow one pellet to dissolve near the site of the ulcer four times a day.

Side effects:
Caution: children under 12 years, pregnant women, and diabetics should consult a doctor before using this product.
Not to be used for: infected areas of the mouth.
Not to be used with:
Contains: hydrocortisone sodium succinate.

Corsodyl
(SmithKline Beecham)

A mouthwash, spray, and dental gel used as an antibacterial treatment for gingivitis, to inhibit plaque formation, and to maintain mouth hygiene. (The mouthwash and dental gel are additionally used to treat thrush, denture stomatitis, mouth ulcers, and for mouth hygiene following dental surgery.)

Dose: rinse mouth with 10 ml mouthwash for one minute, or use up to 12 puffs of spray, or brush with dental gel twice a day. (When treating gingivitis, continue for one month.) Dentures may be soaked in mouthwash for 15 minutes twice a day.
Side effects: irritation, discoloration of teeth and tongue.
Caution: do not swallow. Keep out of eyes and ears. May stain some bleached fabrics.
Not to be used for:
Not to be used with:
Contains: chlorhexidine gluconate.

Cupal Cold Sore Lotion see **Brush Off**
(Seton Healthcare)

Cupal Cold Sore Ointment
(Seton Healthcare)

An ointment used as a local anaesthetic and healing ointment to treat cold sores.

Dose: apply 5-6 times a day.
Side effects:
Caution:
Not to be used for:
Not to be used with:
Contains: diperodon hydrochloride, allantoin, camphor, zinc oxide.

Cymex
(E. C. De Witt)

A cream applied to relieve cold sores and dry cracked lips.

Dose: apply sparingly every hour.
Side effects:
Caution:
Not to be used for:
Not to be used with:
Contains: urea, dimethicone, cetrimide, chlorocresol.

De Witt's Throat Lozenges
(E. C. De Witt)

A lozenge used as antibacterial, antiseptic, and local anaesthetic treatment for inflammation of the mouth and throat.

Dose: 1 lozenge dissolved slowly in the mouth every 3 hours. (Maximum of 8 in 24 hours for adults, and 4 in 24 hours for children over 6 years.)
Side effects:
Caution: avoid hot drinks or food after sucking a lozenge.
Not to be used for: children under 6 years.
Not to be used with:
Contains: benzocaine, cetylpyridinium chloride.

Dentinox Teething Gel
(Dendron)

A sugar-free gel used as an anaesthetic and antiseptic treatment for teething pain.

Dose: apply every 20 minutes when required. (Suitable from birth onwards.)
Side effects:
Caution:
Not to be used for:
Not to be used with:
Contains: lignocaine hydrochloride, cetylpyridinium chloride.

Dentogen
(Dental Health)

A gel and liquid used to give temporary relief of toothache due to decay.

Dose: apply to tooth and repeat as necessary, but do not use continuously. (Seek dental treatment as soon as possible.)
Side effects:
Caution:
Not to be used for:
Not to be used with:
Contains: clove oil.

Dequacaine
(Crookes Healthcare)

An anaesthetic and antibacterial lozenge used to relieve pain and fight infection of severe sore throats.

Dose: 1 lozenge sucked every 2 hours or when required. (Maximum of 8 in 24 hours.)

Side effects:
Caution: avoid hot drinks or food after sucking a lozenge.
Not to be used for: children under 12 years.
Not to be used with:
Contains: dequalinium chloride, benzocaine.

Dequadin
(Crookes Healthcare)

An antibacterial lozenge used to treat throat infections and relieve inflammation.

Dose: 1 lozenge sucked every 2-3 hours. (Maximum of 8 in 24 hours.)
Side effects:
Caution:
Not to be used for: children under 10 years.
Not to be used with:
Contains: dequalinium chloride.

Difflam Oral Rinse
(3M Healthcare)

An oral rinse and spray used as an analgesic and anti-inflammatory treatment for pain and inflammation of the throat and mouth, including mouth ulcers, sore mouth or throat, and post-operative dental pain.

Dose: adults rinse or gargle with 15 ml oral rinse or spray with 4-8 puffs of spray every 1½-3 hours when required, for a maximum of 7 days. (Children aged 6-12 years may use 4 puffs of spray, or children under 6 years up to 4 puffs).
Side effects: numb mouth, stinging.
Caution: do not swallow.
Not to be used for: children under 12 years (oral rinse).
Not to be used with:

Contains: benzydamine hydrochloride.

Elderflower and Peppermint with Composition Essence see entry in 'Respiratory conditions – cough and cold remedies' section (Potters)

Eludril Mouthwash
(Chefaro)

A solution used as an antibacterial treatment for throat and mouth infections, gingivitis, ulcers, and for oral hygiene.

Dose: use 10-15 ml in water as a mouthwash or gargle 2-3 times a day.
Side effects:
Caution: do not swallow.
Not to be used for: infants and children.
Not to be used with:
Contains: chlorhexidine digluconate, chlorbutol hemihydrate.

Eludril Spray
(Chefaro)

A solution supplied in a spray and used as an antibacterial and local anaesthetic treatment for mild mouth and throat conditions, such as ulcers, gingivitis, tonsillitis, pharyngitis, and after dental surgery.

Dose: use 3-4 times a day (or hourly if needed).
Side effects:
Caution: do not swallow. Avoid hot drinks or food after using the spray.
Not to be used for: children under 12 years.
Not to be used with:
Contains: chlorhexidine digluconate, amethocaine.

Frador
(Chemist Brokers)

A tincture supplied with an applicator, and applied to relieve and protect mouth ulcers.

Dose: apply 4 times a day after meals and at bedtime.
Side effects:
Caution: avoid contact with polished surfaces and fabrics.
Not to be used for: children or pregnant women, or for ulcerated throats.
Not to be used with:
Contains: chlorbutol.

Glandosane*
(Fresenius)

An aerosol used to provide artificial saliva for dry mouth and throat.

Dose: spray into the mouth and throat for 1-2 seconds as needed.
Side effects:
Caution:
Not to be used for:
Not to be used with:
Contains: carboxymethylcellulose sodium, sorbitol, potassium chloride, sodium chloride, magnesium chloride, calcium chloride, potassium monohydrogen phosphate.

---

glycerin and thymol compound BP

A liquid (used as a mouthwash or gargle) to clean and deodorize the throat and mouth.

Dose: dilute the liquid with 3 parts of water, then use to rinse

the mouth or to gargle.
Side effects:
Caution:
Not to be used for:
Not to be used with:
Contains: glycerol, thymol.

Halls Soothers
(Warner Wellcome Consumer Healthcare)

A medicated sweet with a liquid centre, used to soothe sore throats.

Dose: 1 dissolved in the mouth when required.
(Maximum of 8 packs in 24 hours for adults, 5 packs for children over 6 years, and 2 packs for children under 6 years.)
Side effects:
Caution:
Not to be used for:
Not to be used with:
Contains: menthol, eucalyptus oil.

---

hydrogen peroxide BP (20 volume)

A liquid used as a deodorant mouthwash and gargle to clean the mouth. (For use as an antiseptic wound cleaner, see 'Antiseptics' section.)

Dose: dilute with 5 parts of water and use to rinse or gargle.
Side effects:
Caution: do not swallow the liquid.
Not to be used for: children under 12 years.
Not to be used with:
Contains: hydrogen peroxide.

Jackson's Antiseptic Throat Lozenge see **Strepsils**
(Ernest Jackson)

Jackson's Antiseptic Throat Pastilles
(Ernest Jackson)

A pastille used as an antiseptic treatment for dry sore throats.

Dose: 1 pastille dissolved in the mouth when required.
Side effects:
Caution:
Not to be used for:
Not to be used with:
Contains: menthol, camphor, benzoic acid.

Jackson's Glycerin Thymol Pastilles
(Ernest Jackson)

A pastille used as a treatment for sore throats.

Dose: a pastille dissolved in the mouth when required.
Side effects:
Caution:
Not to be used for:
Not to be used with:
Contains: glycerin, thymol.

Labosept
(LAB)

A sugar-free pastille used as an antiseptic treatment for mouth and throat infections.

Dose: 1 pastille every 3-4 hours up to a maximum of 8 pastilles in 24 hours.
Side effects:

Caution:
Not to be used for:
Not to be used with:
Contains: dequalinium chloride.

Luborant
(Antigen Pharmaceuticals)

A spray used as an artificial saliva to treat dry mouths.

Dose: use 2-3 sprays up to 4 times a day.
Side effects:
Caution:
Not to be used for:
Not to be used with:
Contains: sorbitol, carmellose sodium, dibasic potassium phosphate, potassium chloride, monobasic potassium phosphate, magnesium chloride, calcium chloride, sodium fluoride.

Lypsyl Cold Sore Gel
(Zyma Healthcare)

A colourless gel used as an astringent, antiseptic, and anaesthetic treatment for cold sores.

Dose: apply 3 or 4 times a day.
Side effects: occasionally skin irritation or allergy.
Caution: avoid contact with eyes. Children under 12 years should consult a doctor before using this product.
Not to be used for:
Not to be used with:
Contains: lignocaine hydrochloride, zinc sulphate, cetrimide.

Mac
(Ernest Jackson)

An antiseptic lozenge used to treat sore throats.

Dose: 1 lozenge sucked slowly. (Maximum of 12 in 24 hours.)
Side effects:
Caution:
Not to be used for:
Not to be used with:
Contains: amylmetacresol, sucrose, and glucose syrup solids.

Mac Extra
(Ernest Jackson)

An antiseptic lozenge used to treat sore throats.

Dose: 1 lozenge sucked slowly every 3 hours or when required. (Maximum of 12 in 24 hours.)
Side effects:
Caution:
Not to be used for: children under 6 years.
Not to be used with:
Contains: hexylresorcinol.

Medijel
(Dendron)

A gel and pastille used as an antiseptic and local anaesthetic treatment for mouth ulcers, sore gums, and denture discomfort.

Dose: apply the gel every 20 minutes when necessary. Dissolve one pastille in the mouth when required.
Side effects:
Caution:

Not to be used for:
Not to be used with:
Contains: aminacrine hydrochloride, lignocaine hydrochloride.

Meggezones see entry in 'Respiratory conditions – cough and cold remedies' section
(Schering-Plough Consumer Health)

Mentholatum Antiseptic Lozenges see entry in 'Respiratory conditions – cough and cold remedies' section
(Mentholatum)

Merocaine
(Marion Merrell Dow)

A lozenge used as an antiseptic and local anaesthetic to treat severe sore throat, as in tonsillitis and pharyngitis.

Dose: 1 lozenge allowed to dissolve in the mouth every 2 hours up to a maximum of 8 lozenges in 24 hours.
Side effects: rarely allergy or burning sensation in the mouth
Caution: avoid hot drinks and food after sucking a lozenge.
Not to be used for: children under 12 years.
Not to be used with:
Contains: cetylpyridinium chloride, benzocaine.

Merocet
(Marion Merrell Dow)

A lozenge and mouthwash/gargle used as an antiseptic to treat infections of the throat and mouth, and sore throats.

Dose: rinse the mouth or gargle with the solution (diluted or undiluted) or suck 1 lozenge, every 3 hours when required.
Side effects: rarely allergy or burning sensation in the mouth.

Caution:
Not to be used for: children under 6 years.
Not to be used with:
Contains: cetylpyridinium chloride.

Merothol see entry in 'Respiratory conditions – cough and cold remedies' section
(Marion Merrell Dow)

Merovit
(Marion Merrell Dow)

A lozenge used as an antiseptic, soothing preparation for sore throats caused by colds.

Dose: 1 lozenge sucked every 3 hours.
Side effects: rarely allergy or burning sensation in mouth.
Caution:
Not to be used for: children under 6 years.
Not to be used with:
Contains: cetylpyridinium chloride, vitamin C.

---

myrrh tincture BPC 1973

A tincture used as an astringent treatment for sore and ulcerated gums.

Dose: apply with finger.
Side effects:
Caution:
Not to be used for:
Not to be used with:
Contains: myrrh, alcohol.

Olbas Pastilles see entry in 'Respiratory Conditions – cough and cold remedies' section'
(Lane)

Orabase
(Convatec)

An ointment used as a mucoprotectant to protect lesions in the mouth, and raw weeping areas.

Dose: apply to the affected area without rubbing in.
Side effects:
Caution:
Not to be used for:
Not to be used with:
Contains: pectin, gelatin, sodium carboxymethylcellulose.

Oragard
(Colgate-Palmolive)

An anaesthetic and antiseptic gel used to relieve mouth ulcers, denture irritation, and teething.

Dose: adults and older children, apply every 3 hours; for babies teething apply to gums and repeat after 20 minutes if necessary. (Maximum of 6 doses in 24 hours.)
Side effects:
Caution:
Not to be used for:
Not to be used with:
Contains: lignocaine hydrochloride, cetylpyridinium chloride.

Oraldene
(Warner-Lambert Healthcare)

A solution used as an antibacterial and antifungal rinse to relieve mouth infections including mouth ulcers, sore or bleeding gums, bad breath, sore throats, and to clean the mouth before or after dental surgery.

Dose: rinse out the mouth or gargle with at least 15 ml 2-3 times a day.
Side effects: local irritation.
Caution: do not dilute. Do not swallow.
Not to be used for: children under 6 years.
Not to be used with:
Contains: hexetidine.

Pickles Toothache Tincture
(Pickles)

A tincture used as a local anaesthetic treatment for toothache.

Dose: apply to the tooth as needed, but do not use continuously. (Seek dental treatment as soon as possible.)
Side effects:
Caution: do not swallow.
Not to be used for:
Not to be used with:
Contains: lignocaine hydrochloride, clove oil.

Potter's Traditional Sore Throat Pastilles see **Jackson's Glycerin Thymol Pastilles**
(Ernest Jackson)

Proctor's Pinelyptus Pastilles
(Ernest Jackson)

A pastille used as an aromatic decongestant to relieve throat irritation, loss of voice, huskiness, and cough.

Dose: 1 pastille dissolved in the mouth when required.

Side effects:
Caution:
Not to be used for:
Not to be used with:
Contains: eucalyptus oil, menthol, pine oil, abietis oil.

Pyralvex
(Norgine)

A liquid supplied with a brush and used as an antiseptic and astringent treatment for mouth ulcers and for irritation from dentures.

Dose: apply to the affected area 3-4 times a day.
Side effects: temporary discoloration.
Caution:
Not to be used for: children under 12 years.
Not to be used with:
Contains: salicylic acid, rhubarb extract.

Rinstead Adult Gel
(Schering-Plough)

A sugar-free gel used as an anaesthetic and antiseptic to treat painful mouth ulcers or other mouth soreness.

Dose: apply up to 6 times a day.
Side effects: irritation, allergy.
Caution:
Not to be used for: children under 12 years.
Not to be used with:
Contains: benzocaine, chloroxylenol.

Rinstead Pastilles
(Schering Plough Consumer Health)

An antiseptic pastille used to relieve pain and help to heal mouth ulcers and other sore mouth conditions.

Dose: 1 pastille sucked every 2 hours.
Side effects:
Caution:
Not to be used for: children under 12 years.
Not to be used with:
Contains: menthol, chloroxylenol.

Rinstead Teething Gel
(Schering Plough Consumer Health)

A sugar-free gel with no artificial colours, used as an antiseptic and pain-relieving gel temporarily to treat teething pain.

Dose: apply every 3 hours when required.
Side effects: allergy.
Caution:
Not to be used for: babies under 3 months.
Not to be used with:
Contains: cetylpyridinium chloride, lignocaine.

Saliva Orthana*
(Nycomed)

A spray (available with or without fluoride) or lozenge used as an artificial saliva to treat dry mouth.

Dose: use 2-3 sprays or suck 1 lozenge when required.
Side effects:
Caution:
Not to be used for:
Not to be used with:
Contains: mucin. (Lozenges also contain xylitol.)

Salivace
(Penn Pharmaceuticals)

A spray used as an artificial saliva to treat dry mouth.

Dose: use 1-2 sprays as required.
Side effects:
Caution:
Not to be used for:
Not to be used with:
Contains: sodium carboxymethylcellulose, xylitol, sodium chloride, calcium chloride, dibasic potassium phosphate, potassium chloride, methyl hydroxybenzoate.

Salivix
(Thames Laboratories)

A sugar-free pastille used to relieve dry mouths.

Dose: 1 pastille sucked when required.
Side effects:
Caution:
Not to be used for:
Not to be used with:
Contains: sodium phosphate, calcium lactate, malic acid.

Sensodyne Search Dental Rinse see **Merocets Mouthwash**
(Stafford-Miller)

Soothake
(Pickles)

A gel used to relieve toothache.

Dose: apply to the tooth as required, but do not use continuously. (Seek dental treatment as soon as possible.)

Side effects:
Caution:
Not to be used for: children.
Not to be used with:
Contains: chlorbutol, clove oil.

Strepsils
(Crookes Healthcare)

An antiseptic lozenge available in various flavours (and with or without vitamin C) and used as a treatment for sore throats and mouth infections.

Dose: suck 1 lozenge every 2-3 hours.
Side effects:
Caution:
Not to be used for:
Not to be used with:
Contains: dichlorobenzyl alcohol, amylmetacresol.

Strepsils Dual Action
(Crookes Healthcare)

A lozenge used as a local anaesthetic and antiseptic treatment for sore throats.

Dose: suck 1 lozenge every 2 hours when needed.
(Maximum of 8 in 24 hours.)
Side effects: allergy.
Caution: avoid hot drinks or food after sucking a lozenge. Pregnant women, nursing mothers, and patients suffering from high fever, headache, nausea, or vomiting should consult a doctor before using this product.
Not to be used for: children under 12 years.
Not to be used with:
Contains: lignocaine, amylmetacresol, dichlorobenzyl alcohol.

T.C.P. Pastilles
(Chemist Brokers)

A pastille used as an antiseptic soothing treatment for sore throats. (The T.C.P. Antiseptic Liquid may be used as a gargle or mouthwash and to treat mouth ulcers – see entry in 'Antiseptics' section.)

Dose: 1 pastille sucked occasionally.
Side effects:
Caution:
Not to be used for:
Not to be used with:
Contains: phenol, sodium salicylate.

Teejel
(Seton Healthcare)

A gel used as an antiseptic, analgesic treatment for teething and other mouth pain

Dose: apply every 3-4 hours.
Side effects:
Caution:
Not to be used for: infants under 4 months.
Not to be used with:
Contains: choline salicylate, cetalkonium chloride.

Tyrocane Junior Antiseptic Lozenges
(Seton Healthcare)

A sugar-free lozenge used as an antiseptic to treat minor throat infections in children aged 6-12 years.

Dose: 1 lozenge sucked slowly when required. (Maximum of 8 in 24 hours.)

Side effects:
Caution:
Not to be used for: children under 6 years.
Not to be used with:
Contains: cetylpyridinium chloride.

Tyrocane Throat Lozenges
(Seton Healthcare)

A sugar-free lozenge used as an antiseptic and local anaesthetic treatment for sore throat, pain and infection in the mouth or throat.

Dose: 1 lozenge sucked slowly every 3-4 hours if needed. (Maximum 7 in 24 hours or 15 in 72 hours.)
Side effects:
Caution: avoid hot drinks or food after sucking a lozenge.
Not to be used for: children under 12 years.
Not to be used with:
Contains: benzocaine, cetylpyridinium chloride, tyrothricin.

Tyrozets
(Centra Healthcare)

A lozenge used as an antibiotic and local anaesthetic to treat mild mouth irritation and sore throat.

Dose: adults 1 lozenge every 3 hours up to a maximum of 8 lozenges in 24 hours; children ½-1 lozenge every 6 hours up to a maximum of 4 lozenges in 24 hours.
Side effects: additional infection, blackening or soreness of mouth and tongue, allergy.
Caution: avoid hot drinks or food after sucking a lozenge.
Not to be used for: children under 3 years.
Not to be used with:
Contains: tyrothricin, benzocaine.

Ulc-Aid Gel
(Seton Healthcare)

A sugar-free gel used to relieve pain from mouth ulcers, teething, and denture irritation.

Dose: apply, then repeat after 20 minutes, and then every 3 hours.
Side effects:
Caution:
Not to be used for: babies under 3 months.
Not to be used with:
Contains: lignocaine hydrochloride, cetylpyridinium chloride.

Ulc-Aid Lozenges see Tyrocane Lozenges
(Seton Healthcare)

Unichem Antiseptic Throat Lozenges
(Unichem)

An antiseptic lozenge used to treat sore throats.

Dose: 1 lozenge sucked slowly. (Maximum of 8 in 24 hours.)
Side effects:
Caution:
Not to be used for: children under 5 years.
Not to be used with:
Contains: amylmetacresol.

Valda Pastilles
(Sterling Health)

A pastille used as an aromatic decongestant to give temporary relief from hoarse, tickly throats, huskiness, and congestion.

Dose: 1 pastille dissolved in the mouth when required.

(Maximum 10 in 24 hours.)
Side effects:
Caution:
Not to be used for: children under 3 years.
Not to be used with:
Contains: eucalyptus oil, menthol, thymol, guaiacol, terpineol.

Vicks Ultra Chloraseptic
(Proctor & Gamble)

A solution supplied with a spray and used as an anaesthetic to treat sore throats.

Dose: use every 2-3 hours. (Children aged 6-12 years, use 1 spray, adults and older children, use 3 sprays.) Maximum of 8 treatments in 24 hours.
Side effects:
Caution: patients with difficulty breathing or swallowing, or with a fever, headache, nausea, or severe persistent sore throat should consult a doctor before using this product. Avoid hot drinks or food after using the spray.
Not to be used for: children under 6 years, or for more than 3 consecutive days.
Not to be used with:
Contains: benzocaine.

Victory V see entry in 'Respiratory conditions – cough and cold remedies' section
(Ernest Jackson)

Vocalzone
(Inphormed)

A pastille used to treat irritation in the throat due to use of the voice, smoking, or colds.

Dose: 1 dissolved in the mouth every 2 hours when required.
Side effects:
Caution:
Not to be used for: children under 12 years.
Not to be used with:
Contains: menthol, peppermint oil, myrrh tincture.

Woodwards Teething Gel see **Calgel**
(Woodwards)

Zovirax Cold Sore Cream
(Wellcome)

A cream used as an anti-viral treatment for cold sores.

Dose: apply five times a day for up to 10 days. Treatment is most effective if started at first sign of cold sore.
Side effects: mild irritation, redness, and drying of skin.
Caution: for use only on the lips and face. Patients taking corticosteroid treatments should consult a doctor before using this product.
Not to be used for: patients with a weak immune system, or for application to the inside of the mouth.
Not to be used with: corticosteroid treatments (see above).
Contains: aciclovir.

Fluoride supplements and decay prevention

The addition of fluoride to drinking water has done much to reduce the incidence of dental decay among the population at large. For children living in areas where fluoride is not added, however, (and, at the discretion of the dentist, for other children who are particularly at risk) a fluoride supplement (usually in the form of sodium fluoride) may be added to the diet. It is important, however, **not** to give fluoride supplements when they are not needed, because a high intake of fluoride can cause permanent discoloration of the teeth. (This can be due to the intake of supplements unnecessarily, or due to children swallowing large amounts of toothpaste containing fluoride.) A dentist should therefore always be consulted before giving fluoride supplements to children.

Other products listed here are of particular use in the reduction of dental decay. Disclosing tablets highlight those areas of the mouth where plaque collects, and teach how to brush until it is removed. Dental health gums (such as Endekay) help to neutralize plaque acids, preventing decay.

Products used to treat other disorders of the mouth are listed separately (see 'Disorders of the mouth and throat' section)

Ceplac
(Rhone-Poulenc Rorer Family Health)

A tablet used as a dental disclosing product, to show areas of plaque.

Dose: 1 tablet crushed in the mouth, and distributed to all tooth surfaces in the saliva with the tongue. (Plaque is then stained red.) Brush teeth until all red colour is removed.
Caution:
Not to be used for:
Contains: erythrosine.

Endekay Daily Fluoride Mouth Rinse
(Stafford Miller)

A mouth rinse used as a fluoride supplement to strengthen tooth enamel to resist decay.

Dose: rinse for 1 minute each day.
Caution: do not swallow.
Not to be used for: children under 6 years.
Contains: sodium fluoride.

Endekay Dental Health Gum
(Stafford Miller)

A chewing gum tablet used to prevent dental decay and relieve dry mouth.

Dose: 1 tablet chewed for 10 minutes after food, or as required, then discarded.
Caution:
Not to be used for:
Contains: urea.

Endekay Fluodrops
(Stafford Miller)

Drops used as a fluoride supplement for children aged 2 weeks to 2 years to strengthen tooth enamel to resist decay.

Dose: 7 drops daily.
Caution: use only if fluoride content of usual drinking water is less than 0.3 ppm.
Not to be used for: infants under 2 weeks of age.
Contains: sodium fluoride.

Endekay Fluotabs
(Stafford Miller)

A tablet available in two strengths for ages 2-4 years and over 4 years, and used as a fluoride supplement to strengthen tooth enamel to resist decay.

Dose: ½-1 tablet daily, depending on age and drinking water fluoride content.
Caution: use only if fluoride content of usual drinking water is less than 0.7 ppm.
Not to be used for:
Contains: sodium fluoride.

Fluor-a-day
(Dental Health)

A chewable tablet available in two strengths for ages up to 4 years and over 4 years, and used as a fluoride supplement to prevent dental decay.

Dose: ½-1 tablet daily, depending on age and drinking water fluoride content.
Caution: use only if fluoride content of usual drinking water is less than 0.7 ppm.

Not to be used for:
Contains: sodium fluoride.

Fluorigard Drops
(Colgate-Palmolive)

Drops used as a fluoride supplement to prevent dental decay.

Dose: 2-8 drops daily according to age and drinking water fluoride content.
Caution: use only if fluoride content of usual drinking water is less than 0.7 ppm.
Not to be used for:
Contains: sodium fluoride.

Fluorigard Gelkam
(Colgate-Palmolive)

A gel used as a toothpaste to prevent dental caries and stop early tooth decay.

Dose: use to brush teeth (after normal brushing) at night.
Caution: do not swallow excess gel.
Not to be used for: children under 6 years.
Contains: stannous fluoride.

Fluorigard Rinse
(Colgate-Palmolive)

A mouth rinse available in two strengths (for daily or weekly use), and used as a fluoride supplement to treat early decay and prevent cavities.

Dose: rinse mouth with 10 ml for 1 minute.
Caution: use only if fluoride content of usual drinking water is less than 0.7 ppm. Do not swallow.

Not to be used for: children under 6 years.
Contains: sodium fluoride.

Fluorigard Tablets
(Colgate-Palmolive)

A chewable tablet available in two strengths, and used as a fluoride supplement to prevent dental caries.

Dose: ½-2 tablets of 0.5 mg strength or ½-1 tablet of 1 mg strength (according to age and drinking water fluoride content) every day.
Caution: use only if fluoride content of usual drinking water is less than 0.7 ppm.
Not to be used for:
Contains: sodium fluoride.

Oral-B Fluoride Tablets see **Fluor-a-day**
(Oral-B Laboratories)

Skin disorders

Because many skin conditions are relatively minor, there is a number of skin preparations available over the counter. Many of these are antiseptics for cleaning infected or sore skin areas (see 'Antiseptics' section). Others are acne lotions, including many unlicensed skin washes and scrubs (which are not listed here), usually containing triclosan or a similar antiseptic, to reduce the bacteria on the skin which cause spots. Treatments for warts and verrucae are also available, often in the form of medicated plasters which are ready to apply. Skin softeners can be used for dry skin conditions. Skin infections (bacterial and fungal) can also be treated (see 'Antiseptics' and 'Antifungal preparations'). Dandruff and other scalp conditions are dealt with in a separate section (see 'Scalp disorders' section).

Mild steroid creams and ointments contain hydrocortisone, and can be used for mild to moderate eczema, dermatitis, and insect bite reactions. There are restrictions on their use without a doctor's supervision, and they should not be purchased for use on a child under 10 years of age, or for use on the face; nor should they be used for more than 7 days (in such cases supply on prescription will be necessary).

E45 cream is a useful general skin softener for dry skin problems. Calamine lotion is useful for itchy skin, and witch hazel for itchy or irritating skin problems. There are a few products licensed for use on burns, but the standard first aid advice to immerse a burn in cold water should always be heeded, and the use of creams on the injury is best avoided. Chilblains may respond to ointments such as Vitathone, and bruises can be treated with heparinoid products such as Lasonil.

Sunscreens are not included here, because many are not licensed, and the contents vary widely. It is useful to point out, however, that skin should be protected against the sun, and those requiring greater protection (such as babies, young children, and people with sensitive skins) should use a product with a high factor number. (SPF 15 will provide extremely high protection, while SPF 25 or higher will give a total sunblock). People with skin conditions such as eczema or allergies should choose a hypoallergenic product with as few additives as possible.

Persistent skin problems, which do not respond to any of these treatments after 14 days, should be seen by a doctor. In particular, bleeding or itchy moles, or moles that change colour, should be seen sooner rather than later because these signs may indicate malignant change. Any skin ulcer that does not heal should also be taken seriously.

Skin rashes are a common side effect to medications, particularly if there is allergy involved. These can progress to more serious urticaria. Local allergy or contact dermatitis often occurs with metals, such as jewellery, or with cosmetics. These will often respond to hydrocortisone preparations. Antihistamine tablets may be used with creams to treat allergic or itchy conditions (see 'Allergic Disorders' section).

Acetoxyl
(Stiefel)

A gel available in two strengths and used as an antibacterial and skin softener to treat acne.

Dose: wash and dry the affected area and apply the gel once a day.
Side effects: irritation, peeling, burning.
Caution: keep away from the eyes, nose, and mouth; use with caution on the neck. Children and new users should use the weaker gel. May bleach dyed fabric.
Not to be used for:
Not to be used with:
Contains: benzoyl peroxide.

Acnaveen
(Bioglan)

A cleansing bar used as a skin softener and antiseptic to treat greasy skin.

Dose: use instead of soap.
Side effects:
Caution:
Not to be used for:
Not to be used with:
Contains: sulphur, salicylic acid.

Acne-Aid
(Stiefel)

A cleansing bar used to treat acne and greasy skin.

Dose: use instead of soap.
Side effects: irritation.

Caution: avoid the eyes.
Not to be used for:
Not to be used with:
Contains: fatty acids, detergents, sulphonated surfactant blend.

Acnecide see **Nericur**.
(Galderma)

Acnegel/Acnegel Forte see **Nericur**
(Stiefel)

Acnidazil
(Cilag)

A cream used as an antibacterial and skin softener to treat acne.

Dose: wash and dry the affected area and apply the cream once a day for the first week, then twice a day for the next 4-8 weeks (then reduce frequency).
Side effects: irritation, peeling, redness.
Caution: keep out of the eyes, nose, and mouth. May bleach dyed clothing.
Not to be used for:
Not to be used with:
Contains: miconazole nitrate, benzoyl peroxide.

After-bite
(E. C. De Witt)

A liquid in a pen applicator used to neutralize insect bites and stings.

Dose: apply when required.
Side effects:

Caution: avoid the mouth and eyes.
Not to be used for: children under 2 years.
Not to be used with:
Contains: ammonia.

Alcoderm
(Galderma)

A cream and lotion used as an emollient to treat dry skin conditions.

Dose: apply as required.
Side effects:
Caution:
Not to be used for:
Not to be used with:
Contains: liquid paraffin, cetylalcohol, stearyl alcohol, sodium lauryl sulphate, carbomer polysorbate 60, triethanolamine, methylparaben, propylparaben.

Alpha-Keri
(Westwood)

A liquid used to treat dry, itchy skin conditions.

Dose: adults and children add 1-2 capsful to the bath, or rub a small amount on to wet skin; infants use half a capful per bath.
Side effects:
Caution:
Not to be used for:
Not to be used with:
Contains: lanolin oil, mineral oil.

Alphosyl
(Stafford-Miller)

A cream and lotion used to treat psoriasis.

Dose: massage thoroughly into the affected area 2-4 times a day.
Side effects: irritation, sensitivity to light, allergy.
Caution: avoid the eyes, and avoid exposure to sunlight after treatment. May stain clothing.
Not to be used for: patients suffering from acute psoriasis.
Not to be used with:
Contains: coal tar extract, allantoin.

Amidose Saline see **Normasol**
(Abatron)

Anethaine
(Crookes Healthcare)

A local anaesthetic cream used to treat bites, stings, and minor rashes.

Dose: apply 2-3 times a day.
Side effects: irritation, inflammation.
Caution: avoid the eyes.
Not to be used for: children under 3 years, or for application to broken skin.
Not to be used with:
Contains: tetracaine hydrochloride.

Anhydrol Forte
(Dermal)

A roll-on solution used to treat excessive sweating of the armpits, hands, or feet.

Dose: apply at night. Wash off in the morning.
Side effects: temporary irritation and redness of skin.

Caution: children to be treated only on feet. Avoid contact with eyes and mucous membranes, clothes, jewellery, metal, or polished surfaces. Do not apply to broken or irritated skin.
Not to be used for:
Not to be used with:
Contains: aluminium hexahydrate.

Aquadrate
(Proctor & Gamble)

A cream used as an emollient to treat dry skin conditions.

Dose: apply twice a day after washing and drying.
Side effects:
Caution:
Not to be used for:
Not to be used with:
Contains: urea.

---

aqueous cream BP

A cream used as an emollient to treat dry skin conditions.

Dose: apply as required.
Side effects:
Caution:
Not to be used for:
Not to be used with:
Contains: emulsifying ointment, phenoxyethanol, purified water.

Aveeno*
(Bioglan)

A range of cleansing and moisturizing products (cleansing bar, bath additives with or without emollient oils, bath oil, cream, emulave bar and fluid) containing oatmeal, and used for delicate skins. (Guard against slipping if products are used in the bath.)

Avoca Wart Treatment
(Bray Health and Leisure)

A treatment kit consisting of a caustic pencil to remove warts, a file, protector pads, and dressings.

Dose: to be applied to the wart a maximum of 3 times at 24 hour intervals. Use only under medical supervision.
Side effects:
Caution: the pencil must not be licked or held other than by its plastic holder.
Not to be used for: areas near the eyes or other sensitive parts of the body.
Not to be used with:
Contains: silver nitrate, potassium nitrate.

Balmosa see entry in 'Joint and muscle disorders' section
(Pharmax Healthcare)

Balneum
(Merck-Whitehall Dermatological)

A lanolin-free bath oil used as an emollient to treat dry skin, including that associated with eczema and dermatitis.

Dose: add to the bath water or apply to wet skin and shower off.
Side effects:
Caution: beware of slipping in the bath. Avoid the eyes.
Not to be used for:
Not to be used with:
Contains: soya vegetable oil.

Balneum Plus
(Merck-Whitehall Dermatological)

A lanolin-free bath oil used as an emollient and anti-itching product to treat itching, irritation, and dry skin (including that associated with eczema and dermatitis).

Dose: add to the bath water or apply to wet skin and shower off. (Effects last for up to 7 hours.)
Side effects:
Caution: beware of slipping in the bath. Avoid the eyes.
Not to be used for:
Not to be used with:
Contains: soya oil, lauromacrogols.

Balneum with Tar
(Merck)

A bath oil used as a medicated emollient to treat eczema, itchy or thickening skin disorders, psoriasis.

Dose: adults 20 ml added to the bath water (children over 2 years use 10 ml) 2-3 times a week.
Side effects: rarely allergy.
Caution: avoid the eyes. Avoid exposure to strong sunlight after using this product. May stain clothing.
Not to be used for: children under 2 years or for patients suffering from wet, weeping, or broken skin.
Not to be used with:
Contains: coal tar, soya oil.

Balsamicum Ointment
(Weleda)

An ointment used as a herbal remedy to aid the healing of abrasions, boils, nappy rash, and minor wounds.

Dose: apply to the skin or on a dry dressing several times a day.
Side effects: allergy.
Caution:
Not to be used for:
Not to be used with:
Contains: marigold, dog's mercury, balsam of Peru, Stibium Metallicum Preparatum.

Balto Foot Balm
(Lane)

A balm used to relieve tired aching feet, excessive perspiration, and hard, cracked skin.

Dose: use twice a day.
Side effects: allergy.
Caution: avoid contact with silver or other jewellery.
Not to be used for:
Not to be used with: homeopathic remedies.
Contains: sulphur, camphor, menthol, zinc oxide.

Bath E45*
(Crookes Healthcare)

A bath oil used as an emollient to soothe and soften dry skin.

Dose: use 15 ml in the bath water, or apply to skin and shower off.
Side effects:
Caution: avoid contact with the eyes. Guard against slipping in the bath or shower.
Not to be used for:
Not to be used with:
Contains: medicinal white oil, cetyl dimethicone.

Bazuka
(Dendron)

A gel supplied with an emery board and applicator, and used as a skin softener to treat verrucae, warts, corns, and calluses.

Dose: apply 1-2 drops each night, and rub down weekly with an emery board. (Treatment may be required for up to 12 weeks.)
Side effects: irritation, tingling, tenderness.
Caution: keep away from the eyes, nose, and mouth, and avoid inhaling the vapour. May damage clothes, jewellery, fabrics, and furniture.
Not to be used for: areas of broken skin, moles, birthmarks, hairy warts or skin problems other than warts, warts on the face, anus, or genital areas, diabetics or patients with circulatory disorders, corns or calluses.
Not to be used with:
Contains: lactic acid, salicylic acid.

Benoxyl
(Stiefel)

A cream and lotion (available in two strengths) and used as an antibacterial and skin softener to treat acne.

Dose: wash and dry the affected area, then apply once a day.
Side effects: irritation, peeling.
Caution: keep out of the eyes, nose, and mouth. Start treatment with the weaker strength and progress to the stronger product only if needed.
Not to be used for:
Not to be used with:
Contains: benzoyl peroxide.

Benzagel see **Nericur**
(Bioglan)

Betadine Scalp and Skin Cleanser see entry in 'Scalp disorders' section
(Seton Healthcare)

Betasept Acne Wash see entry in 'Antiseptics' section
(Seton Healthcare)

Biactol*
(Proctor & Gamble)

A range of medicated products containing antiseptics (as in the face wash) and skin softeners (as in the cleansing pads), used to assist in the treatment of acne.

Blue Flag Root Compound
(Gerard House)

A tablet used as a herbal antiseptic, anti-inflammatory, and anti-itch product to treat the symptoms of minor acne, eczema, and other minor skin conditions.

Dose: 1 tablet after meals 3 times a day.
Side effects:
Caution: pregnant women should consult a doctor before using this product.
Not to be used for: children under 12 years.
Not to be used with:
Contains: blue flag root, burdock, sarsaparilla.

Boots Calamine and Glycerin
(Boots)

A cream applied to the skin to relieve discomfort due to sunburn, windburn, skin irritation, and dry or tender skin.

Dose: massage into skin as required.
Side effects:
Caution:
Not to be used for:
Not to be used with:
Contains: calamine, glycerin, zinc oxide.

Boots Chilblain Cream
(Boots)

A soothing and healing cream applied to chilblains to relieve pain and inflammation.

Dose: apply to chilblains as needed. (Cover with a dressing if chilblain is broken.)
Side effects:
Caution: contains peanut oil.
Not to be used for:
Not to be used with:
Contains: benzyl alcohol, eucalyptus oil, peanut oil.

Boots Corn Paint see Noxacorn
(Boots)

Boots Herbal Skin Tablets
(Boots)

A tablet used as a herbal remedy to relieve skin disorders and eczema.

Dose: adults 2 tablets (children aged 5-12 years 1 tablet) 3 times a day before food.
Side effects: allergy.
Caution:
Not to be used for: children under 12 years, pregnant women, nursing mothers.
Not to be used with:
Contains: echinacea, stinging nettles, burdock root.

Boots Medicated Callous Treatment Plasters see **Carnation Callous Caps**
(Boots)

Boots Medicated Corn Treatment Plasters see **Carnation Corn Caps**
(Boots)

Boots Medicated Talc
(Boots)

A medicated powder used to cool and calm irritated skin, heat rashes, and minor skin troubles.

Dose: apply after washing skin.
Side effects:
Caution:
Not to be used for:
Not to be used with:
Contains: allantoin.

Boots Mediclear*
(Boots)

A range of products (face mask, skin gel, cleansing pads, cleansing lotion, skin wash, cover stick, shower gel, moisturizer, soap) containing antiseptics and used to assist in the treatment of acne. (See *also* 'Boots Mediclear Cream and Lotion'.)

Boots Mediclear Acne Cream and Lotion
(Boots)

A lotion and cream available in two strengths (5% and 10%), used to treat spots and acne.

Dose: apply after washing once a day. Apply only on alternate days to fair skin.
Side effects: irritation, burning, redness, peeling.
Caution: it is advisable to start treatment with the lower-strength preparation and progress to the stronger product if necessary. Avoid contact with eyes, lips, and mouth. These products may bleach coloured fabrics.
Not to be used for: children under 12 years.
Not to be used with:
Contains: benzoyl peroxide.

Boots Pharmacy Skincare no. 1
(Boots)

A cream used as an emollient to treat dry skin conditions, including eczema, nappy soreness, chapping due to weather, and sunburn.

Dose: apply 2-3 times a day.
Side effects:
Caution:
Not to be used for:
Not to be used with:
Contains: lanolin, almond oil.

Boots Pharmacy Skincare no. 3
(Boots)

An ointment used as a steroid treatment for irritant dermatitis, contact allergic dermatitis, and insect bite reactions. (Doctors may prescribe this type of product for other conditions or for longer treatment periods, but self-medication should be restricted to the uses and doses stated here.)

Dose: apply sparingly once or twice a day for a maximum of 7 days.
Side effects: fluid retention, suppression of adrenal glands, thinning of skin.
Caution: pregnant women and nursing mothers should consult a doctor before using this product.
Not to be used for: children under 10 years, or on the face, anus, genital area, or on broken or infected skin conditions.
Not to be used with:
Contains: hydrocortisone acetate.

Boots Pharmacy Skincare no. 4
(Boots)

A local anaesthetic cream used to give temporary relief from itching and irritated skin.

Dose: apply 2-3 times a day for a maximum of 3 days.
Side effects:
Caution:
Not to be used for: children under 3 years, in or near the eyes, on broken skin, or on large areas of skin. Not for prolonged use.
Not to be used with:
Contains: tetracaine hydrochloride.

Boots Sting Relief
(Boots)

A cream used as a soothing, antiseptic treatment for insect bites and stings.

Dose: apply every 2-3 hours when required.
Side effects: irritation, allergy.
Caution: pregnant women and nursing mothers should consult a doctor before using this product.
Not to be used for:
Not to be used with:
Contains: benzyl alcohol, chloroxylenol, eucalyptus oil, zinc oxide.

Boots Verruca Ointment see **Verrugon Ointment**
(Boots)

Boots Wart Remover see **Wartex**
(Boots)

---

borage oil* see **starflower oil***

Brasivol
(Stiefel)

A paste (graded as fine or medium) used as an abrasive to treat acne.

Dose: wet the area, then rub in vigorously for 15-20 seconds, rinse and repeat 1-3 times a day.
Side effects:
Caution: start treatment with no. 1 (fine) and progress to no. 2 (medium) only if necessary after several weeks.
Not to be used for: patients suffering from visible superficial

arteries or veins on the skin.
Not to be used with:
Contains: graded non-silicone abrasive.

Burneze
(Seton Healthcare)

A spray containing a local anaesthetic, used as a first-aid treatment for minor burns and scalds, to reduce pain and blistering.

Dose: spray once, then repeat after 15 minutes if needed.
Side effects:
Caution: patients with known allergy should see a doctor before using this product.
Not to be used for: areas of broken skin, or repeatedly, or on large areas.
Not to be used with:
Contains: benzocaine.

Caladryl see entry in 'Allergic disorders' section
(Warner Wellcome Consumer Healthcare)

---

calamine lotion BP

A lotion used to treat itchy skin conditions. (Also available: calamine lotion oily, calamine cream aqueous, calamine ointment.)

Dose: apply when required.
Side effects:
Caution:
Not to be used for:
Not to be used with:
Contains: calamine.

---

calamine and coal tar ointment BP

An ointment used to treat eczema and psoriasis.

Dose: apply once or twice a day.
Side effects: irritation, allergy, sensitivity to light.
Caution: may stain clothing. Avoid exposure to strong sunlight after treatment.
Not to be used for: patients with acute attacks of psoriasis.
Not to be used with:
Contains: calamine, strong coal tar solution.

Calendolon Ointment
(Weleda)

An ointment used as a herbal antiseptic and anti-inflammatory remedy to treat cuts, minor wounds, and abrasions.

Dose: apply 2-3 times a day to skin or on a dry dressing.
Side effects: redness, itching, allergy.
Caution: pregnant women should consult a doctor before using this product.
Not to be used for: application to infected wounds.
(The surface may heal, sealing in the sepsis.)
Not to be used with:
Contains: marigold.

Calendula Cream
(Nelsons)

A skin salve used as a herbal remedy to treat the symptoms of sore and rough skin.

Dose: apply as needed and rub into skin.
Side effects:
Caution:
Not to be used for:

Not to be used with:
Contains: marigold.

Calendula Lotion
(Weleda)

A lotion used as a herbal antiseptic and anti-inflammatory remedy to treat cuts, minor wounds and abrasions.

Dose: add 5 ml to 200 ml boiled and cooled water, and use to cleanse wounds or as a compress.
Side effects: allergy.
Caution: pregnant women should consult a doctor before using this product.
Not to be used for: application to infected wounds.
(The surface may heal, sealing in the sepsis.)
Not to be used with:
Contains: marigold.

Calmurid
(Galderma)

A cream used as an emollient and skin softener, used to treat dry skin conditions.

Dose: apply twice a day after washing and drying.
Side effects: stinging.
Caution: avoid use on broken or sensitive skin.
Not to be used for:
Not to be used with:
Contains: urea, lactic acid.

Carbo-Dome
(Lagap)

A cream used as a treatment for psoriasis.

Dose: apply to the affected area 2-3 times a day.
Side effects: irritation, sensitivity to light.
Caution: avoid the eyes, and avoid exposure to sunlight after treatment. May stain clothes.
Not to be used for: patients suffering from acute psoriasis.
Not to be used with:
Contains: coal tar.

Carnation Callous Caps
(Cuxson Gerrard)

A medicated plaster used to soften the skin and remove calluses.

Dose: apply and change every 3 days for 6 days.
Side effects:
Caution: children under 16 years and patients suffering from circulation disorders should consult a doctor before using this product. Do not use for more than 14 days except on medical advice.
Not to be used for: diabetics, and on broken or inflamed skin.
Not to be used with:
Contains: salicylic acid.

Carnation Corn Caps
(Cuxson Gerrard)

A medicated plaster used to soften the skin and remove hard corns.

Dose: apply and change every 2 days. Remove corn after 6 days or later. Do not use for more than 10 days, or for more than 3 corns at any one time.
Side effects:
Caution: children under 15 years and patients suffering from circulation disorders should consult a doctor before using this product.

Not to be used for: diabetics, and on broken or inflamed skin.
Not to be used with:
Contains: salicylic acid.

Carnation Verruca Treatment
(Cuxson Gerrard)

A medicated pad used to soften the skin and treat verrucae.

Dose: apply and change every 2 days for up to 10 days. Treatment may be repeated after 28 days.
Side effects:
Caution: children under 6 years and patients suffering from circulation disorders should consult a doctor before using this product.
Not to be used for: diabetics, and on broken or inflamed skin.
Not to be used with:
Contains: salicylic acid.

Ceanel see entry in 'Scalp conditions' section.
(Quinoderm)

Chymol
(Waterhouse)

A balm used as an emollient and analgesic to treat chapped or sore skin, sprains, and bruises.

Dose: apply as required.
Side effects: irritation.
Caution: patients allergic to aspirin should consult a doctor before using this product.
Not to be used for: areas of broken skin.
Not to be used with:
Contains: eucalyptus oil, terpineol, methyl salicylate, phenol.

Clearasil*
(Proctor & Gamble)

A range of medicated products containing antiseptics (e.g. in the lotion and face wash), and skin softeners (as in the nightclear gel and cleansing pads), to assist in the treatment of acne. (See *also* 'Clearasil Medicated Cream' and 'Clearasil Max 10'.)

Clearasil Max 10
(Proctor & Gamble)

A cream used as an antibacterial skin softener to treat acne.

Dose: apply once daily for the first week, then twice daily thereafter if no irritation has developed.
Side effects: irritation, redness, peeling.
Caution: may bleach coloured fabrics.
Not to be used for: children under 12 years.
Not to be used with:
Contains: benzoyl peroxide.

Clearasil Medicated Cream
(Proctor & Gamble)

A cream used as an antiseptic to treat acne.

Dose: apply twice a day.
Side effects: irritation, inflammation.
Caution: may discolour jewellery. Avoid use near the mouth and eyes.
Not to be used for:
Not to be used with:
Contains: triclosan, sulphur.

Clinitar
(Shire)

A cream and shampoo used as a treatment for psoriasis, eczema.

Dose: apply to the affected area 1-2 times a day.
Side effects: sensitivity to light.
Caution: avoid exposure to sunlight after using this product, and avoid the eyes. May stain clothing.
Not to be used for: patients suffering from pustular psoriasis
Not to be used with:
Contains: stantar.

---

coal tar and salicylic acid ointment BP

An ointment used to treat eczema and psoriasis.

Dose: apply once or twice a day.
Side effects: irritation, allergy, sensitivity to light.
Caution: may stain clothing. Avoid exposure to strong sunlight after treatment.
Not to be used for: patients with acute attacks of psoriasis.
Not to be used with:
Contains: coal tar, salicylic acid.

---

coal tar paste BP

A paste used to treat eczema and psoriasis.

Dose: apply once or twice a day.
Side effects: irritation, allergy, sensitivity to light.
Caution: may stain clothing. Avoid exposure to strong sunlight after treatment.
Not to be used for: patients with acute attacks of psoriasis.
Not to be used with:

Contains: compound zinc paste, strong coal tar solution.

Combudoron Lotion
(Weleda)

A lotion used as a herbal remedy to relieve the symptoms of sunburn, insect bites, minor burns, minor rashes, and nettle rash.

Dose: add 5 ml to a cup of boiled water and apply on lint as a compress. Keep moist. Apply undiluted to insect bites.
Side effects:
Caution:
Not to be used for:
Not to be used with:
Contains: small nettle, arnica.

Combudoron Ointment
(Weleda)

An ointment used as a herbal remedy to relieve the symptoms of minor burns and scalds.

Dose: apply directly to skin or on a dry dressing.
Side effects: allergy.
Caution:
Not to be used for:
Not to be used with:
Contains: small nettle, arnica.

---

comfrey*

Commonly called 'knitbone', this herb has been traditionally used for its healing properties, and can be found in skin products for use on insect bites, cuts, and grazes. Used internally, it can be soothing and expectorant in its action on coughs.

Dose: (as specified for each individual product).
Side effects:
Caution:
Not to be used for:
Not to be used with:
Contains: comfrey.

Compeed*
(Sorbothane)

An adhesive dressing applied to the skin to give relief and protect the area from blisters and friction injuries, (by functioning as an extra layer of skin), and to provide a barrier to dirt, and absorb any fluid. (May be used on existing blisters or on areas exposed to friction as a preventative measure.)

Dose: wash and dry the affected area, then apply the dressing to stretched skin and warm with the hand. Leave in place until the dressing loosens naturally. (May be left for several days).
Side effects:
Caution: diabetics should consult a doctor before using this product. Do not cut the dressing.
Not to be used for: inflamed skin areas.
Not to be used with:
Contains:

Compound V
(Whitehall)

A liquid used as a skin softener to treat warts and verrucae.

Dose: apply daily for up to 12 weeks.
Side effects:
Caution: avoid application to normal skin.
Not to be used for:
Not to be used with:

Contains: salicylic acid.

Compound W
(Whitehall)

A liquid used as a skin softener to treat warts and verrucae.

Dose: apply daily for up to 4 weeks.
Side effects:
Caution: children under 6 years should be seen by a doctor before using this product.
Not to be used for: moles, birthmarks, or for hairy, facial or genital warts.
Not to be used with:
Contains: salicylic acid.

Conotrane
(Yamanouchi)

A cream used as an antiseptic and barrier for protecting the skin from water, and for nappy rash, bed sores, and irritations.

Dose: apply to the affected area several times a day.
Side effects:
Caution:
Not to be used for:
Not to be used with:
Contains: benzalkonium chloride, dimethicone.

Cream E45
(Crookes Healthcare)

A cream used as an emollient to treat dry skin conditions, including dry-stage eczema.

Dose: apply 2-3 times a day.

Side effects:
Caution:
Not to be used for:
Not to be used with:
Contains: white soft paraffin, light liquid paraffin, lanolin.

Cupal Verruca Treatment see **Verrugon**
(Seton Healthcare)

Cuplex
(Smith & Nephew)

A gel used as a skin softener to treat warts, corns, callouses, and verrucae.

Dose: apply at night and remove the dried film in the morning. (Usual treatment period 6-12 weeks)
Side effects:
Caution: do not apply to healthy skin.
Not to be used for: infants, or for warts on the face, or on anal and genital areas
Not to be used with:
Contains: salicylic acid, lactic acid, copper acetate, collodion.

Dermacort
(Panpharma)

A steroid cream used to treat mild to moderate eczema, allergic contact dermatitis, irritant contact dermatitis, and insect bites. (Doctors may prescribe this type of product for other conditions or for longer treatment periods, but self-medication should be restricted to the uses and doses stated here.)

Dose: apply sparingly once or twice a day for a maximum of 7 days.
Side effects: fluid retention, suppression of adrenal glands,

thinning of skin.

Caution: pregnant women and nursing mothers should consult a doctor before using this product.

Not to be used for: children under 10 years, or on the face, anus, genital area, or on broken or infected skin conditions.

Not to be used with:

Contains: hydrocortisone.

Dermacreme
(Potters)

A cream used as an antiseptic to treat cuts, grazes, minor burns, and scalds.

Dose: apply as needed.
Side effects:
Caution:
Not to be used for:
Not to be used with:
Contains: menthol, methyl salicylate, phenol, zinc oxide.

Dermamist
(Yamanouchi)

A spray used as an emollient to treat dry skin conditions, including eczema and itching in the elderly.

Dose: use after a bath or shower.
Side effects:
Caution: guard against slipping in the bath or shower. Avoid inhalation.
Not to be used for: application to the face, or near naked flames.
Not to be used with:
Contains: white soft paraffin, liquid paraffin, coconut oil.

Dermatodoron Ointment
(Weleda)

An ointment used as a herbal remedy to relieve the symptoms of eczema.

Dose: apply 3-4 times a day.
Side effects: allergy.
Caution:
Not to be used for:
Not to be used with:
Contains: woody nightshade, loosestrife.

Dermidex
(Seton Healthcare)

A cream used as a local anaesthetic and antiseptic to soothe sore skin due to stings, cuts, grazes, and contact with jewellery, detergents, etc.

Dose: apply every 3 hours for a maximum of 7 days.
Side effects:
Caution:
Not to be used for: children under 4 years, or for sensitive areas of skin (such as the nose, eyes, or genital areas).
Not to be used with:
Contains: lignocaine, chlorbutanol, aluminium chlorhydroxyallantoinate, cetrimide.

Diprobase
(Schering Plough)

A lanolin-free emollient cream or ointment used to treat dry skin conditions.

Dose: apply sparingly when required.

Side effects:
Caution:
Not to be used for:
Not to be used with:
Contains: liquid paraffin, white soft paraffin. (Cream also contains cetostearyl alcohol and cetomacrogol.)

Diprobath
(Schering-Plough)

A bath emollient used to treat dry skin conditions.

Dose: add to the bath water 2-3 times a week.
Side effects:
Caution: take care to avoid slipping.
Not to be used for:
Not to be used with:
Contains: light liquid paraffin, isopropyl myristate, laureth-4.

Dithrocream
(Dermal)

A cream available in 5 strengths (4 available over the counter and 1 only on prescription), and used to treat psoriasis.

Dose: apply to the affected area once a day and wash off after 1 hour. Start with the weakest cream and gradually increase the strength if needed. (Only the two weakest creams should be used without medical supervision.)
Side effects: irritation, allergy, warmth, burning.
Caution: children should be seen by a doctor before using this product. Keep away from eyes and mucous membranes. May stain hair, skin, clothing, plastics, and other materials
Not to be used for: patients suffering from acute psoriasis.
Not to be used with:
Contains: dithranol.

Dithrolan
(Dermal)

An ointment used to treat psoriasis.

Dose: leave on for 1-2 hours at first (until skin feels warm), then gradually increase the contact time.
Side effects: irritation, allergy, burning.
Caution: may stain skin, hair, and clothes. Patients using steroid creams should consult a doctor or pharmacist before using this product.
Not to be used for: patients suffering from acute psoriasis, or for application to normal skin, the eyes, or mucous membranes.
Not to be used with:
Contains: dithranol, salicyclic acid.

Driclor
(Stiefel)

A liquid with roll-on applicator used to treat excessive sweating.

Dose: apply at night initially, then reduce to once or twice a week. Do not apply within 1 hour of bathing.
Side effects: irritation.
Caution:
Not to be used for: broken, irritated or recently shaved skin.
Not to be used with:
Contains: aluminium chloride hexahydrate.

Duofilm
(Stiefel)

A liquid used as a skin softener to treat warts.

Dose: apply the liquid to the wart once or twice a day. (Usual treatment period 6-12 weeks.)

Side effects:
Caution: do not apply to healthy skin.
Not to be used for: children under 2 years, or for warts on the face or anal and genital areas.
Not to be used with:
Contains: salicylic acid, lactic acid, flexible collodion.

---

echinacea*
(licensed product available from Gerard House)

A herbal remedy used either alone or in combination with other herbal ingredients. It is licensed to relieve minor skin conditions (and in combination products to relieve symptoms of catarrh). It is also thought to stimulate the immune system, and possibly to treat (or prevent) common infections. It is believed to be of help in relieving the symptoms of tonsillitis, and may also be taken as an internal skin cleanser. It may be of use in treating insect bites and stings if applied directly to the skin.

Dose: (as specified for each individual product).
Side effects:
Caution: pregnant women should consult a doctor before using this product.
Not to be used for: children under 12 years, or for patients suffering from multiple sclerosis, HIV infection, or AIDS-related illnesses.
Not to be used with:
Contains: echinacea.

Eczema Ointment
(Potters)

An ointment used as a herbal remedy to relieve the symptoms of eczema.

Dose: apply twice a day.

Side effects: allergy.
Caution: avoid contact with jewellery.
Not to be used for: children under 5 years.
Not to be used with:
Contains: chickweed, lanolin, zinc oxide, salicylic acid, benzoic acid.

Emulsiderm
(Dermal)

An emollient liquid used as an aid in the treatment of dry skin conditions (including eczema).

Dose: add to bath water or apply directly to skin.
Side effects:
Caution: keep away from eyes. Take care to avoid slipping in treated bath water.
Not to be used for:
Not to be used with:
Contains: benzalkonium chloride, liquid paraffin, isopropyl myristate.

---

emulsifying ointment BP

An ointment used as an emollient in eczema or other dry skin conditions. (May be used as a soap substitute.)

Dose: use as needed.
Side effects:
Caution:
Not to be used for:
Not to be used with:
Contains: emulsifying ointment.

En-Solv*
(DePuy Healthcare)

A moist wipe used to assist in the removal of adhesive dressings from the skin.

Dose: use when required to remove adhesive from the skin.
Side effects:
Caution:
Not to be used for:
Not to be used with:
Contains: D-limonene.

Eskamel
(Goldshield Healthcare)

A cream used as a skin softener and antiseptic to treat acne.

Dose: apply a little to the affected area once a day.
Side effects: irritation, redness, peeling.
Caution: may tarnish jewellery.
Not to be used for: infected skin, or near eyes or mouth.
Not to be used with:
Contains: resorcinol, sulphur.

Eurax
(Zyma Healthcare)

A cream and lotion used to treat itching skin and skin irritation (e.g. allergy, eczema, sunburn, and dermatitis).

Dose: apply when required. Effect lasts for up to 10 hours
Side effects:
Caution: keep out of the eyes. Infants, pregnant women, nursing mothers, and patients with genital itching should see a doctor before using this product.

Not to be used for: patients suffering from broken or weeping skin.
Not to be used with:
Contains: crotamiton.

Eurax HC
(Zyma Healthcare)

A steroid cream used to treat irritant and allergic contact dermatitis, mild to moderate eczema, and reactions to insect bites. (Doctors may prescribe this product for other conditions or for longer treatment periods, but self-medication should be restricted to the uses and doses stated here.)

Dose: apply sparingly twice a day for a maximum of 7 days.
Side effects: fluid retention, suppression of adrenal glands, thinning of skin, irritation, allergy.
Caution: pregnant women and nursing mothers should consult a doctor before using this product.
Not to be used for: children under 10 years, or on the face, anus, genital area, or on broken or infected skin conditions.
Not to be used with:
Contains: hydrocortisone, crotamiton.

---

evening primrose oil* see entry in 'Women's disorders' section

---

Freezone see **Noxacorn**
(Whitehall)

Frost Cream
(Weleda)

A cream used as a herbal remedy to relieve symptoms of chilblains.

Dose: apply to skin or on a dry dressing several times a day.
Side effects: allergy.
Caution:
Not to be used for:
Not to be used with:
Contains: balsam of Peru, petroleum, rosemary oil, Stibium Metallicum Praep.

Gelcosal
(Quinoderm)

A gel used as a skin softener to treat psoriasis, dermatitis, when the condition is scaling.

Dose: massage into the affected area twice a day.
Side effects:
Caution: avoid the eyes, and avoid exposure to sunlight after treatment. May stain clothing.
Not to be used for:
Not to be used with:
Contains: coal tar solution, tar, salicyclic acid.

Gelcotar
(Quinoderm)

A gel and liquid shampoo used as an antipsoriatic treatment for psoriasis, dermatitis, and dandruff.

Dose: massage gel into the affected area twice a day. Use shampoo twice a week.
Side effects: irritation, sensitivity to light
Caution: avoid the eyes, and avoid exposure to sunlight after treatment. May stain clothing.
Not to be used for: patients suffering from acute psoriasis.
Not to be used with:
Contain: coal tar solution, tar.

Germolene New Skin*
(SmithKline Beecham Consumer)

A liquid used to form a waterproof and germ-proof barrier on the skin, to protect minor damage.

Dose: apply as needed and leave to dry.
Side effects:
Caution:
Not to be used for: deep cuts, severe burns, severe injuries.
Not to be used with:
Contains:

Glutarol
(Dermal)

A solution used as a virucidal, skin-drying agent to treat warts.

Dose: apply the solution to the wart twice a day after soaking.
Side effects: staining of the skin, irritation.
Caution: do not apply to healthy skin. Keep away from the eyes. Avoid contact with linen and clothing.
Not to be used for: warts on the face or anal and genital areas.
Not to be used with:
Contains: glutaraldehyde.

---

glycerin BP

A liquid used as an emollient to treat dryness and retain moisture in the skin. (For use in treating coughs and throat conditions, see 'Respiratory conditions – cough and cold remedies' section.)

Dose: apply as often as needed. (May be diluted with water.)
Side effects:
Caution:

Not to be used for:
Not to be used with:
Contains: glycerin.

HC45
(Crookes Healthcare)

A steroid cream used to treat mild to moderate eczema, allergic contact dermatitis, irritant contact dermatitis, and insect bites. (Doctors may prescribe this type of product for other conditions or for longer treatment periods, but self-medication should be restricted to the uses and doses stated here.)

Dose: apply sparingly once or twice a day for a maximum of 7 days.
Side effects: fluid retention, suppression of adrenal glands, thinning of skin.
Caution: pregnant women and nursing mothers should consult a doctor before using this product.
Not to be used for: children under 10 years, or on the face, anus, genital area, or on broken or infected skin conditions.
Not to be used with:
Contains: hydrocortisone acetate.

Healing Ointment (Calendula)
(Nelsons)

An ointment used as a herbal remedy to treat cuts and rough, sore, sensitive skin.

Dose: apply and cover if necessary.
Side effects:
Caution:
Not to be used for:
Not to be used with:
Contains: calendula.

Heath and Heather Skin Tablets
(Ferrosan Healthcare)

A tablet used as a herbal remedy to relieve symptoms of spots, skin blemishes, and dry eczema.

Dose: 2 tablets 3 times a day.
Side effects: stomach upset.
Caution: pregnant women should consult a doctor before using this product.
Not to be used for: children.
Not to be used with:
Contains: burdock root, wild pansy.

Herbheal Ointment
(Potters)

An ointment used as a herbal anti-itch remedy to relieve the symptoms of skin conditions where itching and irritation are present.

Dose: apply twice a day.
Side effects: allergy.
Caution:
Not to be used for: children under 5 years.
Not to be used with:
Contains: colophony, marshmallow root, chickweed, sulphur, zinc oxide, lanolin.

Hewletts Cream
(Bioglan)

A protecting, healing cream used to treat sore skin and nappy rash.

Dose: use as needed.

Side effects:
Caution: avoid contact with the eyes.
Not to be used for: large areas of broken skin.
Not to be used with:
Contains: zinc oxide, lanolin, white soft paraffin.

Hirudoid
(Panpharma)

A cream and gel used as an anti-inflammatory product to treat bruising.

Dose: apply up to 4 times a day. (Use the gel for a cooling effect.)
Side effects: rash.
Caution: patients with thrombophlebitis are advised to consult a doctor before using any medication.
Not to be used for: children under 5 years, or for large areas of skin, broken or sensitive skin, or mucous membranes.
Not to be used with:
Contains: organo-heparinoid.

Humiderm
(CV Laboratories)

A cream used as an emollient to treat dry skin conditions.

Dose: apply after bathing.
Side effects:
Caution:
Not to be used for:
Not to be used with:
Contains: sodium pyrrolidone carboxylate.

Hydromol
(Quinoderm)

A lanolin-free cream and bath additive used as an emollient to treat dry skin conditions.

Dose: apply cream to skin or add bath additive to bath water when required.
Side effects:
Caution: take care to avoid slipping in the bath.
Not to be used for:
Not to be used with:
Contains: liquid paraffin, isopropyl myristate. (Cream also contains arachis oil, sodium pyrrolidone carboxylate, and sodium lactate.)

---

hydrous ointment BP

An ointment used as an emollient to treat dry skin conditions.

Dose: apply as needed.
Side effects:
Caution:
Not to be used for:
Not to be used with:
Contains: hydrous ointment.

Hypercal
(Nelsons)

A cream and tincture used as a herbal, soothing remedy for cuts and sores.

Dose: apply to affected area. (The tincture should be diluted 1 in 10 with water for larger cuts, but applied undiluted to minor wounds.) Cover if necessary.
Side effects:
Caution:
Not to be used for:

Not to be used with:
Contains: marigold, hypericum.

Hypericum/Calendula Ointment
(Weleda)

An ointment used as a herbal remedy to relieve painful cuts and minor wounds.

Dose: apply directly to skin or on a dry dressing.
Side effects: allergy.
Caution: pregnant women should consult a doctor before using this product.
Not to be used for: infected wounds, or for patients with known sensitivity to light.
Not to be used with:
Contains: hypericum, marigold.

Ionax
(Galderma)

A gel used as an abrasive, antibacterial preparation to clean the skin in the treatment of acne.

Dose: wet the face, then rub for 1-2 minutes and rinse, once or twice a day.
Side effects: redness, drying of skin.
Caution: avoid the eyes.
Not to be used for: children under 12 years.
Not to be used with:
Contains: polyethylene granules, benzalkonium chloride, polyoxyethylene lauryl ether.

Jamaican Sarsaparilla
(Potters)

A liquid used as a herbal remedy to relieve the symptoms of minor skin complaints, blemishes, and rashes.

Dose: 10 ml in water 3 times a day.
Side effects:
Caution: children, pregnant women, and nursing mothers should consult a doctor before using this product.
Not to be used for:
Not to be used with:
Contains: sarsaparilla root.

Jungle Formula Bite and Sting Relief Cream
(Chefaro)

A steroid cream used to treat insect bites and stings. (Doctors may prescribe this type of product for other conditions or for longer treatment periods, but self-medication should be restricted to the uses and doses stated here.)

Dose: apply sparingly once or twice a day for a maximum of 7 days.
Side effects: fluid retention, suppression of adrenal glands, thinning of skin.
Caution: pregnant women and nursing mothers should consult a doctor before using this product.
Not to be used for: children under 10 years, or on the face, anus, genital area, or on broken or infected skin conditions.
Not to be used with:
Contains: hydrocortisone acetate.

Kamillosan
(Norgine)

An ointment used to relieve chapped skin, sore and cracked nipples, and nappy rash.

Dose: adults apply twice a day or after breastfeeding; infants,

apply at each nappy change.
Side effects:
Caution:
Not to be used for:
Not to be used with:
Contains: camomile.

Keri Therapeutic Lotion
(Westwood)

A lotion used as an emollient to treat dry skin, dermatitis and
nappy rash.

Dose: apply 3 times a day or when needed.
Side effects:
Caution:
Not to be used for:
Not to be used with:
Contains: mineral oil.

Kleer Tablets
(Lane)

A tablet used as a herbal remedy to treat skin disorders and
eczema.

Dose: adults 2 tablets (children aged 5-12 years 1 tablet) 3
times a day before meals.
Side effects:
Caution:
Not to be used for: children under 5 years, pregnant women,
or nursing mothers.
Not to be used with:
Contains: echinacea, stinging nettle, burdock root.

Kleer Ti-Tree and Witch Hazel Cream
(Lane)

A cream used as a herbal antiseptic and astringent remedy to relieve minor skin conditions, cuts, and wounds.

Dose: apply when required and at bedtime. (Wash cuts and wounds before treatment.)
Side effects:
Caution:
Not to be used for:
Not to be used with: creams containing benzyl penicillin.
Contains: witch hazel, ti-tree oil, eucalyptus oil, methyl salicylate, camphor, zinc oxide.

La Formule*
(Bioconcepts)

A range of aromatherapy products (skin wash, protective skin shield, and skin pen) used to remove impurities and excess oil from the skin, and combat bacteria.

Dose: use the skin wash twice a day instead of soap; apply the protective skin shield twice a day after cleansing; use the spot pen 4-5 times a day when required according to the instructions.
Side effects:
Caution: avoid the eyes. Do not apply the spot pen before sunbathing. If prone to skin allergies, test the product first on a small patch of skin.
Not to be used for:
Not to be used with:
Contains: skin wash and protective skin shield: oils of lavender, rosemary, thyme. Extracts of camomile, calendula. (The protective skin shield also contains sweet almond oil. The skin wash also contains extracts of thyme, mallow, and lappa.) Spot pen: de-natured alcohol, purified water, oils of lavender,

rosemary, oregano, clove, savory, thyme, and cinnamon.

Lacticare
(Stiefel)

A lotion used to treat dry skin conditions.

Dose: apply as required.
Side effects: temporary mild stinging, irritation.
Caution: avoid use on broken or inflamed skin.
Not to be used for:
Not to be used with:
Contains: lactic acid, sodium pyrrolidone carboxylate.

Lactocalamine
(Schering Plough)

A lotion used to relieve skin irritation, sunburn, insect bites and stings. (An unlicensed cream* formulation with similar ingredients is also available.)

Dose: apply when required.
Side effects:
Caution:
Not to be used for:
Not to be used with:
Contains: calamine, zinc oxide, hamamelis water, phenol.

Lanacane Cream
(Combe International)

A local anaesthetic cream used to give temporary relief from itching and burning due to nettle rash, insect bites and stings, scraped and chafed skin, and rectal or vaginal itching.

Dose: apply up to 3 times a day for a maximum of 1 week.

Side effects: allergy.
Caution: pregnant women should consult a doctor before using this product.
Not to be used for: children under 3 years, or for large areas of skin.
Not to be used with:
Contains: benzocaine.

Lanacane Medicated Body Powder*
(Combe International)

A medicated powder used to disinfect and dry the skin, and assist in the treatment of chapped skin, prickly heat, itching, and sunburn.

Dose: apply when required.
Side effects:
Caution: keep away from babies' eyes and noses.
Not to be used for:
Not to be used with:
Contains: corn starch, zinc oxide, menthol, eucalyptol, triclosan, camphor, aloe.

Lanacort
(Combe International)

A cream or ointment used as a steroid treatment for mild to moderate eczema, irritant dermatitis, contact allergic dermatitis, and insect bite reactions. (Doctors may prescribe this type of product for other conditions or for longer treatment periods, but self-medication should be restricted to the uses and doses stated here.)

Dose: apply sparingly once or twice a day for a maximum of 7 days.
Side effects: fluid retention, suppression of adrenal glands,

thinning of skin.

Caution: pregnant women and nursing mothers should consult a doctor before using this product.

Not to be used for: children under 10 years, or on the face, anus, genital area, or on broken or infected skin conditions.

Not to be used with:

Contains: hydrocortisone acetate.

Lipobase
(Yamanouchi)

An emollient cream used to treat dry skin conditions.

Dose: apply 3-4 times a day.
Side effects:
Caution:
Not to be used for:
Not to be used with:
Contains: cetostearyl alcohol, cetomacrogol, liquid paraffin, white soft paraffin.

Lotion E45*
(Crookes Healthcare)

A lotion used to moisturize dry skin conditions.

Dose: use frequently.
Side effects:
Caution:
Not to be used for:
Not to be used with:
Contains: white soft paraffin, light liquid paraffin, lanolin.

---

magnesium sulphate paste BP

A paste used to treat boils.

Dose: apply under a dressing.
Side effects:
Caution: stir before use.
Not to be used for:
Not to be used with:
Contains: magnesium sulphate, glycerol, phenol.

Masse
(Cilag)

A cream used for nipple care before and after childbirth.

Dose: before birth, apply once or twice a day. After birth, apply after nursing.
Side effects: allergy.
Caution:
Not to be used for:
Not to be used with:
Contains: glycerin, lanolin, arachis oil.

Mentholatum
(Mentholatum)

An ointment used as a soothing treatment for minor skin conditions, such as itching, insect bites, allergic rashes, dry or chapped skin, bruises and chilblains. (For use in treating coughs and colds see 'Respiratory conditions – inhaled remedies' section. For use in treating muscular disorders see 'Joint and muscle disorders' section.)

Dose: apply lightly to the affected area.
Side effects:
Caution: avoid the eyes, nose, and delicate skin.
Not to be used for: children under 1 year.
Not to be used with:
Contains: menthol, camphor, methyl salicylate.

Metanium
(Syntex Pharmaceuticals)

A soothing and protective ointment used to treat and prevent nappy rash.

Dose: apply at each nappy change.
Side effects:
Caution:
Not to be used for:
Not to be used with:
Contains: titanium dioxide, titanium peroxide, titanium salicylate, silicone.

Morhulin
(Seton Healthcare)

An ointment used as a barrier to treat minor skin conditions, including pressure sores and nappy rash.

Dose: apply as needed.
Side effects:
Caution:
Not to be used for:
Not to be used with:
Contains: cod liver oil, zinc oxide.

Nericur
(Schering)

A gel available in 2 strengths (5% and 10%) and used as an antibacterial skin softener to treat acne.

Dose: wash and dry the affected area, then apply the gel once a day.
Side effects: irritation, peeling.

Caution: keep out of the eyes, nose, mouth. May bleach dyed fabric. Start treatment with the weaker-strength product and progress to the stronger product only if necessary.
Not to be used for: children.
Not to be used with:
Contains: benzoyl peroxide.

Normasol see entry in 'Eye conditions' section
(Seton Healthcare)

Noxacorn
(Cox)

A liquid used as a skin softener to treat corns and calluses.

Dose: apply every night (or every 2nd night) for 3-6 nights.
Side effects:
Caution: avoid application to normal skin.
Not to be used for: children under 6 years.
Not to be used with:
Contains: salicylic acid.

Nutraplus see **Aquadrate**
(Galderma)

Occlusal
(Euroderma)

A paint used as a skin softener to treat warts and verrucae.

Dose: apply, allow to dry and re-apply. Repeat treatment daily.
Side effects: irritation.
Caution: avoid contact with eyes, mucous membranes, damaged skin. Pregnant women should consult a doctor or pharmacist before using this product.

Not to be used for: diabetics and patients with impaired circulation, or on moles, birthmarks, facial warts, or hairy warts.
Not to be used with:
Contains: salicylic acid.

Odaban*
(Bracey's Pharmaceuticals)

A spray used as an antiperspirant to reduce sweating.

Dose: apply at bedtime (usually once a week).
Side effects:
Caution: avoid contact with the eyes and mouth, and with clothes and polished or metal surfaces.
Not to be used for: broken skin.
Not to be used with:
Contains: aluminium chloride, silicone.

Oilatum cream
(Stiefel)

A cream used as an emollient to treat dry skin and eczema.

Dose: apply when required.
Side effects:
Caution:
Not to be used for:
Not to be used with:
Contains: arachis oil.

Oilatum emollient
(Stiefel)

An emollient liquid used to treat dry, itching, and irritated skin, including eczema and psoriasis.

Dose: add to bath water [2 capsful to 8 inches (20 cm) of bath water, or ½-2 capsful in a basin for infants], or apply to skin and rinse off.
Side effects: rash, irritation.
Caution: beware of slipping in the bath.
Not to be used for:
Not to be used with:
Contains: light liquid paraffin, lanolin.

Oilatum Gel
(Stiefel)

A shower gel used to treat dry skin conditions, such as eczema and dermatitis.

Dose: apply to wet skin, massage, then rinse and dry.
Side effects:
Caution: beware of slipping in the bath or shower.
Not to be used for:
Not to be used with:
Contains: light liquid paraffin.

Oilatum Plus
(Stiefel)

A liquid used as an antiseptic emollient to treat eczema, including eczema at risk from infection.

Dose: add to bath water [2 capsful to 8 inches (20 cm) of bath water, or 1 ml to an infant's bath].
Side effects: irritation.
Caution: avoid contact with eyes. Beware of slipping in the bath.
Not to be used for: infants under 6 months.
Not to be used with: soap.
Contains: light liquid paraffin, benzalkonium chloride, triclosan.

Oilatum Skin Therapy*
(Stiefel)

An emollient bath oil used to moisturize and soothe dry, sensitive skin.

Dose: 2 capsful added to the bath (or 1 capful to a basin).
Side effects:
Caution: guard against slipping.
Not to be used for:
Not to be used with:
Contains: light liquid paraffin, lanolin.

Oilatum Soap*
(Stiefel)

A soap used to cleanse dry, sensitive skins.

Dose: use as a soap.
Side effects:
Caution:
Not to be used for:
Not to be used with:
Contains: liquid paraffin.

---

oily cream see **hydrous ointment BP**

Ointment for Burns
(Nelsons)

An ointment used as a herbal remedy to treat burns.

Dose: apply and cover when needed.
Side effects:
Caution:
Not to be used for:

Not to be used with:
Contains: calendula, urtica urens, echinacea, hypericum.

---

omega 3 fish oils*

See entry in 'Miscellaneous' section.

Oxy*
(SmithKline Beecham Consumer)

A range of medicated products containing antiseptics (as in the cleanser, face wash, and cleansing pads) and skin softeners (as in the medicated cream and cleansing pads), used to assist in the treatment of acne. (See *also* '**Oxy 5 and Oxy 10**').

Oxy 5 and Oxy 10
(SmithKline Beecham Consumer)

A lotion available in two strengths (5% and 10%), and used to treat acne.

Dose: apply once daily for the first week, then twice daily thereafter if no irritation has developed.
Side effects: irritation, swelling, redness, peeling.
Caution: it is advisable to start treatment with the lower-strength preparation, and progress to the stronger product if necessary. Avoid the eyes, lips, and mouth. May bleach coloured fabrics.
Not to be used for: more than 3 months.
Not to be used with:
Contains: benzoyl peroxide.

Panda Baby Cream
(Thornton & Ross)

A cream used as a soothing and protective cream to relieve

the symptoms of chapped skin and nappy rash.

Dose: apply as needed.
Side effects:
Caution:
Not to be used for:
Not to be used with:
Contains: zinc oxide, castor oil, lanolin.

Panoxyl see **Nericur**
(Stiefel)

Panoxyl Aquagel see **Nericur**
(Stiefel)

Panoxyl Wash
(Stiefel)

A lotion used as a skin softener to treat acne.

Dose: once a day, use to wash the skin after wetting, then rinse.
Side effects:
Caution: avoid the eyes, mouth, and mucous membranes.
Not to be used for:
Not to be used with:
Contains: benzoyl peroxide.

Papulex
(Euroderma)

A gel used as an anti-inflammatory treatment for acne.

Dose: apply twice a day after washing. (Reduce to once a day or once every other day if side effects are a problem.)

Side effects: dryness, irritation, peeling, reddening, burning, itching.

Caution: keep away from mucous membranes, including mouth and nose. Pregnant women and nursing mothers should consult a doctor before using this product.

Not to be used for:

Not to be used with:

Contains: nicotinamide (vitamin B_3).

Pickles Ointment

(Pickles)

An ointment used as a skin softener to treat corns, calluses, and hard skin.

Dose: apply at night for 3-4 nights.

Side effects:

Caution: diabetics should consult a doctor before using this product.

Not to be used for:

Not to be used with:

Contains: salicylic acid.

Pixol

(Thames)

A liquid used as a medicated bath oil treatment for psoriasis, eczema, dermatitis, dandruff and flaky scalp conditions.

Dose: use 20-30 ml in bath water and soak the skin for up to 20 minutes. (For use on the scalp, apply 5-15 ml as a shampoo and rinse off after 2-3 minutes.)

Side effects:

Caution: avoid contact with the eyes. Guard against slipping in the bath. Avoid exposure to strong sunlight after treatment.

Not to be used for:

Not to be used with:
Contains: coal tar solution, cade oil, pine tar.

Polytar Emollient
(Stiefel)

A liquid used as a medicated bath treatment for psoriasis, eczema, and itchy skin conditions.

Dose: 2-4 capsful added to an 8-inch (20-cm) deep bath.
Side effects: irritation.
Caution: avoid contact with the eyes. Guard against slipping in the bath. Avoid exposure to strong sunlight after treatment.
Not to be used for:
Not to be used with:
Contains: tar, coal tar, arachis oil, cade oil, liquid paraffin.

Psoradrate
(Procter and Gamble Pharmaceuticals)

A cream available in 2 strengths, used to treat psoriasis.

Dose: wash and dry the area, then apply the cream twice a day.
Side effects: irritation, allergy.
Caution: may stain skin and clothing.
Not to be used for: pustular psoriasis.
Not to be used with:
Contains: dithranol, urea.

Psorasolv
(Potters)

An ointment used as a herbal antiseptic and anti-inflammatory remedy to relieve the symptoms of mild psoriasis.

Dose: apply up to 4 times a day.
Side effects:
Caution: remove jewellery. Do not apply on top of another product.
Not to be used for:
Not to be used with: other remedies – see above.
Contains: poke root, clivers, sulphur, zinc oxide.

Psoriderm
(Dermal)

A bath emulsion, cream, and scalp lotion used to treat psoriasis.

Dose: add 30 ml of the emulsion to the bath water and soak for 5 minutes. The cream is applied twice daily, and the scalp lotion is used as a shampoo.
Side effects: irritation, sensitivity to light.
Caution: avoid the eyes, and avoid exposure to sunlight after treatment. Clothing may be stained.
Not to be used for: patients suffering from acute psoriasis.
Not to be used with:
Contains: coal tar.

Psorigel
(Galderma)

An emollient gel used as a treatment for psoriasis and eczema to relieve the itching and flaking.

Dose: rub into the affected area and allow to dry 1-2 times a day. Remove any excess.
Side effects: irritation, sensitivity to light.
Caution: avoid the eyes, and avoid exposure to sunlight after treatment. Clothing may be stained.
Not to be used for: patients suffering from acute psoriasis, or on very inflamed or broken skin.

Not to be used with:
Contains: coal tar solution.

Psorin
(Thames)
An ointment and scalp gel used as an antipsoriatic skin softener to treat psoriasis.

Dose: apply ointment to the affected area twice a day. Use scalp gel for 10-20 minutes before washing off.
Side effects: irritation, sensitivity to light.
Caution: keep out of the eyes, and avoid direct sunlight after treatment. Clothing may be stained. (It is advisable to test the skin for sensitivity before using full treatment.)
Not to be used for: patients suffering from unstable psoriasis.
Not to be used with:
Contains: coal tar, dithranol, salicyclic acid.

Pyrethrum
(Nelsons)

A liquid or spray used as a herbal treatment for insect bites and stings.

Dose: apply as soon as possible after bite or sting.
Side effects:
Caution:
Not to be used for:
Not to be used with:
Contains: tinctures of hypericum, rumex crispus, echinacea, ledum palustre, calendula, arnica, pyrethrum.

Quinoderm
(Quinoderm)

A cream (available in 2 strengths) and lotio-gel (available in the weaker strength) used as an antibacterial skin softener to treat acne.

Dose: massage into the affected area 1-3 times a day.
Side effects: irritation, peeling, redness.
Caution: keep out of the eyes, nose, mouth. May bleach dyed fabrics. New users are advised to use the weaker-strength products and progress to the stronger cream only if necessary.
Not to be used for: patients suffering from rosacea (a disease that reddens the face).
Not to be used with: other similar products.
Contains: potassium hydroxyquinolone sulphate, benzoyl peroxide.

Rotersept
(Crookes Holland)

An aerosol used as a disinfectant to treat sore nipples when breastfeeding.

Dose: spray on to the breast before and after feeding.
Side effects:
Caution: may cause staining in contact with chlorine-containing detergents and bleaches.
Not to be used for: children.
Not to be used with:
Contains: chlorhexidine gluconate.

---

royal jelly* see entry in 'Vitamins and minerals' section

Salactol
(Dermal)

A paint used as a skin softener to treat warts, verrucae, corns, and calluses.

Dose: apply at night.
Side effects: inflammation.
Caution: do not apply to healthy skin. Keep away from eyes and mucous membranes. Do not inhale the vapour.
Not to be used for: warts on the face or anal and genital areas, or for moles, birthmarks, or other skin blemishes. Not to be used by diabetics nor patients with poor circulation.
Not to be used with:
Contains: salicyclic acid, lactic acid, flexible collodion.

Salatac
(Dermal)

A gel supplied with an emery board, and used as a skin softener to treat warts, corns, and calluses.

Dose: apply daily, and rub down weekly with the emery board.
Side effects:
Caution:
Not to be used for: moles or skin problems other than warts, corns, or calluses.
Not to be used with:
Contains: lactic acid, salicylic acid, camphor, pyroxylin, ethanol, ethyl acetate.

Savlon Bath Oil
(Zyma Healthcare)

A bath oil used as an emollient to moisturize dry skin conditions.

Dose: 2 capsful added to a bath.
Side effects:
Caution: guard against slipping in the bath.
Not to be used for:
Not to be used with:
Contains: liquid paraffin, acetylated wool alcohols.

Savlon Dry Skin*
(Zyma Healthcare)

A lanolin-free cream and lotion used as an emollient to treat dry, flaking, rough, and chapped skin, including dry-stage eczema.

Dose: apply when required.
Side effects:
Caution: avoid the eyes.
Not to be used for:
Not to be used with:
Contains: cream: white soft paraffin, light liquid paraffin; lotion: purified water, petrolatum, glycerol.

Savlon Nappy Rash Cream
(Zyma Healthcare)

A cream used as a barrier and antiseptic to treat and prevent nappy rash.

Dose: apply as required.
Side effects:
Caution:
Not to be used for:
Not to be used with:
Contains: dimethicone, cetrimide.

Scholl Blister Treatment
(Scholl)

A dressing applied to blisters to soothe and promote healing, and to absorb moisture.

Dose: apply to affected area, and leave in place for several days if needed.

Side effects:
Caution:
Not to be used for:
Not to be used with:
Contains: hydrocolloid absorbent dressing.

Scholl Corn and Callous Removal Products
(Scholl)

A range of medicated products (plasters and liquids) used to soften the skin and remove the corn or callus.

Dose: plasters are applied every day (liquid – applied twice a day) until corn or callus can be removed. Maximum treatment period: 2 weeks.
Side effects: irritation, allergy.
Caution: children under 16 years, diabetics, and patients with poor circulation should consult a doctor before using these products.
Not to be used for: normal skin, inflamed or broken skin.
Not to be used with:
Contains: salicylic acid.

Scholl Toenail Softening Solution*
(Scholl)

A liquid applied to hard or sharp toenails to soften them and reduce discomfort.

Dose: apply twice a day until discomfort is relieved.
Side effects:
Caution: avoid contact with the eyes.
Not to be used for: diabetics, patients with circulatory disorders, broken skin.
Not to be used with:
Contains: sodium thiosulphate.

Scholl Verruca Removal System
(Scholl)

A medicated disc (supplied with a covering plaster) and used as a skin softener to treat verrucae.

Dose: apply disc to verruca and cover with plaster. Leave in place for 48 hours, then replace. Treat for up to 12 weeks.
Side effects:
Caution: diabetics and patients with circulatory disorders should consult a doctor before using this product.
Not to be used for: babies under 4 weeks, of for patients allergic to aspirin, or for inflamed, broken, or normal skin. Do not apply to moles, birthmarks, hairy warts, facial or genital warts, or mucous membranes.
Not to be used with:
Contains: salicylic acid.

Siopel
(Zeneca)

An antiseptic barrier cream used to treat nappy rash and other similar disorders where the skin needs to be protected from water-soluble irritants.

Dose: apply up to 5 times a day at first, then once or twice a day.
Side effects:
Caution: avoid eyes and ears.
Not to be used for: very inflamed or weeping skin.
Not to be used with:
Contains: dimethicone, cetrimide.

Skin Clear Ointment
(Potters)

An ointment used as an astringent and mild antiseptic to relieve the symptoms of mild acne, mild dry eczema, and difficult skin conditions.

Dose: apply twice a day.
Side effects:
Caution: remove jewellery.
Not to be used for: children under 5 years.
Not to be used with:
Contains: sulphur, zinc oxide, tea tree oil.

Skin Clear Tablets
(Potters)

A tablet used as a herbal remedy to relieve symptoms of minor skin conditions and blemishes.

Dose: 2 tablets 3 times a day.
Side effects:
Caution:
Not to be used for: children, pregnant women, or nursing mothers.
Not to be used with:
Contains: echinacea.

Skin Eruptions Mixture
(Potters)

A mixture used as a herbal remedy to treat the symptoms of mild eczema, psoriasis, and other skin diseases.

Dose: adults 5 ml 3 times a day; children over 8 years 5 ml every 12 hours.
Side effects:
Caution: pregnant women and nursing mothers are advised to consult a doctor before using this product.
Not to be used for: children under 8 years.

Not to be used with:
Contains: blue flag, burdock root, yellow dock, sarsaparilla, cascara, buchu leaf.

Skintex
(Aimee Lloyd)

A cream used to soothe chapped or split hands, sunburn, corns, and calluses.

Dose: apply 3-4 times a day for up to 10 days.
Side effects:
Caution: pregnant women and nursing mothers should consult a doctor before using this product.
Not to be used for:
Not to be used with:
Contains: chloroxylenol, camphor.

Snowfire
(Pickles)

An emollient ointment tablet used to treat chapped hands and chilblains.

Dose: apply when required.
Side effects:
Caution:
Not to be used for:
Not to be used with:
Contains: benzoin, citronella, thyme oil, clove oil, cade oil.

Solarcaine
(Schering-Plough)

A spray, cream, and moisturizing lotion used as an antiseptic and local anaesthetic to give temporary relief from itching and pain due to minor injury, insect bites, or sunburn.

Dose: apply 3-4 times a day.
Side effects:
Caution: avoid using spray on the face or sensitive areas of skin.
Not to be used for: children under 3 years, or on deep wounds or serious burns, or for prolonged periods.
Not to be used with:
Contains: benzocaine, triclosan.

Sprilon
(Perstorp Pharma)

A spray used as a barrier product to protect the skin and assist in the treatment of eczema, splits in the skin, and bedsores.

Dose: spray on to the skin for 2-3 seconds.
Side effects:
Caution:
Not to be used for:
Not to be used with:
Contains: dimethicone, zinc oxide.

---

starflower oil* see entry in 'Women's disorders' section

Stingose
(Chancellor)

An astringent spray used to treat insect bites and stings.

Dose: apply as soon as possible, and repeat as necessary.
Side effects:
Caution: keep out of eyes.
Not to be used for:
Not to be used with:

Contains: aluminium sulphate.

Sudocrem
(Tosara)

An antiseptic healing cream used to treat nappy rash, eczema, bedsores, acne, minor wounds and burns, sunburn, and chilblains.

Dose: apply when required.
Side effects:
Caution:
Not to be used for:
Not to be used with:
Contains: zinc oxide, benzyl alcohol, benzyl benzoate, benzyl cinnamate, lanolin.

Steripod Blue see entry in 'Eye conditions' section
(Seton Healthcare)

---

surgical spirit BP

A liquid used to disinfect or clean the skin, or to harden skin on the feet.

Dose: apply as needed, but avoid over-use.
Side effects:
Caution: avoid inhaling the vapour.
Not to be used for:
Not to be used with:
Contains: surgical spirit.

---

talc dusting powder BP

A powder used to prevent friction of skin surfaces (in folds of skin, etc.).

Dose: apply when required.
Side effects:
Caution:
Not to be used for:
Not to be used with:
Contains: starch, sterilized purified talc.

___

tea tree oil*

A herbal product, often incorporated into creams or other skin products, and used for its antiseptic properties.

Dose: (as specified for each individual product).
Side effects:
Caution:
Not to be used for:
Not to be used with:
Contains: tea tree oil (also known as ti-tree oil).

___

Torbetol
(Torbet Laboratories)

A lotion used as an antibacterial treatment for acne.

Dose: apply to the affected area up to 3 times a day.
Side effects: irritation.
Caution: avoid contact with the eyes, lips, and mouth.
Not to be used for: babies.
Not to be used with:
Contains: cetrimide, chlorhexidine gluconate.

___

Trinity Ointment see **zinc cream BP**
(Thornton and Ross)

___

Ultra Clearasil see **Quinoderm Cream**
(Procter & Gamble)

Ultrabase see **Diprobase**
(Schering Health Care)

Unguentum Merck
(Whitehall)

A cream used as a lanolin-free emollient, to treat soreness
and itching of dry skin problems, including eczema and
dermatitis.

Dose: apply when required.
Side effects:
Caution:
Not to be used for:
Not to be used with:
Contains: silicic acid, liquid paraffin, white soft paraffin,
cetostearyl alcohol, polysorbate 40, glycerol monostearate.

Valderma
(Roche Consumer Health)

An antibacterial cream used to treat spots.

Dose: apply 2-3 times a day after washing.
Side effects:
Caution:
Not to be used for:
Not to be used with:
Contains: potassium hydroxyquinoline sulphate, chlorocresol.

Valpeda
(Roche Consumer Health)

A cream used as an antibacterial and antifungal treatment for foot infections, such as athlete's foot.

Dose: apply twice a day.
Side effects:
Caution:
Not to be used for:
Not to be used with:
Contains: halquinol.

Varicose Ointment
(Potters)

An ointment used as a mainly herbal remedy to relieve skin conditions of the lower limbs where there is irritation due to varicosity.

Dose: apply twice a day.
Side effects:
Caution:
Not to be used for: children.
Not to be used with:
Contains: cade oil, witch hazel, zinc oxide.

Vaseline Dermacare Lotion*
(Elida Gibbs)

A lotion used as an emollient to relieve symptoms of dry skin. (Cream* form also available.)

Dose: apply 2-3 times a day.
Side effects:
Caution:
Not to be used for:

Not to be used with:
Contains: white soft paraffin, mineral oil, dimethicone.

Vasogen
(Pharmax)

A cream used as a soothing, antiseptic barrier cream to treat nappy rash, bedsores, and sore hands.

Dose: use regularly.
Side effects:
Caution:
Not to be used for:
Not to be used with:
Contains: dimethicone, zinc oxide, calamine.

Veracur
(Typharm)

A gel used as a skin softener to treat warts and verrucae.

Dose: apply twice a day.
Side effects:
Caution: do not apply to healthy skin.
Not to be used for: warts on the face or anal and genital areas, or on broken skin.
Not to be used with:
Contains: formaldehyde.

Verrugon
(Pickles)

An ointment supplied with felt rings and plasters used as a skin softener to treat verrucae.

Dose: apply a felt ring arround the verruca, apply the ointment, and cover with a plaster. Repeat daily. Treatment is usually required for several weeks.
Side effects:
Caution: do not apply to healthy skin.
Not to be used for: broken or infected areas of skin.
Not to be used with:
Contains: salicyclic acid.

Verucasep
(Galen)

A gel used as a virucidal, skin-drying treatment for viral warts.

Dose: apply twice a day, and cover.
Side effects: stains the skin.
Caution: do not apply to healthy skin.
Not to be used for: warts on the face or anal and genital regions.
Not to be used with:
Contains: glutaraldehyde.

Vitathone
(Seton Healthcare)

An ointment used to relieve the itching of chilblains.

Dose: apply every 2-3 hours.
Side effects:
Caution:
Not to be used for: children.
Not to be used with:
Contains: methyl nicotinate.

Wartex
(Pickles)

An ointment used as a skin softener to treat warts.

Dose: apply daily for several days.
Side effects:
Caution: avoid normal skin.
Not to be used for: diabetics and patients with impaired circulation, or on moles, birthmarks, facial warts, or hairy warts.
Not to be used with:
Contains: salicylic acid.

Wash E45*
(Crookes Healthcare)

A wash cream used to clean and soften dry skin.

Dose: apply to the dry skin and rinse off.
Side effects:
Caution: avoid contact with the eyes. Guard against slipping in bath or shower.
Not to be used for:
Not to be used with:
Contains: zinc oxide, mineral oils.

Wasp-eze see entry in 'Allergic disorders' section
(Seton Healthcare)

WCS Dusting Powder
(Weleda)

A powder used as a herbal remedy to treat minor burns and wounds that need to be kept dry.

Dose: dust the area and cover with a dry dressing. Change the dressing twice a day.
Side effects:

Caution:
Not to be used for: patients with a deep infection. (May heal the surface and seal in sepsis.)
Not to be used with:
Contains: arnica, marigold, echinacea, silica, Stibium Metallicum Praep.

Witch Doctor
(E. C. De Witt)

A gel used as an astringent treatment for itching, insect bites and stings, bruises, grazes, skin irritations, minor burns, and excess oil on the skin.

Dose: apply to the affected area as needed.
Side effects:
Caution:
Not to be used for: application to the eyes.
Not to be used with:
Contains: witch hazel.

---

witch hazel

A liquid used to soothe sore, irritated skin and to relieve the discomfort of bruises and sprains.

Dose: apply to the skin as needed.
Side effects:
Caution:
Not to be used for:
Not to be used with:
Contains: witch hazel.

Witch Stik
(E. C. De Witt)

A stick used as an astringent treatment for minor skin infections, spots, cuts, insect bites, and irritations.

Dose: apply when needed.
Side effects:
Caution:
Not to be used for:
Not to be used with:
Contains: witch hazel.

Zeasorb
(Stiefel)

A dusting powder used to absorb excess moisture in the skin-fold areas (such as armpits, groin, etc.).

Dose: apply to dry skin.
Side effects:
Caution: avoid inhalation and contact with eyes or broken skin.
Not to be used for:
Not to be used with:
Contains: chloroxylenol, aluminium dihydroxyallantoinate.

---

zinc and castor oil ointment BP

An ointment used as an emollient and astringent to treat and protect sore skin (as in nappy rash).

Dose: apply as needed.
Side effects:
Caution:
Not to be used for:
Not to be used with:
Contains: zinc oxide, castor oil.

---

zinc and coal tar paste BP

A paste used to treat eczema and psoriasis.

Dose: apply once or twice a day.
Side effects: irritation, allergy, sensitivity to light.
Caution: may stain clothing. Avoid exposure to strong sunlight after treatment.
Not to be used for: patients with acute attacks of psoriasis.
Not to be used with:
Contains: zinc oxide, coal tar.

---

zinc cream BP

A cream used to relieve nappy rash and eczema conditions.

Dose: apply as needed.
Side effects:
Caution:
Not to be used for:
Not to be used with:
Contains: zinc oxide, arachis oil.

---

zinc ointment BP

An ointment used to treat nappy rash and eczema conditions.

Dose: apply as needed.
Side effects:
Caution:
Not to be used for:
Not to be used with:
Contains: zinc oxide.

---

zinc, starch and talc dusting powder BP

A powder used to prevent friction of skin surfaces (in folds of skin, etc.).

Dose: apply when required.
Side effects:
Caution:
Not to be used for:
Not to be used with:
Contains: zinc oxide, starch, sterilized purified talc.

Zoff Adhesive Remover Wipes*
(Smith & Nephew Medical)

A moist wipe used to assist in the removal of adhesive dressings from the skin.

Dose: squeeze wipe at edge of adhesive, pull off dressing, then wash and dry.
Side effects:
Caution: avoid the eyes. Use with adequate ventilation.
Not to be used for:
Not to be used with:
Contains: p.naphtha, 1,1,1-trichloroethane.

Scalp disorders

Dandruff and other scaly scalp disorders are relatively common, and often respond to one of the products listed below. Tar-based products are useful in relieving irritated scalps due to eczema, dermatitis, or other disorders. Infections of the scalp should be seen by a doctor.

Oil-based products are useful to treat cradle-cap in infants because the oil gently lifts the scales from the scalp. Cradle-cap is not harmful in itself, however, but merely unsightly. Treatment is not essential, therefore.

Minoxidil (Regaine) has been introduced recently to treat hair loss. It is important to remember that treatment with this product must continue for the benefit to persist. (If it is stopped, then the hair loss will probably recur.)

Products for treating head lice are included in the 'Anti-infestation preparations' section.

Adiantine
(Potters)

A liquid used as a herbal remedy to improve the hair condition and eliminate dandruff.

Dose: massage into scalp night and morning.
Side effects:
Caution:
Not to be used for: children.
Not to be used with:
Contains: southernwood, bay oil, rosemary oil, witch hazel.

Alphosyl Shampoo 2-in-1
(Stafford-Miller)

A liquid used as a medicated, conditioning shampoo to treat itchy and scaly scalps, dandruff, and psoriasis.

Dose: apply every 2-3 days as a shampoo.
Side effects: irritation.
Caution: avoid contact with the eyes.
Not to be used for:
Not to be used with:
Contains: coal tar, conditioner.

Baltar
(Merck)

A liquid used as a medicated shampoo to treat psoriasis, dandruff, eczema, seborrhoea, and other itchy scalp disorders.

Dose: shampoo the hair with the liquid 1-3 times a week.
Side effects:
Caution: keep out of the eyes.
Not to be used for: children under 2 years or for patients

suffering from wet or weeping scalp disorders or where the skin is badly broken.
Not to be used with:
Contains: coal tar.

Betadine Scalp and Skin Cleanser
(Seton Healthcare)

A solution used as an antiseptic and detergent to treat scalp conditions and acne on the face and neck.

Dose: use as a shampoo (or apply directly to the skin and rinse) twice a week until improved.
Side effects: allergy, irritation.
Caution: jewellery may be discoloured.
Not to be used for: children under 2 years, or on broken skin.
Not to be used with:
Contains: povidone-iodine.

Betadine Shampoo see Betadine Scalp and Skin Cleanser
(Seton Healthcare)

Betasept Shampoo
(Seton Healthcare)

An antiseptic shampoo used to treat flaky scalp conditions, excess dandruff, itching, scaling, inflammation and reddening of the scalp.

Dose: use as a shampoo twice a week until condition improves, then once a week.
Side effects:
Caution: pregnant women, nursing mothers, and patients with thyroid or kidney disorders should avoid regular use.
Not to be used for: children under 2 years or patients with allergy to iodine.

Not to be used with: lithium treatment.
Contains: povidone-iodine.

Boots Cradle Cap Cream
(Boots)

A cream applied to the scalp to relieve cradle cap and scurf.

Dose: massage on to scalp 2-3 times a day.
Side effects: rash.
Caution:
Not to be used for:
Not to be used with:
Contains: almond oil, lanolin.

Capasal
(Dermal)

A shampoo used to treat dry scaly scalp conditions.

Dose: use daily if needed.
Side effects: irritation.
Caution: avoid the eyes.
Not to be used for:
Not to be used with:
Contains: salicylic acid, coconut oil, coal tar.

Capitol
(Dermal)

A gel used as an antibacterial treatment for dandruff and other scaly scalp disorders.

Dose: use as a shampoo.
Side effects:
Caution:

Not to be used for:
Not to be used with:
Contains: benzalkonium chloride.

Ceanel
(Quinoderm)

A liquid used as an antibacterial, antifungal treatment for psoriasis, seborrhoeic inflammation of the scalp, and dandruff.

Dose: use as a shampoo 3 times a week at first and then twice a week, or apply directly to other areas of the skin as needed.
Side effects:
Caution: keep out of the eyes. Pregnant women should consult a doctor before using this product.
Not to be used for:
Not to be used with:
Contains: phenylethyl alcohol, undecanoic acid, cetrimide.

Clinitar see entry in 'Skin disorders' section
(Shire)

Cocois
(Bioglan)

An ointment used for dry and scaly scalp conditions.

Dose: apply a thin ribbon of ointment to the scalp. Wash out after 1 hour. For severe conditions use initially for 3-7 days, then intermittently as required. (For less severe conditions, use weekly).
Side effects: irritation, sensitivity to sunlight.
Caution: avoid the eyes. Pregnant women, patients with psoriasis and children aged 6-12 years should consult a doctor before using this product. May stain fabrics and jewellery.
Not to be used for: children under 6 years, or for infected

scalp conditions.
Not to be used with:
Contains: coal tar solution, salicylic acid, sulphur, coconut oil.

Denorex
(Whitehall)

A shampoo, available with or without conditioner added, and used as a medicated treatment for dandruff, and to soothe irritation of the scalp.

Dose: use on alternate days for 10 days, then 2-3 times a week thereafter.
Side effects: irritation.
Caution: avoid contact with the eyes.
Not to be used for:
Not to be used with:
Contains: coal tar solution, menthol.

Dentinox Cradle Cap Treatment Shampoo
(Dendron)

A shampoo used as a treatment for cradle cap in infants.

Dose: apply twice at each bath time until condition clears, then use as needed.
Side effects:
Caution: keep out of the eyes.
Not to be used for:
Not to be used with:
Contains: sodium lauryl ether sulphosuccinate.

Gelcotar see entry in 'Skin disorders' section
(Quinoderm)

Genisol
(Roche Consumer Health)

A liquid used as a treatment for dandruff.

Dose: shampoo once a week or as needed.
Side effects: irritation, sensitivity to light.
Caution: dilute before use. Avoid exposure to sunlight after treatment. May stain clothing.
Not to be used for: patients suffering from acute psoriasis.
Not to be used with:
Contains: coal tar, sodium sulphosuccinated undecylenic monoalkylolamide.

Ionil T
(Galderma)

A shampoo used as a treatment for dandruff.

Dose: use as a shampoo once or twice weekly.
Side effects: irritation, sensitivity to light.
Caution: avoid contact with the eyes.
Not to be used for: patients suffering from acute psoriasis.
Not to be used with:
Contains: coal tar solution, salicyclic acid, benzalkonium chloride.

Lenium see Selsun
(Cilag)

Medicated Extract of Rosemary.
(Potters)

A liquid used as a herbal remedy to improve hair condition.

Dose: massage gently into scalp twice a day.

Side effects:
Caution:
Not to be used for: children.
Not to be used with:
Contains: rosemary oil, rosegeranium oil, methyl salicylate, bay oil.

Meted
(Euroderma)

A shampoo used as an antiseptic and skin-softening treatment for psoriasis and scaly scalp conditions.

Dose: use as a shampoo twice a day.
Side effects: irritation.
Caution: avoid the eyes.
Not to be used for:
Not to be used with:
Contains: sulphur, salicylic acid.

Pentrax
(Euroderma)

A shampoo used as a treatment for psoriasis and scaly scalp conditions.

Dose: use as a shampoo, then re-apply and leave on scalp for 10 minutes before washing off.
Side effects: irritation.
Caution: avoid the eyes.
Not to be used for:
Not to be used with:
Contains: coal tar, conditioner.

Pixol see entry in 'Skin disorders' section
(Thames)

Polytar Liquid
(Stiefel)

A liquid used as a medicated treatment for dandruff and other scaly scalp conditions.

Dose: use as a shampoo once or twice a week.
Side effects:
Caution:
Not to be used for:
Not to be used with:
Contains: tar, cade oil, coal tar, arachis oil, oleyl alcohol.

Polytar 3-in-1
(Stiefel)

A medicated scalp cleanser and conditioner for the treatment of itching, flaking scalps and severe dandruff.

Dose: (as directed on the product pack).
Side effects: irritation.
Caution: avoid the eyes.
Not to be used for:
Not to be used with:
Contains: tar blend, oleyl alcohol.

Polytar AF
(Stiefel)

A medicated scalp cleanser for the treatment of scaling scalp disorders including seborrhoeic dermatitis and dandruff.

Dose: use 2-3 times a week for at least 3 weeks, or until cleared.

(For prevention, use once weekly.)
Side effects: irritation, rash, skin which is sensitive to light.
Caution: avoid contact with the eyes.
Not to be used for:
Not to be used with:
Contains: tar blend, zinc pyrithione.

Polytar Plus
(Stiefel)

A liquid used as a medicated, conditioning treatment for itchy and flaking scalps, psoriasis, and dandruff.

Dose: use as shampoo once or twice a week.
Side effects: irritation.
Caution: avoid the eyes.
Not to be used for:
Not to be used with:
Contains: hydrolysed animal protein, tar, oleyl alcohol, arachis oil, coal tar solution, crude coal tar.

Psoriderm Scalp Lotion see entry in 'Skin disorders' section
(Dermal)

Psorin Scalp Gel see entry in 'Skin disorders' section
(Thames)

Regaine
(Upjohn)

A liquid used as a hair restorer to treat hair loss in men and women.

Dose: apply to bald area twice a day for 4 months. Treatment must be continued if hair loss is to be prevented.

Side effects: irritation, allergy, palpitations, dizziness, chest or arm pain, indigestion, swelling of hands, stomach, face, or ankles. Initially hair loss may increase (after 2-6 weeks of use).
Caution: children should not be treated, except under the supervision of a doctor. Keep away from the eyes and mouth. Patients with heart disease, angina, high or low blood pressure, and those taking any other medication should consult a doctor before using this product.
Not to be used for: pregnant women, nursing mothers, or on areas of broken skin.
Not to be used with:
Contains: minoxidil.

Selsun
(Abbott)

A suspension used as a treatment for dandruff.

Dose: shampoo twice a week initially, then use when required
Side effects: irritation.
Caution: keep out of the eyes or broken skin; do not use within 48 hours of using waving or colouring substances. Avoid contact with hairgrips, jewellery, or metal.
Not to be used for: children under 5 years, or for women in the first 3 months of pregnancy
Not to be used with:
Contains: selenium sulphide.

T-Gel
(Neutrogena)

A shampoo used as a treatment for itchy, flaky scalp disorders, such as dandruff, psoriasis, and seborrhoeic dermatitis. (An unlicensed conditioner for the hair is also available in the T-Gel range.)

Dose: use as shampoo when required.
Side effects: irritation, discoloration of blond, bleached, or tinted hair.
Caution: avoid contact with the eyes.
Not to be used for: patients suffering from inflamed or broken skin.
Not to be used with:
Contains: coal tar extract.

Antiseptics

Included below is a wide variety of antiseptic creams, lotions, and solutions that are available over the counter. Products containing antiseptics and other ingredients will be found in the general skin section of this book (see 'Skin disorders'). Many people are familiar with products, such as Savlon, TCP, and Germolene, and these skin disinfectants all do essentially the same job in the treatment of wounds, burns, nappy rash, or ulcers that may have an infective component. Your pharmacist will be able to advise which of these is appropriate in any particular situation but, in general, liquid applications (which dry quickly) are preferred because creams can encourage infections to develop owing to the increased moisture content of the area treated. Severe skin infection (cellulitis) may develop into lymphangitis, with red streaks appearing under the skin. These need antibiotic therapy and must be seen by the physician. Deep-seated boils will also need antibiotic treatment, although magnesium sulphate paste can be tried on smaller boils to draw out the pus.

Acriflex
(Seton Healthcare)

A cream used as an antiseptic treatment for minor burns and scalds, minor wounds, sunburn, blisters, and infected or cracked skin.

Dose: apply when required.
Side effects:
Caution:
Not to be used for:
Not to be used with:
Contains: chlorhexidine gluconate.

Anaflex Cream
(Geistlich)

A cream used as an antibacterial and antifungal treatment for skin infections.

Dose: apply the cream to the affected area 1-2 times a day.
Side effects:
Caution:
Not to be used for: application to deep wounds.
Not to be used with:
Contains: polynoxylin.

Betadine Ointment
(Seton Healthcare)

An ointment used as an antiseptic to treat or prevent infection in minor wounds.

Dose: apply to the affected area and cover once a day.
Side effects: irritation, allergy.
Caution:

Not to be used for: children under 2 years.
Not to be used with:
Contains: povidone-iodine.

Betadine Paint
(Seton Healthcare)

A liquid used as an antiseptic to prevent infection in cold sores and minor wounds.

Dose: apply twice a day.
Side effects: irritation, allergy.
Caution:
Not to be used for:
Not to be used with:
Contains: povidone-iodine.

Betadine Scalp and Skin Cleanser see entry in 'Scalp conditions' section.
(Seton Healthcare)

Betadine Skin Cleanser
(Seton Healthcare)

A liquid used as an antiseptic and cleansing treatment for acne and other skin conditions.

Dose: use to wash the skin twice a day, reducing to once daily when improved.
Side effects: allergy, irritation.
Caution: may discolour jewellery.
Not to be used for: children under 2 years.
Not to be used with:
Contains: povidone-iodine.

Betadine Spray
(Seton Healthcare)

A dry powder spray used as an antiseptic to treat and prevent infection in cuts, wounds, and burns.

Dose: spray on to the affected area once a day or as needed, and cover.
Side effects: allergy, irritation.
Caution: keep out of the eyes, and avoid inhaling the spray.
Not to be used for: children under 2 years.
Not to be used with:
Contains: povidone-iodine.

Betasept Acne Wash
(Seton Healthcare)

An antiseptic face wash used to treat acne on the face and neck.

Dose: use to wash the skin twice a day.
Side effects: allergy, irritation.
Caution: pregnant women and nursing mothers should avoid regular use of this product. May discolour jewellery.
Not to be used for: patients with allergy to iodine or with thyroid disorders.
Not to be used with:
Contains: povidone-iodine.

Betasept Antiseptic Gargle and Mouthwash Concentrate
see entry in 'Diseases of the mouth and throat' section.
(Seton Healthcare)

Betasept Shampoo see entry in 'Scalp disorders' section.
(Seton Healthcare)

Boots Antiseptic Cream
(Boots)

A cream used as a soothing and healing treatment for minor wounds, insect bites, and spots.

Dose: apply 2-3 times a day.
Side effects:
Caution:
Not to be used for:
Not to be used with:
Contains: dichlorobenzyl alcohol, cetrimide, allantoin.

Boots Antiseptic Disinfectant Wipes*
(Boots)

A wipe impregnated with antiseptic, for personal use (to clean minor wounds, insect bites, or stings, or to disinfect the hands), and around the home.

Dose: use as required.
Side effects: irritation.
Caution: avoid contact with the mouth.
Not to be used for:
Not to be used with:
Contains: cetrimide, bronopol.

Boots Antiseptic Wipes
(Boots)

A moist wipe impregnated with antiseptic, used to clean minor wounds and prevent re-infection.

Dose: wipe the wound to clean, when required.
Side effects: irritation.
Caution:

Not to be used for: areas near the eyes.
Not to be used with:
Contains: cetrimide.

Boots Extra Protection Antiseptic Disinfectant* see Savion Liquid*
(Boots)

Brulidine
(Rhone-Poulenc Rorer Family Health)

A cream used as an antiseptic and antifungal treatment for minor wounds and burns, scalp ringworm and other fungal infections, and nappy rash.

Dose: adults apply 2-3 times a day.
Side effects:
Caution:
Not to be used for:
Not to be used with:
Contains: dibromopropamidine isethionate.

Cepton
(Zyma Healthcare)

An antiseptic lotion and skin wash, used to treat and tone oily skin (lotion) and treat or prevent acne (skin wash).

Dose: apply skin wash to clean skin and leave for one minute before washing off. Apply lotion as required.
Side effects:
Caution: keep out of eyes and ears.
Not to be used for:
Not to be used with:
Contains: chlorhexidine gluconate.

Cetavlex
(Zeneca)

A cream used as an antiseptic to treat minor wounds, burns, and nappy rash.

Dose: apply as needed.
Side effects: irritation.
Caution: keep out of the eyes and ears.
Not to be used for:
Not to be used with:
Contains: cetrimide.

Cetrimide Cream see **Cetavlex**
(Waterhouse)

Co-op Antiseptic Cream
(Co-op)

A cream used as an antiseptic to treat minor wounds, spots, pimples, and rashes.

Dose: apply 2-3 times a day. (If necessary, clean wound first).
Side effects:
Caution:
Not to be used for:
Not to be used with:
Contains: allantoin, cetrimide, dichlorobenzyl alcohol.

DDD
(DDD Ltd)

A medicated cream and lotion used as an antiseptic to treat spots and minor skin problems.

Dose: apply twice a day (or more frequently for the lotion if

needed).
Side effects:
Caution:
Not to be used for:
Not to be used with:
Contains: chlorbutol, menthol, thymol, methyl salicylate. (The cream also contains titanium dioxide. The lotion also contains glycerin, alcohol, and salicylic acid.)

Dettol Antiseptic Cream
(Reckitt & Colman)

An antiseptic cream used to treat minor wounds, insect bites, and stings.

Dose: apply when required.
Side effects:
Caution:
Not to be used for:
Not to be used with:
Contains: chloroxylenol, triclosan, edetic acid.

Dettol Fresh
(Reckitt & Colman)

A liquid used as an antiseptic to treat minor wounds, insect bites, stings, spots, and as an antiseptic bath additive.

Dose: dilute as directed, then bathe affected area or add to bath water.
Side effects:
Caution: babies under 9 months should not be bathed in water containing this product unless a doctor is first consulted. Do not use this product undiluted.
Not to be used for: areas of eczema.
Not to be used with:

Contains: benzalkonium chloride.

Dettol Liquid
(Reckitt & Colman)

A liquid used as an antiseptic to treat minor wounds, insect bites, stings, dandruff, spots, and as an antiseptic bath additive.

Dose: dilute as directed, then bathe affected area or add to bath water.
Side effects:
Caution: babies under 9 months should not be bathed in water containing this product unless a doctor is first consulted. Do not use this product undiluted.
Not to be used for: areas of eczema.
Not to be used with:
Contains: chloroxylenol.

Germolene Antiseptic Cream
(SmithKline Beecham Consumer)

A cream used as an antiseptic and local anaesthetic to treat minor wounds and burns, scalds, blisters, insect bites, stings, spots, and chapped skin.

Dose: apply when required.
Side effects:
Caution:
Not to be used for:
Not to be used with:
Contains: phenol, chlorhexidine gluconate.

Germolene Antiseptic Ointment
(SmithKline Beecham Consumer)

An antiseptic, soothing, and protective ointment used to treat minor wounds, burns and scalds, blisters, and sore skin. (For use in treating aching muscles, see entry in 'Joint and muscle disorders' section.)

Dose: apply to affected area when required.
Side effects:
Caution:
Not to be used for:
Not to be used with:
Contains: lanolin, white soft paraffin, yellow soft paraffin, light liquid paraffin, starch, zinc oxide, methyl salicylate, octaphonium chloride, phenol.

Germolene Antiseptic Wipes*
(SmithKline Beecham Consumer)

A wipe impregnated with antiseptic, used to clean the skin and help protect from infection.

Dose: use when required.
Side effects:
Caution:
Not to be used for:
Not to be used with:
Contains: benzalkonium chloride, chlorhexidine gluconate.

Hioxyl
(Quinoderm)

A cream used as a disinfectant to treat minor wounds, infections, bed sores, and leg ulcers.

Dose: apply freely as needed and cover with a dressing.
Side effects:
Caution: avoid contact with dyed fabrics. Leg ulcers should be treated only under medical supervision.

Not to be used for:
Not to be used with: other skin medications.
Contains: hydrogen peroxide.

hydrogen peroxide BP (20 volume)

A liquid used to clean and disinfect wounds. (For use as a mouthwash and gargle, see 'Diseases of the mouth' section.)

Dose: dilute with an equal amount of water and wash the wound to clean.
Side effects:
Caution:
Not to be used for:
Not to be used with:
Contains: hydrogen peroxide.

Neo Baby Cream
(Neo)

An antiseptic cream used to treat nappy rash.

Dose: apply when required.
Side effects:
Caution:
Not to be used for:
Not to be used with:
Contains: cetrimide, benzalkonium chloride.

Permitabs
(Bioglan)

A tablet used to make a solution of potassium permanganate, for use as an antiseptic. (See **potassium permanganate solution**.)

Dose: dissolve 1 tablet in 4 litres of water to make a 0.01% solution.

Side effects: irritation of mucous membranes.

Caution: tablets are not to be swallowed – for external use only. Will stain skin and clothing.

Not to be used for:

Not to be used with:

Contains: potassium permanganate.

Phiso-Med
(Sanofi Winthrop)

A solution used as a disinfectant to treat acne, and to disinfect skin.

Dose: lather on to wet skin for 1 minute, then rinse.

Side effects:

Caution: in newborn infants dilute 10 times. Avoid the ears and eyes. May stain bleached fabrics.

Not to be used for:

Not to be used with:

Contains: chlorhexidine gluconate.

Pickles Antiseptic Cream see **Brulidine**
(Pickles)

---

potassium permanganate solution

A solution used as an antiseptic to cleanse and deodorize weeping eczema and wounds.

Dose: apply as a wet dressing, or soak the affected part in a 0.01% solution.

Side effects: irritation of mucous membranes.

Caution: stains skin and clothing.

Not to be used for:

Not to be used with:
Contains: potassium permanganate.

Savlon Antiseptic Wound Wash
(Zyma Healthcare)

An alcohol-free liquid spray used as a first-aid treatment to clean and disinfect minor wounds.

Dose: spray to flood the wound.
Side effects: irritation.
Caution: keep out of eyes.
Not to be used for:
Not to be used with: soap.
Contains: chlorhexidine gluconate.

Savlon Cream
(Zyma Healthcare)

An antiseptic cream used to help prevent infection and soothe and heal cuts, grazes, insect bites, and stings.

Dose: apply when required.
Side effects: irritation.
Caution:
Not to be used for:
Not to be used with:
Contains: cetrimide, chlorhexidine gluconate.

Savlon Dry
(Zyma Healthcare)

A dry spray used as an antiseptic first-aid treatment for minor wounds, burns, and scalds.

Dose: apply as required.

Side effects: irritation, allergy.
Caution: keep away from eyes and nose. Pregnant women and nursing mothers should consult a doctor before using this product.
Not to be used for: newborn or low birth-weight infants, or for patients allergic to iodine.
Not to be used with:
Contains: povidone-iodine.

Savlon Liquid*
(Zyma Healthcare)

A liquid used as an antiseptic to treat minor wounds and burns, insect bites and stings, and for use as a bath additive.

Dose: dilute before use, and follow directions on bottle.
Side effects: irritation.
Caution: keep out of the ears and eyes.
Not to be used for: areas of eczema.
Not to be used with:
Contains: chlorhexidine gluconate, cetrimide.

Scholl Antiseptic Foot Balm
(Scholl)

An antiseptic balm used to relieve foot discomfort, soothe sore areas, heal blisters and cracks, relieve itching due to chilblains, reduce tenderness due to sweating, and guard against infection.

Dose: apply twice a day.
Side effects:
Caution: diabetics should consult a doctor before using this product.
Not to be used for:
Not to be used with:
Contains: menthol, halquinol, methyl salicylate.

Secaderm
(Roche Consumer Health)

A salve used as an antiseptic and analgesic ointment to treat boils and minor skin infections.

Dose: apply once or twice a day, and cover.
Side effects:
Caution:
Not to be used for:
Not to be used with:
Contains: colophony, turpentine oil, melaleuca oil, terebene, phenol.

Solarcaine see entry in 'Skin disorders' section
(Schering-Plough)

Sudocrem see entry in 'Skin disorders' section
(Tosara)

TCP Antiseptic Ointment
(Chemist Brokers)

An antiseptic ointment used to treat pain and itching due to piles, minor wounds and burns, scalds, spots, insect bites and stings.

Dose: apply twice a day (for spots or piles) or when required for other conditions.
Side effects:
Caution:
Not to be used for:
Not to be used with:
Contains: TCP liquid antiseptic, iodine, methyl salicylate, sulphur, tannic acid, camphor, salicylic acid.

TCP First Aid Antiseptic Cream
(Chemist Brokers)

A cream used as an emollient and antiseptic to soothe minor wounds, insect bites, stings, blisters, and spots.

Dose: apply when required.
Side effects:
Caution:
Not to be used for:
Not to be used with:
Contains: chloroxylenol, triclosan, TCP liquid antiseptic, sodium salicylate.

TCP Liquid
(Chemist Brokers)

A liquid used as an antiseptic to treat sore throats, mouth ulcers, minor wounds, insect bites, stings, and spots.

Dose: for use as gargle, mouthwash, or first-aid cleanser, dilute before use. To treat mouth ulcers or spots, apply undiluted.
Side effects:
Caution:
Not to be used for:
Not to be used with:
Contains: phenol, halogenated phenols.

Vesagex see **Cetavlex**.
(Rybar)

Medicated dressings

To treat injuries, dressings may be obtained impregnated with various chemicals (for example, antiseptics to help prevent wound infections). The commonly used ones are listed below, although others are available (usually used by doctors and nurses) to dress leg ulcers and more serious wounds.

Bactigras
(Smith & Nephew Medical)

A sterile gauze dressing impregnated with an antiseptic and used to dress minor wounds where bacterial infection is (or may be) present.

Contains: chlorhexidine acetate, white soft paraffin.

Inadine
(Johnson & Johnson Medical)

A non-adherent dressing impregnated with a slow-releasing antiseptic, used to dress minor injuries and burns.

Contains: povidone-iodine.

Jelonet
(Smith & Nephew Medical)

A sterile gauze dressing impregnated with soft paraffin, and used to dress minor wounds and burns.

Contains: white soft paraffin.

Kaltostat
(Britcair)

A dressing used to help stop bleeding when applied to minor wounds.

Contains: calcium alginate.

Paratulle see **Jelonet**
(Seton Healthcare)

Serotulle see **Bactigras**
(Seton Healthcare)

Sorbsan see **Kaltostat**
(Pharma-Plast)

Unitulle see **Jelonet**
(Roussel)

Antifungal preparations

Fortunately, there is a number of antifungal preparations available over the counter, and those for external or oral use are described below. (For internal vaginal antifungal treatments, see 'Women's disorders' section.)

Athlete's foot is caused by a fungus infection, as is Dhobi itch, where the sufferer has a red ring in the groin area. Circular skin complaints are often due to fungus infections, and one particular type causes depigmentation (pale circles) in people who are suntanned. Treatment of a fungus infection with a steroid will prolong or worsen the symptoms, so hydrocortisone should never be used on these problems. If in doubt, consult a doctor, but relatively little harm can be caused by trial and error when using antifungal agents.

Fungus infections can occur after a repeated course of antibiotics, or in those who have low immunity, sometimes due to steroids. (Oral thrush in the mouth is often seen in asthmatic patients using steroid inhalers.) Internal fungus infections (other than vaginal infections) can be treated only by prescription medicines. Fungus infections of the nails can be persistent and may need prescribed medication.

benzoic acid compound ointment BP

An ointment used as an antifungal preparation to treat fungal infections such as ringworm and athlete's foot.

Dose: apply twice a day.
Side effects:
Caution:
Not to be used for:
Not to be used with:
Contains: benzoic acid, salicylic acid, emulsifying ointment.

Boots Athlete's Foot Spray
(Boots)

A spray used to treat and prevent athlete's foot.

Dose: apply night and morning. (Continue treatment for at least one week after symptoms disappear.)
Side effects:
Caution: avoid inhaling the spray.
Not to be used for:
Not to be used with:
Contains: triclosan, dichlorophen.

Boots Dual Action Athlete's Foot Cream
(Boots)

A cream used to treat and prevent athlete's foot.

Dose: apply twice a day to existing infection. (Continue treatment for at least one week after symptoms disappear.) Apply once daily to prevent infection.
Side effects:
Caution:
Not to be used for:

Not to be used with:
Contains: benzalkonium chloride, tolnaftate.

Boots Dual Action Athlete's Foot Powder
(Boots)

A powder applied to the feet to treat and prevent athlete's foot infections. (The use of Boots Dual Action Athlete's Foot Cream in conjunction with this product is recommended.)

Dose: apply twice a day to existing infection. (Continue treatment for at least one week after symptoms disappear.) Apply once daily to prevent infection.
Side effects:
Caution:
Not to be used for:
Not to be used with:
Contains: chlorhexidine hydrochloride, tolnaftate.

Boots Pharmacy Skincare no. 2 see Canesten Cream
(Boots)

Brulidine see entry in 'Antiseptics' section
(Rhone-Poulenc Rorer Family Health)

Canesten
(Bayer)

A cream, spray, powder, and solution used as an antifungal treatment for fungal infection of the skin (such as athlete's foot and ringworm). The solution is also used to treat fungal infections of the outer ear. The powder is used alone to prevent recurrence of infection, or with the cream or spray to treat existing infection.

Dose: 2-3 applications a day until 14 days after the symptoms have gone.

Side effects: irritation, mild burning.

Caution: pregnant women should consult a doctor before using this product.

Not to be used for:

Not to be used with:

Contains: clotrimazole.

Daktarin
(Janssen)

A cream, powder, and spray used as an antifungal treatment for infections of the skin and nails, such as athlete's foot, dhobi itch, and infected nappy rash.

Dose: apply twice a day until 10 days.after the symptoms have gone.

Side effects:

Caution: avoid the eyes, nostrils, and body orifices. Pregnant women should consult a doctor before using this product.

Not to be used for: hairy areas. The spray should not be used on broken skin.

Not to be used with:

Contains: miconazole nitrate.

Daktarin Oral Gel
(Janssen)

A sugar-free gel used as an antifungal treatment for fungal infections of the mouth and pharynx (such as oral thrush).

Dose: children under 6 years apply twice a day; older children and adults apply 4 times a day. Continue until 2 days after the symptoms have gone.

Side effects: mild stomach upset.

Caution: pregnant women should consult a doctor before using

this product.
Not to be used for:
Not to be used with: anticoagulants, some antidiabetic and anti-epileptic drugs.
Contains: miconazole.

Ecostatin see **Pevaryl**
(Squibb)

Germolene Medicated Foot Spray
(SmithKline Beecham Consumer Healthcare)

A spray used as an antifungal treatment for athlete's foot and foot odour.

Dose: apply up to 6 times a day.
Side effects:
Caution:
Not to be used for: children under 3 years.
Not to be used with:
Contains: triclosan, dichlorophen.

Healthy Feet
(Pickles)

A cream used as an antifungal and antihistamine treatment for athlete's foot and hot, tired, and aching feet.

Dose: use as needed.
Side effects:
Caution:
Not to be used for:
Not to be used with:
Contains: undecylenic acid, dibromopropamidine isethionate.

Masnoderm see **Canesten Cream**
(Cusi)

Monphytol
(LAB)

A paint used as an antifungal treatment for athlete's foot.

Dose: paint on twice a day.
Side effects: stinging.
Caution: children under 12 years, pregnant women, and nursing mothers should consult a doctor before using this product. May damage clothing, plastics, and other items.
Not to be used for: bleeding areas.
Not to be used with:
Contains: chlorbutol, methyl undecylenate, salicylic acid, methyl salicylate, propyl salicylate, propyl undecylenate.

Mycil
(Crookes Healthcare)

An ointment, powder, and spray used as an antifungal to treat and prevent fungal infections such as athlete's foot and dhobi itch.

Dose: apply twice a day until a week after symptoms have disappeared. (Use the powder in conjunction with the cream or spray to treat an infection, or use it alone to prevent infection.)
Side effects:
Caution:
Not to be used for:
Not to be used with:
Contains: tolnaftate. (The ointment also contains benzalkonium chloride. The powder also contains chlorhexidine.)

Mycil Gold see **Canesten Cream**
(Crookes Healthcare)

Mycota
(Seton Healthcare)

A cream, powder, and spray used as an antifungal to treat and prevent athlete's foot.

Dose: apply twice a day until 1 week after symptoms have disappeared.
Side effects:
Caution: avoid inhalation of spray.
Not to be used for:
Not to be used with:
Contains: undecenoic acid. (The cream and powder also contain zinc undecenoate. The spray also contains dichlorophen.)

Pevaryl
(Cilag)

A cream and lotion used as an antifungal product to treat fungal infections of the skin.

Dose: apply twice a day.
Side effects: irritation.
Caution: avoid contact with eyes and mucous membranes.
Not to be used for:
Not to be used with:
Contains: econazole nitrate.

Phytex
(Pharmax)

A paint used as an antifungal treatment for skin and nail infections.

Dose: apply twice a day for up to 10 days.
Side effects:
Caution:
Not to be used for: children under 5 years or pregnant women. Not for use on broken skin.
Not to be used with:
Contains: tannic acid, boric acid, salicylic acid.

Quinoped
(Quinoderm)

A cream used as an antifungal and skin softener to treat athlete's foot and other related fungal infections.

Dose: massage into the affected area twice a day.
Side effects: reddening or irritation of the skin.
Caution: may bleach dyed fabric.
Not to be used for:
Not to be used with:
Contains: potassium hydroxyquinolone sulphate, benzoyl peroxide.

Scholl Athlete's Foot Treatments see Tinaderm/Tinaderm Plus
(Scholl)

Tinaderm
(Schering-Plough)

A cream (Tinaderm) used as an antifungal treatment for athlete's foot. The powder and spray (Tinaderm Plus) may be used with the cream to assist in treatment of the condition, or used alone to prevent recurrence.

Dose: apply to affected skin twice a day. (The powder and spray may also be applied inside socks and shoes.) Continue treatment for 2 weeks after symptoms have disappeared.
Side effects:
Caution: keep away from the eyes.
Not to be used for:
Not to be used with:
Contains: tolnaftate.

Valpeda see entry in 'Skin disorders' section
(Roche Consumer Health)

Whitfield's Ointment see **benzoic acid compound ointment**

Anti-infestation preparations

Conditions such as lice and scabies are caused by infestations with insects. These can be picked up from infested bedding, often in poorly cleaned rooms. Overseas climates, which are warm and moist, encourage the growth of these insects. In the United Kingdom, the most commonly seen infestations are head lice in children, and pubic lice, which can be transmitted venereally. Scabies is more common in patients with poor general health and nutrition.

Head lice are a common source of worry to parents, because they are so easily transmitted between children at school and at play. If treatment is carried out properly, there should be no problem with eradicating the lice, but recontamination is common. Many of the products will suggest that protection from re-infestation will be provided for some time after treatment but, in practice, this cannot be guaranteed, because the use of heat on the hair (from hair dryers) or contact with chlorine (as in a swimming pool) may inactivate any residual effect. Hence, it must be recognized that re-infestation may occur almost immediately, and, unless contacts are traced and also treated, the cycle will continue. If possible, treatment should always be with a lotion because this will kill live lice and eggs. (Shampoo treatment should be reserved only for those unable to tolerate treatment with lotions.) Asthmatics may react to alcohol-based lotions, but there are now water-based lotions and hair rinses available to overcome this difficulty. Once treatment has been carried out, it is not essential to remove eggs from the hair because they should have been killed by the treatment. For cosmetic purposes, however, some people prefer to remove them, and a product is now available specifically for this purpose (Step-2), or they can be combed out with a fine dust comb. A repellent is also available (Rappell) which makes the hair more slippery to deter lice from passing to the treated head.

Ascabiol
(Rhone-Poulenc Rorer)

An emulsion used as an insect-destroying preparation to treat scabies and lice.

Dose: apply once, and repeat if needed. (For children dilute with water as directed.)
Side effects: irritation.
Caution: keep out of the eyes. Pregnant women should consult a doctor before using this product.
Not to be used for: nursing mothers.
Not to be used with:
Contains: benzyl benzoate.

---

benzyl benzoate application BP

A lotion used to treat scabies.

Dose: apply to whole body (except head and neck). Repeat after 24 hours (without washing), and wash off after a further 24 hours. (A third application is sometimes needed.)
Side effects: irritation, rash, burning sensation.
Caution: pregnant women and nursing mothers should consult a doctor before using this product. Avoid contact with eyes and mucous membranes such as the mouth.
Not to be used for: children, or for areas of broken or infected skin.
Not to be used with:
Contains: benzyl benzoate.

Carylderm
(Seton Healthcare)

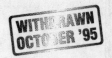

A shampoo and alcoholic lotion used to treat lice in the head and pubic areas.

Dose: rub lotion into the hair, leave on for at least 2 hours (preferably overnight), then wash out. The shampoo should be used only for people unable to tolerate treatment with the lotion. (For maximum effect, use shampoo 3 times at 3-day intervals.)
Side effects: irritation. (Lotion may aggravate asthma or eczema.)
Caution: keep out of the eyes. Do not use artificial heat to dry hair after using lotion. Permed, bleached, or coloured hair may be affected.
Not to be used for: infants under 6 months. Lotion should not be used for anyone suffering from asthma or eczema.
Not to be used with:
Contains: carbaryl.

Clinicide
(E. C. De Witt)

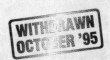

A liquid used to treat lice in the head and pubic areas.

Dose: apply to the hair and allow to dry, then shampoo the following day. Treatment may be repeated after 7 days if re-infestation occurs.
Side effects: irritation.
Caution: keep out of the eyes. Infants under 6 months should be seen by a doctor before using this product.
Not to be used for:
Not to be used with:
Contains: carbaryl.

Derbac-C
(Napp Consumer)

A liquid and shampoo used to treat head lice.

Dose: rub lotion into the hair and leave on for 12 hours, then wash out. The shampoo should be used only for those patients

unable to tolerate the lotion. (Use shampoo 3 times at 3-day intervals for maximum effect.)
Side effects: irritation.
Caution: avoid eyes. Permed, bleached, or coloured hair may be affected.
Not to be used for: children under 6 months.
Not to be used with:
Contains: carbaryl.

Derbac-M
(Seton Healthcare)

A liquid used to treat scabies, lice in the head, eyebrows, eyelashes, and pubic areas.

Dose: apply liberally and then wash out after 24 hours (for scabies), 12 hours (for head lice), or 1-12 hours (for pubic lice).
Side effects: irritation.
Caution: keep out of the eyes. Permed, bleached, or coloured hair may be affected.
Not to be used for: infants under 6 months.
Not to be used with:
Contains: malathion.

Full Marks
(Napp Consumer)

An alcoholic lotion used to treat lice in the head and pubic areas.

Dose: rub into hair and leave on for at least 2 hours (or preferably overnight), then wash out.
Side effects: irritation, aggravation of eczema or asthma.
Caution: avoid eyes. Do not use artificial heat to dry the hair. Permed, bleached, or coloured hair may be affected.
Not to be used for: children under 6 months, asthmatics, or for patients suffering from eczema.

Not to be used with:
Contains: phenothrin.

Lyclear Creme Rinse
(Wellcome)

A conditioning lotion applied to the head to treat head lice.

Dose: shampoo hair, then saturate hair and scalp with lotion. Leave for 10 minutes, rinse and dry.
Side effects: occasionally itching.
Caution: consult a doctor before using on children under 2 years, pregnant women, or nursing mothers.
Not to be used for:
Not to be used with:
Contains: permethrin.

Lyclear Dermal Cream
(Wellcome)

A cream applied to the skin to eradicate scabies.

Dose: Apply to the whole body (except face and head in adults and children over 2 years). Wash off after 8-24 hours.
Side effects: burning, stinging, itching, redness, rash.
Caution: children under 2 years, pregnant women, nursing mothers, and patients over 70 years should consult a doctor before using this product. Avoid the eyes and mouth.
Not to be used for: children under 2 months and patients known to be allergic to chrysanthemums.
Not to be used with:
Contains: permethrin.

Prioderm
(Seton Healthcare)

A shampoo and alcoholic lotion used to treat scabies, and lice in the head and pubic areas.

Dose: apply lotion and leave on for at least 2 hours (preferably overnight) for lice, and for 12 hours for scabies, then wash out. (Repeat the treatment for lice after 7-9 days.) The shampoo should be used only for those patients unable to tolerate treatment with lotion, and only to treat lice. (For maximum effect, use shampoo 3 times at 3-day intervals.)
Side effects: irritation. (Lotion may aggravate eczema and asthma.)
Caution: keep out of the eyes. Bleached, permed, or coloured hair may be affected. Do not use artificial heat to dry hair.
Not to be used for: infants under 6 months. (Lotion not to be used for patients suffering from asthma or eczema.)
Not to be used with:
Contains: malathion.

Quellada Application PC
(Stafford-Miller)

A liquid used as a shampoo to eradicate head lice and pubic lice.

Dose: apply to the dry hair and nearby skin, leave for 4 minutes, then lather and rinse.
Side effects:
Caution: infants, pregnant women, and nursing mothers should be seen by a doctor before using this product.
Not to be used for:
Not to be used with:
Contains: lindane.

Quellada Lotion
(Stafford-Miller)

A lotion used to treat scabies.

Dose: apply as directed to whole body except face and scalp.
Wash off after 24 hours. Repeat after 7 days if needed.
Side effects:
Caution: pregnant women, nursing mothers, and infants under
6 months should be seen by a doctor before using this product.
Supervise children constantly to ensure that the lotion is not
ingested.
Not to be used for: infants under 1 month, or for application
to broken skin or mucous membranes.
Not to be used with:
Contains: lindane.

Rappell*
(Charwell Health Care)

A pump spray containing a liquid which, when applied to the
hair, repels head lice. N. B. this product does NOT kill head
lice. Use only as a preventative.

Dose: spray hair after styling, and allow to dry naturally.
Side effects: sensitive skin and asthma may be aggravated.
Caution: avoid spraying the face and eyes. Children under 2
years should see a doctor before using this product.
Not to be used for:
Not to be used with:
Contains:

Step 2 Lice Egg Removal System*
(DDD)

A lotion applied after treatment for head lice, to remove dead
eggs from the hair. N. B. this product does NOT kill head lice.

Dose: apply after rinsing the treatment out of hair. Leave for 10 minutes, then comb out the dead eggs.
Side effects:
Caution: avoid contact with eyes.
Not to be used for:
Not to be used with:
Contains:

Suleo-C
(Seton Healthcare)

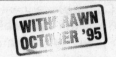

A lotion and shampoo used to treat head lice.

Dose: apply lotion to scalp, allow to dry naturally and shampoo off after 12 hours. The shampoo should be used only for patients unable to tolerate the lotion. (Use shampoo 3 times at 3-day intervals.)
Side effects: irritation.
Caution: keep out of the eyes.
Not to be used for: infants under 6 months.
Not to be used with:
Contains: carbaryl.

Suleo-M
(Seton Healthcare)

A lotion used to treat head lice.

Dose: apply to scalp, allow to dry naturally, and shampoo off after 12 hours.
Side effects: irritation.
Caution: keep out of the eyes.
Not to be used for: infants under 6 months.
Not to be used with:
Contains: malathion.

Antimalarials

Malaria is a feverish disease which can be caught in many areas of Africa, Asia, and Central and South America if you are bitten by an infected mosquito. It is best to avoid being bitten by mosquitoes by covering arms and legs, and by using mosquito nets and insect repellents (see 'Insect repellents' section). If you are planning to travel to any country within the risk areas, however, ask your doctor or pharmacist for advice. There are resistant strains of malaria in some areas, so you will need to be given the correct medication for the area you will be visiting. Your doctor or pharmacist may need to check which is suitable for your destination, or may refer you to a central authority if your itinerary is complicated. (Some products are available only on prescription, so you may need to see your doctor.)

Medication should be started before travelling (the exact time varies for different products) and should be continued while you are abroad and for a few weeks (usually 4–6) after returning from overseas. Any influenza-like condition should be regarded as potential malaria in someone who has returned from an area where malaria is endemic. Medication alone is no guarantee that malaria will not be contracted, so the additional precautions (as outlined above) are strongly recommended. Never forget that malaria can be fatal, and all possible precautions should be taken.

Avloclor
(Zeneca)

A tablet used as an antimalarial drug for the prevention of malaria. (This product may be prescribed by doctors for other conditions.)

Dose: adults 2 tablets once a week (on the same day each week), starting 2 weeks before entering malarious area, and continuing for at least 4 weeks after leaving. (Children should use reduced doses.)

Side effects: headache, stomach upset, skin eruptions, hair loss, eye disorders, blood disorders, loss of pigment, convulsions.

Caution: pregnant women, nursing mothers, and patients suffering from porphyria (a rare blood disorder), psoriasis, severe stomach disorder, nervous or blood disorder, or with a history of epilepsy should consult a doctor before using this product. Check with your doctor, a pharmacist, or MASTA whether this product is suitable for the country to be visited.

Not to be used for:

Not to be used with:

Contains: chloroquine phosphate.

Daraprim
(Wellcome)

A tablet used as an antimalarial drug for the prevention of malaria.

Dose: adults and children over 10 years 1 tablet a week; children 5-10 years half adult dose. Start 1 week before entering malarious area. Continue until 4 weeks after leaving area.

Side effects: rash, anaemia.

Caution: pregnant women, nursing mothers, and patients suffering from blood diseases should consult a doctor before using this product. Check with your pharmacist, doctor, or with

MASTA that this product is suitable for the area to be visited.
Not to be used for: children under 5 years.
Not to be used with: some antibiotics, some sedatives.
Contains: pyrimethamine.

Nivaquine
(Rhone-Poulenc Rorer)

A tablet or liquid used as an antimalarial drug for the prevention of malaria. (This product may be prescribed by doctors for other conditions.)

Dose: adults 2 tablets once a week (on the same day each week), starting 2 weeks before entering malarious area, and continuing for at least 4 weeks after leaving. (Children should use reduced doses in liquid form.)
Side effects: headache, stomach upset, skin eruptions, hair loss, eye disorders, blood disorders, loss of pigment, convulsions.
Caution: pregnant women, nursing mothers, and patients suffering from porphyria (a rare blood disorder), psoriasis, severe stomach disorder, nervous or blood disorder, or with a history of epilepsy should consult a doctor before using this product. Check with your doctor, a pharmacist, or MASTA whether this product is suitable for the country to be visited.
Not to be used for:
Not to be used with:
Contains: chloroquine sulphate.

Paludrine
(Zeneca)

A tablet used as an antimalarial drug for the prevention of malaria.

Dose: adults 2 tablets every day, starting at least 24 hours before entering malarious area, and continuing for at least 4 weeks after leaving. Reduced doses are recommended for children – consult a pharmacist for advice.

Side effects: stomach upset, skin reactions, hair loss, mouth ulcers.

Caution: pregnant women should consult a doctor before using this product. Check with your doctor, a pharmacist, or MASTA whether this product is suitable for the country to be visited.

Not to be used for:

Not to be used with:

Contains: proguanil hydrochloride.

Insect repellents

Insect repellents are not generally licensed as medicinal products, but are included here to emphasize the importance of using repellents to avoid insect bites, particularly in areas where malaria is a problem. The recommended ingredient is diethyltoluamide (DEET), although heavy repeated use of this is not recommended for children, and some products are not suitable at all for youngsters. Insect repellents are also sometimes included in sunscreen products (such as those made by Maws, Boots, Jungle Formula, and Gurkha), but these are not included below. (Combined products such as these are particularly useful where repellent activity is required in a sunny environment, when sunscreen protection is also needed).

Products used to treat insect bites are included elsewhere (see 'Skin disorders' and 'Allergic disorders' sections).

Autan*
(Scholl Consumer Products)

A cream, gel, spray, or stick applied to the skin to repel insects.

Dose: apply to exposed skin. Effect lasts for up to 8 hours.
Side effects:
Caution: avoid contact with eyes, nose, mouth, plastic, synthetic materials, varnished surfaces.
Not to be used for: heavy repeated use on children under 6 years.
Not to be used with:
Contains: diethyltoluamide (DEET).

Autan Fresco* see Autan*
(Scholl Consumer Products)

Ban the Bug*
(Three 'Es)

A band impregnated with insect repellent, supplied in a resealable bag and worn on the wrist to repel mosquitoes and many other flying insects.

Dose: effects last for 60 hours-14 days once outside the resealable bag.
Side effects:
Caution:
Not to be used for:
Not to be used with:
Contains: natural fragrances and essential oils.

Boots Repel-Plus*
(Boots)

A gel, spray, or roll-on used to repel mosquitoes, midges, and other biting insects.

Dose: apply when required.
Side effects:
Caution: avoid lips and eyes. Avoid contact with contact lenses, spectacles, plastics, rayon, acetate, and polished or painted surfaces.
Not to be used for: children under 6 years.
Not to be used with:
Contains: diethyltoluamide (DEET), permethrin.

Buzpel*
(Torbet Laboratories)

A moist wipe impregnated with an insect repellent to deter midges, mosquitoes, and other biting insects.

Dose: apply to exposed areas of skin. Effects last for up to 8 hours.
Side effects:
Caution:
Not to be used for:
Not to be used with:
Contains: pyrethrum.

---

citronella oil*

An oil used as an insect repellent.

Dose: apply a few drops to clothing.
Side effects:
Caution:
Not to be used for:
Not to be used with:
Contains: citronella oil.

Jungle Formula*
(Chefaro)

An aerosol, liquid, gel, or roll-on, used to repel mosquitoes, midges, and other biting insects.

Dose: apply to exposed areas of skin. Effects last for up to 8 hours (or up to 10 hours for liquid).
Side effects:
Caution: avoid lips and eyes. Keep away from acetates, leather, rayon, plastic, and varnished or painted surfaces.
Not to be used for: repeated use on children under 6 years, or on broken or sensitive skin.
Not to be used with:
Contains: diethyltoluamide (DEET).

Jungle Formula Junior*
(Chefaro)

A roll-on product used to repel mosquitoes, midges, and other biting insects.

Dose: apply to exposed areas of skin. Effects last for up to 5 hours.
Side effects:
Caution: avoid lips and eyes. Keep away from acetates, leather, rayon, plastic, and varnished or painted surfaces.
Not to be used for: children under 2 years.
Not to be used with:
Contains: diethyltoluamide (DEET).

Mosiguard*
(Robinsons Healthcare)

A roll-on, spray, or stick suitable for adults and children, and used to repel mosquitoes and other biting insects.

Dose: apply to exposed areas of skin. Effects last for up to 7 hours (or 10 hours for roll-on.)
Side effects: rash.
Caution: avoid lips and eyes.
Not to be used for:
Not to be used with:
Contains:

Mosquito Milk*
(Parlour Products)

A milk or gel used to repel mosquitoes.

Dose: apply to exposed areas of skin. Effects last for up to 8 hours, but re-apply after 4 hours if sweating or in high humidity.
Side effects:
Caution: avoid lips, eyes, and mucous membranes.
Not to be used for: broken or sensitive skin.
Not to be used with:
Contains: diethyltoluamide (DEET).

Prevent*
(Agropharm)

A spray used to repel flying and crawling insects.

Dose: apply directly to the body, or use as a fly spray.
Side effects:
Caution:
Not to be used for:
Not to be used with:
Contains: refined pyrethrum.

Protec*
(Ceuta)

An odour-free insect-repellent body lotion used to protect against mosquito bites.

Dose: apply to exposed areas of skin. Safe for use on damaged skin (e.g. sunburn).
Side effects:
Caution:
Not to be used for:
Not to be used with:
Contains: dioctyl adipate.

S-care*
(Munro Wholesale)

A spray, containing diethyltoluamide (DEET), applied to clothing to repel insects. Other products in the range are applied to tents and caravans (**S-camper***), inner tents and bed-nets (**S-cote***), and rugs and groundsheets (**S-mat***), and contain permethrin.

Shoo*
(Rolas Distributors)

A water-resistant, odourless, and non-greasy lotion or wipe used to repel mosquitoes, midges, and other biting insects.

Dose: apply to exposed areas of skin. Effects last for 6-8 hours.
Side effects:
Caution:
Not to be used for:
Not to be used with:
Contains: dimethylphthalate.

Ultrathon*
(3M Health Care)

A water-resistant cream and spray used to repel mosquitoes and other biting insects.

Dose: spray exposed areas of skin (effect lasts for up to 8 hours) or apply cream (effect lasts for up to 12 hours).
Side effects:
Caution: avoid heavy repeated use on children under 6 years. May damage synthetic materials, plastic, or painted and varnished surfaces.
Not to be used for: areas near the mouth or eyes, or on broken and irritated skin.
Not to be used with:
Contains: diethyltoluamide (DEET).

Women's disorders

Cystitis and thrush (Candida) are the most common women's disorders, and it is reassuring to see that some preparations are available over the counter for these conditions.

The subject of cystitis is covered in the 'Bladder and other urinary tract disorders' section. Vaginal thrush responds to antifungal preparations, such as Canesten, but there are restrictions on the sale of such products if they are for use inside the vagina. First-time sufferers of thrush, and children under 16 years or women over 60 years, should not self-medicate but should see a doctor. Similarly, pregnant women, women who have (or whose partner has) a history of sexually transmitted disease, and patients who have had more than two attacks of thrush in the last six months, or who have bladder or abdominal pain should also consult a doctor before self-medicating. Many women who suffer thrush occasionally, however, perhaps due to antibiotic therapy or the contraceptive pill, will be able to use these treatments successfully.

Vaginal dryness is a common problem, and several lubricating products are listed below. Older women experiencing discomfort through dryness should consult a doctor. Allergic reactions to bath oils can occur in the genital area, and calamine is soothing in these cases.

Any unexpected vaginal bleeding or blood in the urine, even if associated with thrush or cystitis, should be reported to a doctor. Some vaginal medications can damage the latex used in condoms and diaphragms. If barrier contraceptives are being used, beware of using creams or pessaries that may affect the device, as pregnancy may then be a real risk.

Period pain is commonly experienced in younger women, and many pain-killing products are available. (See 'Simple pain killers' section for simple analgesics.) Some, such as Feminax, have added antispasm ingredients to help with the cramps. (Buscopan is a product with just the antispasm ingredient). Any older woman experiencing period pain for the first time (or unusually severe period pain) should consult a doctor without delay. The possibility of menopause and thus oestrogen deficiency should be considered and a doctor consulted. Some non-steroidal inflammatory drugs are particularly effective in relieving period pain.

Water retention is common for the week or two before a period is due. This can be treated with herbal diuretics or products such as Aqua-ban, but often the most effective treatment is found to be evening primrose oil. (This is unlikely to have any side effects, and should help to relieve the problem). It is important not to self-medicate if the water retention is permanent (i.e. not connected with the menstrual cycle) or if swelling occurs in the ankles or legs. (In these cases, consult a doctor). Products specifically for premenstrual use are included in this section. More general diuretics are included in the 'Bladder and other urinary tract disorders' section.

Premenstrual tension is another common disorder for women, and is best treated either with vitamin B6 (see 'Vitamin preparations' section) or by a doctor.

Aqua-ban
(Thompson Medical)

A tablet used as a mild diuretic to relieve water retention before a period.

Dose: 2 tablets 3 times a day for 4-5 days before period is due.
Side effects: abdominal pain, nausea.
Caution:
Not to be used for: children.
Not to be used with: excess tea or coffee.
Contains: ammonium chloride, caffeine.

Athera
(Lane)

A tablet used as a herbal diuretic, tonic, and laxative to treat the symptoms of the menopause.

Dose: 2-3 tablets 3 times a day after meals.
Side effects: diarrhoea.
Caution:
Not to be used for: children, pregnant women, nursing mothers, or for patients with intestinal disease.
Not to be used with:
Contains: parsley, vervain, clivers, senna.

Betadine vaginal products
(Seton Healthcare)

A vaginal cleansing kit, vaginal gel, and pessary with applicator used as an antiseptic and antifungal treatment for vaginal infections.

Dose: 1 pessary inserted into the vagina night and morning, or

1 application of gel to be inserted at night, or the cleansing kit used in the morning.

Side effects: irritation, allergy, redness, swelling.

Caution: these products are spermicidal – do not use if trying to become pregnant. Underwear will be stained.

Not to be used for: children, pregnant women, nursing mothers.

Not to be used with:

Contains: povidone-iodine.

Boots Herbal Menopause Tablets
(Boots)

A tablet used as a herbal remedy to relieve minor conditions associated with the menopause.

Dose: 2-3 tablets 3 times a day after food.

Side effects: diarrhoea.

Caution:

Not to be used for: children, pregnant women, nursing mothers.

Not to be used with:

Contains: parsley root, vervain, clivers, senna.

Boots Herbal Menstrual Comfort Tablets
(Boots)

A tablet used as a herbal remedy to relieve the symptoms of painful menstrual cramps.

Dose: for discomfort, 2 tablets 3 times a day after food if required.

Side effects:

Caution:

Not to be used for: children, pregnant women, and nursing mothers.

Not to be used with:
Contains: dry extract raspberry leaf.

Buscopan see entry in 'Stomach disorders' section
(Windsor Healthcare)

Canesten-1
(Bayer)

A vaginal tablet plus applicator, supplied at a strength of 500
mg and used as an antifungal treatment for vaginal candidiasis
(thrush).

Dose: 1 tablet inserted into the vagina at night.
Side effects: mild burning or irritation, allergy.
Caution: pregnant women, patients under 16 or over 60, first-
time sufferers, patients who are allergic to any antifungal
treatments, women who have (or whose partner has) a history
of sexually transmitted disease, and patients who have had
more than two attacks of thrush in the last six months, or who
have bladder or abdominal pain should consult a doctor before
using this product.
Not to be used for: children.
Not to be used with:
Contains: clotrimazole.

Canesten 10% VC
(Bayer)

A white vaginal cream plus applicator used as an antifungal
treatment for vaginal candidiasis (thrush).

Dose: one application of cream into the vagina at night.
Side effects: mild burning or irritation, allergy.
Caution: pregnant women, patients under 16 or over 60 first-
time sufferers, patients who are allergic to any antifungal

treatments, women who have (or whose partner has) a history of sexually transmitted disease, and patients who have had more than two attacks of thrush in the last six months, or who have bladder or abdominal pain should consult a doctor before using this product.

Not to be used for: children.
Not to be used with:
Contains: clotrimazole.

Canesten Combi
(Bayer)

A vaginal tablet and cream used as an antifungal treatment for vaginal candidiasis (thrush) and associated external infection in women, and to treat sexual partners to avoid re-infection.

Dose: 1 tablet inserted into the vagina at night. The cream applied twice a day to external areas around the vagina, and to the partner's penis.
Side effects: mild burning or irritation, allergy.
Caution: pregnant women, patients under 16 or over 60 years of age, first-time sufferers, patients who are allergic to any antifungal treatments, women who have (or whose partner has) a history of sexually transmitted disease, and patients who have had more than two attacks of thrush in the last 6 months, or who have bladder or abdominal pain should consult a doctor before using this product.
Not to be used for: children.
Not to be used with:
Contains: clotrimazole.

Cascade
(Lane)

A tablet used as a herbal diuretic remedy to relieve premenstrual water retention in women.

Dose: 2 tablets 3 times a day before meals.
Side effects: constipation.
Caution: pregnant women and nursing mothers should consult a doctor before using this product.
Not to be used for: children under 12 years.
Not to be used with:
Contains: burdock root, uva ursi, clivers.

Cymalon see entry in 'Bladder and other urinary tract disorders' section
(Sterling Health)

Cystemme see entry in 'Bladder and other urinary tract disorders' section
(Abbott)

Cystoleve see entry in 'Bladder and other urinary tract disorders' section
(Seton Healthcare)

Cystopurin see entry in 'Bladder and other urinary tract disorders' section
(Roche Consumer Health)

Effercitrate see entry in 'Bladder and other urinary tract disorders' section
(Typharm)

---

evening primrose oil*

Evening primrose oil contains a substance used by the body to make prostaglandins which regulate many body functions. Food supplements containing evening primrose oil are available as capsules or chewable tablets, and are thought to be of help in promoting healthy skin, supple joints, cell growth and hormone balance. (Women may find it useful to treat premenstrual bloating.) Creams are also available for direct application to the skin. High-strength products are available on prescription to treat breast pain and eczema, but these conditions are not suitable for self-medication with evening primrose oil, and over-the-counter preparations are not appropriate.

Dose: as specified for each individual product. Women using the product for premenstrual bloating will require approximately 1000 mg (1 g) per day while symptoms persist.
Side effects: indigestion, headache.
Caution: pregnant women and patients with epilepsy (or receiving anti-epileptic medication) should consult a doctor before using these products.
Not to be used for:
Not to be used with: anti-epileptic medication (see above).
Contains: gamma linolenic acid (GLA).

Femeron
(Janssen)

A soft pessary and a cream used as an antifungal treatment for vaginal candidiasis (thrush).

Dose: 1 pessary inserted into the vagina once (at night) to treat internal infection, and the cream applied twice a day for external infection.
Side effects: mild burning or irritation, allergy.
Caution: pregnant women, patients under 16 or over 60, first-time sufferers, patients who are allergic to any antifungal treatments, women who have (or whose partner has) a history of sexually transmitted disease, and patients who have had more than two attacks of thrush in the last six months, or who have bladder or abdominal pain should consult a doctor before using this product.

Not to be used for: children.
Not to be used with: rubber contraceptives (condoms, diaphragms, etc.).
Contains: miconazole nitrate.

Feminesse*
(Unipath)

A vaginal gel (supplied in an applicator for single use), applied internally and used to eliminate vaginal odour.

Dose: apply internally when required. (One application lasts for up to 3 days.)
Side effects:
Caution:
Not to be used for:
Not to be used with:
Contains: purified water, glycerin, mineral oil.

Heath & Heather Water Relief
(Ferrosan Healthcare)

A tablet used as a herbal diuretic to relieve the symptoms of premenstrual water retention.

Dose: 1-2 tablets up to 3 times a day for up to 7 days before an expected period.
Side effects:
Caution: pregnant women should consult a doctor before using this product.
Not to be used for: children.
Not to be used with:
Contains: bladderwrack, clivers, ground ivy, burdock root.

K-Y*
(Johnson and Johnson)

A non-irritating jelly and lubricating pessary used to provide additional vaginal lubrication.

Dose: apply a little jelly to the vagina, or insert a pessary high into the vagina.
Side effects:
Caution: allow 10 minutes for pessary to melt.
Not to be used for:
Not to be used with:
Contains:

Melissa Compound see entry in 'Bowel disorders' section
(Weleda)

---

potassium citrate mixture see entry in 'Bladder and other urinary tract disorders' section

---

Prementaid
(Potters)

A tablet used as a sedative, diuretic, and antispasmodic herbal remedy to relieve the symptoms of bloating and abdominal discomfort associated with premenstrual tension.

Dose: 2 tablets 3 times a day on uncomfortable days. (Take the tablets regularly for several days for maximum effect.)
Side effects: possible drowsiness.
Caution:
Not to be used for: children or pregnant women.
Not to be used with: other sedating medicines, alcohol.
Contains: vervain, motherwort, wild anemone, uva ursi, valerian.

Raspberry Leaf
(Potters)

A tablet used as a herbal toning and relaxing remedy to relieve painful menstrual cramps.

Dose: 2 tablets 3 times a day after meals.
Side effects:
Caution:
Not to be used for: children or pregnant women (except where labour has begun).
Not to be used with:
Contains: raspberry leaf.

Replens
(Unipath)

A fragrance-free, non-staining vaginal moisturizer supplied in a pre-filled applicator to treat dryness inside the vagina.

Dose: insert one application 3 times a week. (The effect will last for several days.)
Side effects:
Caution:
Not to be used for: children, pregnant women, or for those who have recently had a baby.
Not to be used with:
Contains: purified water.

Senselle*
(LRC Products)

An unperfumed moisturizer for temporary relief of vaginal dryness.

Dose: apply to the entrance of the vagina when required.

Side effects:
Caution:
Not to be used for:
Not to be used with:
Contains:

---

starflower oil*

Unlicensed food supplement capsules containing starflower oil (borage oil) are available (often in combination with other vitamins or minerals), and are thought to be of help in promoting healthy skin, supple joints, and hormone balance. (Women may find it useful to treat premenstrual bloating.) The oil is richer in gamma linolenic acid than evening primrose oil.

Dose: as specified for each individual product.
Side effects: indigestion, headache.
Caution: pregnant women and patients with epilepsy (or receiving anti-epileptic medication) should consult a doctor before using these products.
Not to be used for:
Not to be used with: anti-epileptic medication (see above).
Contains: gamma linolenic acid (GLA).

Uvacin
(Kallo Foods)

A tablet used as a herbal diuretic to disinfect the urinary tract and bladder, and relieve bladder discomfort in women.

Dose: 2 tablets 3 times a day.
Side effects:
Caution:
Not to be used for: men, children under 16 years, pregnant women, or nursing mothers.
Not to be used with:

Contains: extract of dandelion root, uva ursi, peppermint.

Vagisil*
(Combe International)

A powder and washing lotion used to deodorize the vaginal area. (See *also* 'Vagisil Cream'.)

Vagisil Cream
(Combe International)

A cream used as a local anaesthetic to relieve feminine itch, burning, and irritation of the external areas around the vagina.

Dose: apply 3-4 times a day for a maximum of one week.
Side effects: allergy.
Caution: pregnant women should consult a doctor before using this product.
Not to be used for: children under 3 years, or on extensive areas of skin.
Not to be used with:
Contains: lignocaine.

Wellwoman
(Potters)

A tablet and herbal teabag used as a herbal sedative remedy to promote the well-being of middle-aged women.

Dose: 2 tablets 3 times a day, or 2 teabags infused 3 times a day. Take as a 6-day course for best effects.
Side effects: possible drowsiness.
Caution:
Not to be used for: children or pregnant women.
Not to be used with: other sedating medicines, alcohol.
Contains: yarrow, scullcap, lime flowers. (The tablets also

contain motherwort and valerian. The teabags also contain uva ursi.)

Contraceptives

The chemical contraceptives that may be purchased without prescription are spermicidal pessaries, creams, foams, and gels. Used alone, these are not very effective, but are useful as a extra precaution when using barrier methods of contraception – diaphragms, cervical caps, or condoms (sheaths). None of the products listed here will affect the latex used in condoms or diaphragms, but other products (particularly oil-based preparations used as simple lubricants or vaginal medications) may damage the structure of the rubber, making the barrier less effective.

Contraceptive pessaries normally need to be inserted at least 10 minutes before intercourse, to allow time for the pessary to melt and the spermicide to be released. (The use of one pessary inside the diaphragm or cap, and another inside the vagina may be recommended.) Jellies and creams may be spread over the surface and rim of a cap or inserted directly into the vagina using an applicator. (Delfen foam is supplied with an applicator for ease of insertion.).

There are usually no side effects from the use of these products, except for occasional allergy to either the active ingredient or to a perfume included in the formulation.

Delfen
(Cilag)

A spermicidal foam for vaginal use in conjunction with barrier methods of contraception. (Supplied with applicator.)

Contains: nonoxynol-9.

Double Check
(F. P. Sales)

A spermicidal pessary for vaginal use in conjunction with barrier methods of contraception.

Contains: nonoxynol-9.

Duracreme
(LRC Products)

A spermicidal cream for vaginal use in conjunction with barrier methods of contraception. (Applicator available separately.)

Contains: nonoxynol-9.

Duragel
(LRC Products)

A spermicidal jelly for vaginal use in conjunction with barrier methods of contraception. (Applicator available separately.)

Contains: nonoxynol-9.

Gynol II
(Cilag)

A non-scented spermicidal jelly. (Applicator available separately.)

Contains: nonoxynol-9.

Orthocreme
(Cilag)

A spermicidal cream. (Applicator available separately.)

Contains: nonoxynol-9.

Orthoforms
(Cilag)

A spermicidal pessary.

Contains: nonoxynol-9.

Orthogynol
(Cilag)

A spermicidal jelly. (Applicator available separately.)

Contains: diisobutylphenoxypolyethoxyethanol.

Staycept
(Syntex)

A spermicidal jelly and pessary.

Contains: nonoxynol-9.

Bowel disorders

Constipation, diarrhoea, and irritable bowel syndrome are three bowel conditions for which over-the-counter preparations are available. Simple remedies for diarrhoea include adsorbent formulations (such as kaolin), but the use of such products is no longer recommended. The importance of oral rehydration (with products such as Dioralyte) cannot be overstated, particularly for children, the elderly, or debilitated people. This is the treatment of choice for diarrhoea, (and the only treatment recommended for children under 6 years), although other products (such as Imodium) can be useful in adults.

Various laxatives are available but, in general, their use (particularly on a long-term basis) is to be discouraged. Stimulant types can cause abdominal cramps, and prolonged use can cause the large bowel to stop functioning. (Phenolphthalein is particularly strong, and should be used only if other measures have failed.) Liquid paraffin laxatives can interfere with the absorption of some vitamins from the diet, and can cause a form of pneumonia and anal irritation. Anyone with persistent abdominal pain, difficulty swallowing, or a need for laxatives every day or repeatedly should consult a doctor.

Finally, there are some medications available over the counter that are used to treat haemorrhoids (piles) and anal problems. The best known of these are Preparation H and Anusol. Anusol-Plus is a steroid treatment with certain restrictions attached to its sale (see product entry below).

Significant changes in bowel habit, passing blood, or weight loss should be reported to a doctor.

Agarol
(Warner Wellcome Consumer Healthcare)

An emulsion used as a lubricant and stimulant laxative to give temporary relief from constipation.

Dose: adults 5-15 ml at bedtime (or twice a day); children 5-12 years 5 ml at bedtime (or after breakfast).
Side effects: allergy, pink urine.
Caution: patients who require a laxative every day, or who have persistent abdominal pain or difficulty swallowing should consult a doctor before using this product.
Not to be used for: children under 5 years, or for repeated use.
Not to be used with:
Contains: liquid paraffin, phenolphthalein, agar.

Alophen
(Warner Wellcome Consumer Healthcare)

A brown pill used as a stimulant laxative to treat constipation.

Dose: 1-3 pills at bedtime.
Side effects: allergy, pink urine.
Caution: patients suffering from nausea, vomiting, abdominal pain, persistent symptoms, or those taking any other medication should consult a doctor before using this product.
Not to be used for: children.
Not to be used with:
Contains: aloin, phenolphthalein.

Anacal
(Panpharma)

A suppository and rectal ointment (supplied with applicator) used as an anti-inflammatory treatment for haemorrhoids (piles).

Dose: 1 application of ointment or 1 suppository used once or twice a day. (Ointment may be required up to 4 times a day.)
Side effects:
Caution:
Not to be used for: children under 5 years.
Not to be used with:
Contains: heparinoid, oxypolyethoxydodecane.

Andrews Liver Salts
(Sterling Health)

A white effervescent powder used to treat constipation. (For use as an antacid see 'Stomach preparations' section.)

Dose: adults 2 teaspoonsful or 2 sachets in water, children over 3 years half the adult dose.
Side effects:
Caution: patients with abdominal pain, or requiring laxatives regularly or for long periods should consult a doctor before using this product.
Not to be used for: children under 3 years.
Not to be used with: some antibiotics or tablets coated to protect the stomach.
Contains: sodium bicarbonate, citric acid, magnesium sulphate.

Anodesyn
(Seton Healthcare)

Ointment or suppositories used as an anaesthetic, soothing, and astringent treatment for the symptoms of haemorrhoids (piles).

Dose: to be used twice a day and after each bowel movement.
Side effects:
Caution: this product should not be used for more than 14

days without consulting a doctor.
Not to be used for: children under 12 years.
Not to be used with:
Contains: lignocaine hydrochloride, allantoin.

Anusol Cream/Ointment
(Warner Wellcome Consumer Healthcare)

A cream or ointment used as a soothing, antiseptic, astringent treatment for haemorrhoids (piles) and anal itching.

Dose: apply night and morning, and after each bowel motion.
Side effects: occasionally mild irritation or burning.
Caution: patients with rectal bleeding should consult a doctor.
Not to be used for: children.
Not to be used with:
Contains: bismuth oxide, zinc oxide, Peru balsam. (Ointment also contains bismuth subgallate.)

Anusol Plus HC
(Warner Wellcome Consumer Healthcare)

An ointment (supplied with an applicator for internal use) or suppository used as a steroid and soothing treatment for haemorrhoids (piles) and anal itching.

Dose: use 1 suppository or apply the ointment twice a day and after each bowel movement. (Maximum of 3 suppositories in 24 hours.) Maximum treatment period 7 days.
Side effects: allergy, temporary burning.
Caution: pregnant women and patients with rectal bleeding should consult a doctor before using this product.
Not to be used for: children or adults under 18 years, or for infected conditions.
Not to be used with:
Contains: hydrocortisone acetate, benzyl benzoate, bismuth

subgallate, bismuth oxide, Peru balsam, zinc oxide.

Anusol Suppositories
(Warner Wellcome Consumer Healthcare)

A suppository used as an soothing, antiseptic, astringent treatment for internal haemorrhoids (piles).

Dose: 1 suppository inserted into the rectum night and morning, and after each bowel motion.
Side effects: occasionally mild irritation or burning.
Caution: patients with rectal bleeding should consult a doctor.
Not to be used for: children.
Not to be used with:
Contains: bismuth oxide, zinc oxide, Peru balsam, bismuth subgallate.

Arret see Imodium
(Janssen)

Beechams Pills
(SmithKline Beecham Consumer Healthcare)

A pill used as a stimulant laxative to relieve constipation.

Dose: 1-2 tablets at night if required.
Side effects:
Caution: patients requiring laxatives every day, or who have abdominal pain or difficulty swallowing should consult a doctor before using this product.
Not to be used for: children under 12 years.
Not to be used with:
Contains: aloin.

Bellocarb see entry in 'Stomach preparations' section
(Sinclair Pharmaceuticals)

Bonomint
(Intercare)

A chewing gum used as a laxative to treat constipation.

Dose: adults 1 piece (children aged 6-12 years ½-1 piece)
chewed before bedtime.
Side effects: pink urine, skin rash.
Caution: pregnant women, nursing mothers, and patients who
need laxatives every day, or who have persistent abdominal
pain should see a doctor before using this product.
Not to be used for: children under 6 years.
Not to be used with:
Contains: yellow phenolphthalein.

Boots Cream of Magnesia see **magnesium hydroxide
mixture**
(Boots)

Boots Diareze see **Imodium**
(Boots)

Boots Diarrhoea Mixture
(Boots)

A liquid used as an adsorbent treatment for occasional
diarrhoea.

Dose: 5-20 ml up to 4 times a day when required (according to
age).
Side effects:
Caution: this product is not a substitute for oral rehydration

therapy. Drink plenty of fluids during treatment. See note at start of chapter concerning the use of adsorbent medications.
Not to be used for: children under 1 year, or for more than 24 hours.
Not to be used with:
Contains: attapulgite.

Boots Diarrhoea Mixture for Children
(Boots)

A liquid used as an adsorbent treatment for upset stomach and diarrhoea.

Dose: 5-10 ml every 4 hours if required.
Side effects:
Caution: this product is not a substitute for oral rehydration therapy. Drink plenty of fluids during treatment. See note at start of chapter concerning the use of adsorbent medications.
Not to be used for: infants under 3 months, or for more than 24 hours.
Not to be used with:
Contains: light kaolin.

Boots Health Salts
(Boots)

An effervescent powder used as a laxative to treat occasional constipation. (For use as an antacid, see entry in 'Stomach disorders' section.)

Dose: 3-4 teaspoonsful in water in the morning, for a maximum of 5 days.
Side effects:
Caution: patients with abdominal pain, or who require the use of laxatives regularly or for prolonged periods should consult a doctor before using this product.

Not to be used for: children under 12 years.
Not to be used with: some antibiotics or tablets coated to protect the stomach.
Contains: sucrose, sodium bicarbonate, magnesium sulphate, citric acid, tartaric acid, sodium chloride.

Boots Oral Rehydration Treatment see **Glucolyte**
(Boots)

Boots Suppositories for Haemorrhoids
(Boots)

A suppository used as a soothing treatment for the pain, irritation, and discomfort of haemorrhoids (piles).

Dose: 1 suppository inserted into the rectum twice a day and after each bowel motion.
Side effects:
Caution: pregnant women should consult a doctor before using this product.
Not to be used for:
Not to be used with:
Contains: glycol monosalicylate, benzyl alcohol, methyl salicylate, zinc oxide.

Boots Syrup of Figs see **Califig California Syrup of Figs**
(Boots)

Brooklax
(Intercare)

A chocolate piece or tablet used as a strong laxative to treat constipation.

Dose: adults ½-2 chocolate tablets (children over 6 years ¼-1

chocolate tablet) at bedtime.
Side effects: skin rash, pink urine.
Caution: pregnant women, nursing mothers, and patients who need laxatives every day, or who have persistent abdominal pain should see a doctor before using this product.
Not to be used for: children under 6 years.
Not to be used with:
Contains: yellow phenolphthalein.

Califig California Syrup of Figs
(Sterling Health)

A dark brown liquid used as a stimulant laxative to treat constipation.

Dose: 2.5-30 ml at bedtime, according to age.
Side effects:
Caution: patients needing laxatives regularly or for long periods should consult a doctor before using this product.
Not to be used for: children under 1 year, or for patients with abdominal pain.
Not to be used with:
Contains: senna extract.

Calsalettes
(Torbet)

A coated or uncoated tablet used as a stimulant laxative to treat constipation.

Dose: 1 tablet at bedtime. (Maximum of 4 in 24 hours.)
Side effects:
Caution: patients requiring laxatives every day, or who have abdominal pain or difficulty swallowing should consult a doctor before using this product.
Not to be used for: children under 12 years.

Not to be used with:
Contains: aloin.

Carter's Little Pills
(Carter Wallace)

A pill used as a stimulant laxative to treat constipation.

Dose: 1-2 pills before bedtime.
Side effects: pink urine, skin rash.
Caution: pregnant women, nursing mothers, and patients who need laxatives every day, or who have persistent abdominal pain should see a doctor before using this product.
Not to be used for: children.
Not to be used with:
Contains: aloin, phenolphthalein.

---

charcoal tablets see entry in 'Stomach disorders' section

Clairo Tea
(Weleda)

A tea used as a herbal stimulant laxative and calming remedy to relieve the symptoms of occasional or non-persistent constipation.

Dose: adults use 2.5 ml tea added to 200 ml boiling water and allow to simmer for 1 minute. Filter before drinking. (For a milder action, add the tea to water which has already boiled and leave to stand for 5 minutes.) Use this dose once daily in the evening. (Children over 6 years may use half adult dose in the morning.)
Side effects:
Caution: not for prolonged use. Pregnant women should consult a doctor before using this product.
Not to be used for: children under 6 years, or for patients with

inflamed bowel conditions, severe abdominal pain, or who require laxatives regularly.
Not to be used with: homeopathic remedies.
Contains: aniseed, clove, peppermint, senna.

Cleansing Herb
(Potters)

A herb mixture used as a stimulant laxative to treat the symptoms of occasional constipation.

Dose: 2.5 ml twice a day when required. (Add boiling water, allow to stand for 15 minutes, then drink all of it.) Vary the dose if required.
Side effects: harmless discoloration of urine or stools.
Caution: patients requiring laxatives regularly should consult a doctor.
Not to be used for: children, pregnant women, nursing mothers, or for patients with intestinal disorders.
Not to be used with:
Contains: senna leaves, buckthorn bark, psyllium seeds.

Colpermin
(Pharmacia)

A capsule, coated to resist stomach acid, used as an anti-spasm treatment to relieve symptoms of irritable bowel syndrome, or intestinal spasm due to other causes (such as diverticular disease).

Dose: 1-2 capsules 3 times a day.
Side effects: allergy, burning in back passage, slow pulse, muscle tremor, lack of co-ordination.
Caution: pregnant women and patients taking indigestion remedies should consult a doctor before using this product. Do not chew the capsules.

Not to be used for: children.
Not to be used with: antacids, homeopathic remedies.
Contains: peppermint oil.

Correctol
(Schering-Plough)

A tablet used as a stimulant laxative to treat constipation.

Dose: 1 at bedtime or in the morning.
Side effects: skin rash, pink urine.
Caution: pregnant women, nursing mothers, and patients who need laxatives every day, or who have persistent abdominal pain should see a doctor before using this product.
Not to be used for: children.
Not to be used with:
Contains: phenolphthalein, dioctyl sodium sulphosuccinate.

Cranesbill
(Gerard House)

A tablet used as a herbal astringent treatment for short-term relief of diarrhoea.

Dose: adults 1-2 tablets when needed 3 times a day; children over 12 years 1 tablet twice a day.
Side effects:
Caution: pregnant women are advised to consult a doctor before using this product.
Not to be used for: children under 12 years.
Not to be used with:
Contains: cranesbill.

Diasorb see **Imodium**
(Baker-Norton)

Diocalm Dual Action
(SmithKline Beecham Consumer)

A chewable tablet used as an opiate and adsorbent treatment for diarrhoea.

Dose: adults 2 tablets every 2-4 hours, (children aged 6-12 years half the adult dose). Maximum 6 doses in 24 hours.
Side effects: constipation, dependence.
Caution: asthmatics should consult a doctor or pharmacist before using this product. If diarrhoea continues for 48 hours, a doctor should be consulted. Body fluids should be replaced while diarrhoea persists. See note at start of chapter concerning the use of adsorbent medications.
Not to be used for: children under 6 years.
Not to be used with: MAOIs.
Contains: morphine hydrochloride, attapulgite.

Diocalm Ultra see Imodium
(SmithKline Beecham Consumer)

Diocalm Replenish see Dioralyte
(SmithKline Beecham Consumer)

Dioctyl
(Schwarz)

A capsule, adult solution, and paediatric solution used to prevent and treat constipation.

Dose: adults up to 5 capsules (or 50 ml adult solution) to be taken each day (in divided doses). Children use paediatric solution. The dose should be reduced as the condition improves.
Side effects:
Caution: pregnant women, nursing mothers, and patients with stomach pains or who need laxatives regularly should see a

doctor before using this product.

Not to be used for: infants under 6 months or for patients suffering from abdominal pain, nausea, vomiting, or blocked intestine.

Not to be used with: mineral oil.

Contains: docusate sodium.

Dioralyte
(Rhone-Poulenc Rorer)

A powder (available in various flavours and supplied in sachets) or effervescent tablet (available in various flavours), used as a fluid and electrolyte replacement to treat acute watery diarrhoea and/or vomiting.

Dose: adults 2 sachets or 4 tablets (children aged 1-12 years 1 sachet or 2 tablets) after each loose bowel motion. Bottle-fed infants should be given the same volume of the reconstituted sachet solution in place of feeds.

Side effects:

Caution: infants under 12 months should be seen by a doctor. Reconstitute the powder or dissolve the tablets before use. Consult a doctor if diarrhoea lasts for more than 36 hours.

Not to be used for: patients who require a low-sodium diet.

Not to be used with:

Contains: glucose, sodium chloride, potassium chloride. (Tablets also contain sodium bicarbonate and citric acid. Sachets also contain disodium hydrogen citrate.)

Dual-lax
(Lane)

A tablet, available in normal or extra strengths, used as a herbal stimulant laxative to relieve temporary constipation.

Dose: adults 1-3 normal or 1-2 extra-strong tablets at night.

(Children aged 7-14 years may take 1 normal-strength tablet at night.)

Side effects: harmless red discoloration of urine.

Caution: pregnant women and patients who need laxatives regularly should consult a doctor before using this product.

Not to be used for: children under 7 years, women in the early stages of pregnancy, or nursing mothers. Children should not use the extra-strength product.

Not to be used with:

Contains: senna leaf, aloes, cascara.

Dulcolax
(Windsor Healthcare)

A tablet or suppository (in two strengths) used as a stimulant laxative to treat constipation.

Dose: adults 1-2 tablets at night or 1 suppository in the morning; children under 10 years 1 children's suppository in the morning.

Side effects:

Caution: children under 10 years, pregnant women, and patients requiring a laxative every day (or who have persistent abdominal pain) should consult a doctor before using this product.

Not to be used for:

Not to be used with: tablets not to be used with antacids.

Contains: Bisacodyl.

Duphalac see lactulose solution
(Duphar)

Duphalac Dry
(Duphar Laboratories)

A powder, supplied in sachets, and used as a laxative to treat constipation.

Dose: adults and children over 10 years 1 sachet (children aged 5-10 years ½ sachet) twice a day.
Side effects:
Caution:
Not to be used for: children under 5 years.
Not to be used with:
Contains: lactulose.

Electrolade see **Glucolyte**
(Eastern Pharmaceuticals)

Enterosan
(Monmouth)

A chewable tablet used as an adsorbent, opiate, and anti-spasm treatment for diarrhoea and stomach upset.

Dose: 4 tablets to start, then 2 tablets every 3-4 hours if required. Continue until 24 hours after symptoms have gone.
Side effects: constipation, dependence.
Caution: asthmatics should consult a doctor or pharmacist before using this product. Avoid solid food, and drink plenty of fluids. See note at start of chapter concerning the use of adsorbent medications.
Not to be used for: children, pregnant women, nursing mothers.
Not to be used with: MAOIs.
Contains: light kaolin, morphine hydrochloride, belladonna.

Entrotabs
(Monmouth)

A tablet used as an adsorbent, antacid treatment for stomach upset and diarrhoea.

Dose: adults 4 tablets immediately, then 2 every 3-4 hours.

(Children aged 6-12 years take 1 tablet every 4 hours.)
Side effects:
Caution: drink plenty of fluids. See note at start of chapter concerning the use of adsorbent medications.
Not to be used for: children under 6 years.
Not to be used with: some antibiotics or tablets coated to protect the stomach.
Contains: attapulgite, aluminium hydroxide, pectin.

Epsom salts

An osmotic laxative for occasional use to treat constipation by rapid evacuation of the bowels.

Dose: adults 5-10 g in water on an empty stomach.
Side effects:
Caution: children and pregnant women should consult a doctor before using this product.
Not to be used for: patients suffering from abdominal pain, nausea, vomiting, or blocked intestine.
Not to be used with:
Contains: magnesium sulphate.

Exlax
(Intercare)

A chocolate piece or pill used as a strong laxative to treat constipation.

Dose: adults 1 chocolate tablet or pill (children over 6 years ½-1 chocolate tablet or 1 pill) at bedtime.
Side effects: skin rash, pink urine.
Caution: pregnant women, nursing mothers, and patients who need laxatives every day, or who have persistent abdominal pain should see a doctor before using this product.
Not to be used for: children under 6 years.

255

Not to be used with:
Contains: yellow phenolphthalein.

Fam-lax
(Torbet Laboratories)

A chewable tablet used as a strong laxative to treat constipation.

Dose: ½-1 tablet at bedtime.
Side effects: skin rash, pink urine.
Caution: pregnant women, nursing mothers, and patients who need laxatives every day, or who have persistent abdominal pain should see a doctor before using this product.
Not to be used for: children under 12 years.
Not to be used with:
Contains: yellow phenolphthalein.

Fybogel
(Reckitt & Colman)

A sachet of effervescent granules (plain or flavoured) used for conditions requiring a high-fibre diet (e.g. constipation, diverticular disease, irritable colon).

Dose: adults 1 sachet twice a day. Children aged 6-12 years 2.5-5 ml twice a day. Mix with water before taking.
Side effects:
Caution: children under 6 years should be seen by a doctor before using this product. Do not take a dose immediately before going to bed. Drink plenty of fluids.
Not to be used for: patients suffering from blocked intestine, or who have difficulty swallowing.
Not to be used with:
Contains: ispaghula husk.

Fynnon Salts
(Seton Healthcare)

A salt used as a laxative to treat constipation.

Dose: 5 ml once or twice a day in water.
Side effects:
Caution: children under 12 years, and patients requiring regular use of laxatives should consult a doctor before using this product.
Not to be used for:
Not to be used with:
Contains: sodium sulphate.

Germoloids
(SmithKline Beecham Consumer Healthcare)

An ointment, cream, or suppository used as a local anaesthetic and soothing preparation to treat the symptoms of haemorrhoids (piles) and anal itching.

Dose: apply cream/ointment (or insert 1 suppository into the rectum) twice a day and after bowel movements. (Maximum of 4 applications per day.)
Side effects:
Caution:
Not to be used for: children.
Not to be used with:
Contains: lignocaine hydrochloride, zinc oxide.

Gladlax
(Gerard House)

A tablet used as a herbal laxative to relieve occasional or non-persistent constipation.

Dose: 1-2 tablets at bedtime if required.

Side effects:
Caution:
Not to be used for: children under 12 years, pregnant women, or nursing mothers.
Not to be used with: other laxatives.
Contains: cape aloes, fennel, valerian, holy thistle.

Glauber's salt BP see **Fynnon Salts**

Glucolyte
(Seton Healthcare)

A powder supplied in sachets and used to replace fluids during episodes of diarrhoea.

Dose: adults 1-2 sachets (children aged 1-12 years 1 sachet) after each loose bowel motion. Infants should be given the same volume of solution in place of feeds, or given the appropriate amount before breastfeeding.
Side effects:
Caution: infants under 12 months should be seen by a doctor. Reconstitute the powder before use.
Not to be used for: patients who require a low-sodium diet.
Not to be used with:
Contains: sodium bicarbonate, glucose, sodium chloride, potassium chloride.

Haemorrhoid Cream
(Nelsons)

A cream used as a soothing herbal remedy to treat the symptoms of haemorrhoids (piles).

Dose: apply when needed.
Side effects:

Caution:
Not to be used for:
Not to be used with:
Contains: horse chestnut, calendula, witch hazel, paeonia officinalis.

Heath and Heather Inner Fresh Tablets
(Ferrosan Healthcare)

A tablet used as a stimulant herbal laxative to relieve occasional constipation.

Dose: 1-2 tablets before bedtime.
Side effects: griping pain, harmless discoloration of urine.
Caution: pregnant women and patients with a history of serious bowel disorder should consult a doctor before using this product.
Not to be used for: children.
Not to be used with:
Contains: frangula bark.

Heemex
(Lane)

An ointment supplied with an applicator, used as an astringent and soothing remedy to relieve the discomfort and irritation of internal and external haemorrhoids (piles).

Dose: apply night and morning and after each bowel movement.
Side effects: allergy.
Caution:
Not to be used for: children.
Not to be used with:
Contains: witch hazel, benzoin tincture, zinc oxide.

Hemocane
(Intercare)

A non-staining, odourless cream (supplied with an applicator) and suppository used as an anaesthetic, antiseptic, and soothing treatment for haemorrhoids (piles).

Dose: insert 1 suppository into the rectum (for internal piles) or apply the cream (internally or externally) morning and night and after each bowel movement.
Side effects: allergy.
Caution: patients with rectal bleeding are advised to consult a doctor.
Not to be used for: children.
Not to be used with:
Contains: lignocaine hydrochloride, benzoic acid, cinnamic acid, zinc oxide, bismuth oxide.

Herbulax
(English Grains)

A herbal remedy used as a stimulant laxative to relieve symptoms of occasional constipation.

Dose: adults 1 tablet before bedtime, increasing to 2 tablets if needed. (Children aged 5-12 years half adult dose.)
Side effects:
Caution: patients with abdominal pain or who need laxatives every day should consult a doctor before using this product. This product is intended for short-term use only.
Not to be used for: children under 5 years or for nursing mothers.
Not to be used with:
Contains: frangula bark, dandelion root.

Imodium
(Centra Healthcare)

A capsule used as a treatment for diarrhoea.

Dose: 2 capsules initially, then one capsule after each loose bowel motion. (Maximum 8 in 24 hours.)
Side effects: abdominal cramps, nausea, vomiting, drowsiness, dizziness, dry mouth, skin reaction.
Caution: rehydration therapy should also be used with this product. Pregnant women and nursing mothers should consult a doctor before using this product.
Not to be used for: children under 12 years, or for patients with a swollen abdomen or suffering from colitis.
Not to be used with:
Contains: loperamide hydrochloride.

Isogel
(Charwell Health Care)

Granules used as a bulking agent to treat occasional constipation, diarrhoea associated with diverticular disease, and to assist in the treatment of irritable bowel syndrome and the management of colostomies.

Dose: to treat constipation, adults 10 ml once or twice a day in water or carbonated water. (Children aged 6-12 years half adult dose.) To treat diarrhoea, adults 5 ml 3 times a day.
Side effects:
Caution: Drink plenty of fluids. Do not take a dose immediately before going to bed.
Not to be used for: patients suffering from blocked intestine, or who have difficulty swallowing.
Not to be used with:
Contains: ispaghula husk.

Jaap's Health Salt see entry in 'Stomach preparations' section
(Askit Laboratories)

J. Collis Browne's
(Napp Consumer)

A mixture or chewable tablet used as an opiate treatment for
diarrhoea and stomach upsets. (The tablets are also an
adsorbent treatment.)

Dose: adults 2-3 tablets or 10-15 ml mixture (children aged 6-
10 years 5 ml mixture or 1 tablet, children aged 10-12 years 2-
3 tablets or 5 ml mixture) every 4 hours.
Side effects: constipation, dependence.
Caution: asthmatics should consult a doctor or pharmacist
before using this product. Drink plenty of fluids. See note at
start of chapter concerning the use of adsorbent medications.
Not to be used for: children under 6 years.
Not to be used with: MAOIs. (Mixture should also not be used
with homeopathic remedies.)
Contains: morphine hydrochloride. (Mixture also contains peppermint
oil. Tablets also contain light kaolin and calcium carbonate.)

Junior Kao-C
(Torbet Laboratories)

A sugar-free suspension used as an adsorbent treatment for
diarrhoea.

Dose: 5-20 ml (according to age) 3 times a day.
Side effects:
Caution: see note at start of chapter concerning the use of
adsorbent medications.
Not to be used for: children under 1 year.
Not to be used with:
Contains: light kaolin, calcium carbonate.

Juno Junipah Salts
(Torbet Laboratories)

A powder used as a laxative to treat constipation.

Dose: 10 ml once or twice a day.
Side effects:
Caution: children under 12 years, and patients requiring regular use of laxatives should consult a doctor before using this product.
Not to be used for:
Not to be used with: some antibiotics or tablets coated to protect the stomach.
Contains: sodium sulphate, sodium phosphate, sodium bicarbonate, juniper berry oil.

Juno Junipah Tablets
(Torbet Laboratories)

A tablet used as a stimulant laxative to treat constipation.

Dose: 2-4 tablets at night.
Side effects: pink urine, skin rash.
Caution: children under 12 years, pregnant women, nursing mothers, and patients who need laxatives every day, or who have persistent abdominal pain should see a doctor before using this product.
Not to be used for:
Not to be used with:
Contains: sodium sulphate, sodium chloride, sodium phosphate, phenolphthalein, juniper berry oil.

Kaodene
(Boots)

A liquid used as an adsorbent and opiate anti-spasm treatment for diarrhoea.

Dose: adults 20 ml (children over 5 years 10 ml) 3-4 times a day.
Side effects: constipation, dependence.
Caution: asthmatics should consult a doctor or pharmacist before using this product. See note at start of chapter concerning the use of adsorbent medications.
Not to be used for: children under 5 years.
Not to be used with: MAOIs.
Contains: light kaolin, codeine phosphate.

---

kaolin mixture BP

An adsorbent treatment for occasional diarrhoea.

Dose: 10-20 ml every 4 hours in water.
Side effects: constipation.
Caution: see note at start of chapter concerning the use of adsorbent medications.
Not to be used for: children.
Not to be used with:
Contains: light kaolin, light magnesium carbonate, sodium bicarbonate.

---

kaolin and morphine mixture BP

An adsorbent and opiate treatment for occasional diarrhoea.

Dose: 10 ml every 4 hours in water.
Side effects: constipation, dependence, drowsiness.
Caution: asthmatics should consult a doctor or pharmacist before using this product. See note at start of chapter concerning the use of adsorbent medications.
Not to be used for: children.
Not to be used with: MAOIs.
Contains: light kaolin, morphine tincture.

Kaopectate
(Upjohn)

A sugar-free suspension used as an adsorbent treatment for diarrhoea.

Dose: 5-30 ml (according to age) every 4 hours.
Side effects:
Caution: see note at start of chapter concerning the use of adsorbent medications. Drink plenty of fluids.
Not to be used for: children under 1 year, or for patients with intestinal obstruction.
Not to be used with:
Contains: light kaolin.

Kest
(Torbet Laboratories)

A tablet used as a stimulant laxative to treat constipation.

Dose: 1-2 tablets at night.
Side effects: skin rash, pink urine.
Caution: children under 12 years, pregnant women, nursing mothers, and patients who need laxatives every day, or who have persistent abdominal pain should see a doctor before using this product.
Not to be used for:
Not to be used with:
Contains: phenolphthalein, magnesium sulphate.

KLN
(Roche Consumer Health)

A suspension used as an adsorbent treatment for diarrhoea in children.

Dose: 5-20 ml (according to age) after each bowel movement,

265

for a maximum of 24 hours.
Side effects:
Caution: see note at start of chapter concerning the use of adsorbent medications.
Not to be used for: children with fever.
Not to be used with: homeopathic remedies.
Contains: light kaolin, pectin, peppermint oil, sodium citrate.

Konsyl
(Eastern Pharmaceuticals)

A powder supplied in sachets and available as a sugar-free higher-strength sachet or an orange-flavoured or dextrose version (with added glucose) in the normal-strength sachets, and used to treat occasional constipation, (and diarrhoea associated with diverticular disease).

Dose: to treat constipation, adults 1 sachet up to 3 times a day in water. (Children aged 6-12 years, half adult dose, or less.) To treat diarrhoea, adults 1 sachet in water 3 times a day.
Side effects:
Caution: children under 6 years should be seen by a doctor before using this product. Do not take a dose immediately before going to bed.
Not to be used for: patients with intestinal obstruction or difficulty swallowing.
Not to be used with:
Contains: ispaghula husk.

---

lactulose solution

A liquid used as a laxative to relieve constipation.

Dose: initially, adults 15 ml (children 2.5-10 ml according to age) twice a day. It may take 2-3 days for this product to have the desired effect.

Side effects: wind, cramp, abdominal discomfort.
Caution: children requiring a laxative should be seen by a doctor before starting treatment.
Not to be used for: patients suffering from galactosaemia (an inherited disorder) or blocked intestines.
Not to be used with:
Contains: lactulose.

Laxoberal
(Windsor Healthcare)

A sugar-free liquid used as a stimulant laxative to treat constipation.

Dose: 2.5-15 ml at night, according to age.
Side effects:
Caution: children under 12 years, pregnant women, nursing mothers, and patients who need laxatives every day, or who have persistent abdominal pain should see a doctor before using this product.
Not to be used for:
Not to be used with:
Contains: sodium picosulphate.

Laxose see **lactulose solution**
(Berk Pharmaceuticals).

Lion Cleansing Herb Tablets
(Potters)

A tablet used as a herbal stimulant laxative to relieve occasional constipation.

Dose: 1-2 tablets at bedtime when necessary.
Side effects:
Caution:

Not to be used for: children or pregnant women.
Not to be used with:
Contains: senna, aloes, cascara, dandelion root, fennel.

___

liquid paraffin

A liquid used as a laxative for occasional use to relieve constipation.

Dose: adults 10-30 ml daily (reduced doses for children).
Side effects: anal irritation, vitamin deficiencies, seepage of paraffin into lungs and out from anus.
Caution: patients requiring laxatives every day, or who have abdominal pain or difficulty swallowing should consult a doctor before using this product.
Not to be used for: children under 3 years, or for prolonged use.
Not to be used with:
Contains: liquid paraffin.

___

Lusty's Herbalene
(Lane)

A herb mixture used as a stimulant laxative to relieve the symptoms of temporary or occasional constipation.

Dose: adults 2.5-5 ml twice a day. (The herbs are placed on the tongue and washed down with water.) Children aged 7-14 years half adult dose.
Side effects:
Caution:
Not to be used for: children under 7 years.
Not to be used with:
Contains: senna, frangula, elder leaves, fennel.

___

magnesium hydroxide mixture BP

A liquid used as a laxative to treat constipation.

Dose: adults 30-45 ml at bedtime.
Side effects:
Caution: patients with persistent abdominal pain, or a regular need for laxatives should consult a doctor before using this product.
Not to be used for:
Not to be used with:
Contains: magnesium hydroxide.

Manevac
(Galen)

A granule used as a fibre and stimulant laxative to relieve constipation.

Dose: adults 5-10 ml once or twice a day; pregnant women 5-10 ml once daily; children aged 5-12 years 5 ml once daily. Place the granules on the tongue and swallow with liquid.
Side effects:
Caution: do not chew the granules.
Not to be used for: children under 5 years.
Not to be used with:
Contains: plantago ovata fibre, tinnevelly senna pods.

Melissa Compound
(Weleda)

A liquid used as a herbal remedy to relieve the symptoms of nausea, upset stomach, occasional diarrhoea, and period pains.

Dose: adults 10-20 drops in a little water every hour as required, up to 8 times a day; children over 8 years half adult dose.

Side effects:
Caution: children under 8 years should be treated with caution because of the alcohol content of the product. Pregnant women should consult a doctor before using this product.
Not to be used for:
Not to be used with: some homeopathic remedies.
Contains: archangelica, cinnamon, clove, coriander, lemon oil, lemon balm, nutmeg, alcohol.

Milk of Magnesia
(Sterling Health)

A liquid used as a laxative to treat constipation. (For use as an antacid, see 'Stomach preparations' section.)

Dose: adults 30-45 ml at bedtime, reducing dose as soon as possible. (Children aged 3-12 years, 5-10 ml at bedtime.)
Side effects:
Caution: children under 3 years and patients with persistent abdominal pain, or a regular need for laxatives should consult a doctor before using this product.
Not to be used for: patients suffering from abdominal pain, nausea, vomiting or blocked intestine.
Not to be used with: some antibiotics or tablets coated to protect the stomach.
Contains: magnesium hydroxide.

Mil-par
(Sterling Health)

A liquid used as a lubricating laxative to relieve constipation.

Dose: adults 15-30 ml each day. (Children 5-15 ml daily, according to age.)
Side effects: anal irritation, pneumonia, and loss of vitamins (with long-term use).

Caution: patients with persistent abdominal pain, difficulty swallowing, or a regular need for laxatives should consult a doctor before using this product.
Not to be used for: children under 3 years.
Not to be used with:
Contains: magnesium hydroxide mixture, liquid paraffin.

Mintec
(Monmouth Pharmaceuticals)

A capsule, coated to resist stomach acid, used as an anti-spasm treatment to relieve the symptoms of irritable bowel syndrome (trapped wind, abdominal bloating, and pain).

Dose: 1 capsule 3 times a day before meals.
Side effects: heartburn, allergy.
Caution: pregnant women should consult a doctor before using this product. Do not chew the capsules.
Not to be used for: children or for patients suffering from heartburn.
Not to be used with: antacids, homeopathic remedies.
Contains: peppermint oil.

Normacol
(Norgine)

A granule used as a bulking agent to treat constipation.

Dose: adults 1 sachet (or 5 ml granules) once or twice a day after food, with a drink. (Children over 6 years, half adult dose.)
Side effects: irritation.
Caution: do not chew the granules.
Not to be used for: children under 6 years, or for patients with obstructed bowel or suffering from inflammatory bowel disorder.
Not to be used with:
Contains: sterculia.

Normacol Plus
(Norgine)

A granule used as a bulking agent and stimulant to treat constipation.

Dose: adults 1 sachet (or 5 ml granules) once or twice a day after food, with a drink.
Side effects: irritation.
Caution: do not chew the granules. Children should be seen by a doctor before using this product.
Not to be used for: patients with obstructed bowel or suffering from inflammatory bowel disorder.
Not to be used with:
Contains: sterculia, frangula.

Nupercainal
(Zyma Healthcare)

An ointment (supplied with an applicator) and used to relieve the pain and irritation of haemorrhoids (piles).

Dose: apply up to 3 times a day.
Side effects:
Caution: sufferers of haemorrhoids are advised to consult a doctor.
Not to be used for:
Not to be used with:
Contains: cinchocaine.

Nylax
(Crookes Healthcare)

A tablet used as a stimulant laxative to treat constipation.

Dose: 1-2 at bedtime for a maximum of 2 weeks.

Side effects: skin rash, pink urine.
Caution: patients who need laxatives every day, or who have persistent abdominal pain should see a doctor before using this product.
Not to be used for: children, pregnant women, nursing mothers, or for patients with blocked intestines.
Not to be used with:
Contains: yellow phenolphthalein, bisacodyl, senna.

Opazimes
(Rybar)

A chewable tablet used as an adsorbent, antacid, opiate and anti-spasm treatment for upset stomach and diarrhoea.

Dose: adults 2 tablets (children over 6 years 1 tablet), sucked or chewed, every 4 hours. (Maximum of 4 doses in 24 hours.)
Side effects: constipation, dependence.
Caution: asthmatics should consult a doctor or pharmacist before using this product. See note at start of chapter concerning the use of adsorbent medications.
Not to be used for:
Not to be used with: MAOIs, some antibiotics or tablets coated to protect the stomach.
Contains: aluminium hydroxide, light kaolin, belladonna dry extract, morphine hydrochloride.

Out of Sorts Tablets
(Potters)

A tablet used as a herbal laxative to relieve the symptoms of occasional constipation and bloatedness.

Dose: 1-2 tablets at bedtime when needed.
Side effects:

Caution: patients needing laxatives repeatedly or persistently should consult a doctor before using this product.
Not to be used for: children, pregnant women, or nursing mothers.
Not to be used with:
Contains: senna, cape aloes, cascara, dandelion root, fennel.

---

peppermint* see entry in 'Stomach preparations' section

Pepto-Bismol
(Procter & Gamble)

A sugar-free liquid used to treat diarrhoea, stomach discomfort, indigestion, and nausea.

Dose: adults 30 ml (children 10-20 ml) every ½-1 hour (up to 8 times in 24 hours). Maximum treatment period 2 days.
Side effects: dark stools.
Caution: pregnant women and patients suffering from diabetes, gout, or with allergy to aspirin should consult a doctor before using this product.
Not to be used for: children under 6 years.
Not to be used with: aspirin.
Contains: bismuth subgallate.

Pileabs
(Lanes)

A tablet used as a soothing and laxative herbal remedy to relieve temporary constipation and the symptoms of haemorrhoids (piles).

Dose: 2 tablets 3 times a day with food.
Side effects: harmless red discoloration of urine.
Caution:
Not to be used for: children, women in early stages of

pregnancy, or for patients with digestive disorders. (Pregnant women should consult a doctor before using this product.) If a laxative is needed repeatedly, seek medical advice.
Not to be used with:
Contains: slippery elm bark, cascara.

Piletabs
(Potters)

A tablet used as a herbal laxative and astringent remedy to relieve the symptoms of haemorrhoids (piles) which are aggravated by constipation.

Dose: 2 tablets 3 times a day. (Elderly patients should use 2 tablets twice a day.)
Side effects:
Caution: patients who need laxatives regularly or repeatedly should consult a doctor.
Not to be used for: children or pregnant women.
Not to be used with:
Contains: pilewort, agrimony, cascara, stone root.

Pilewort Compound
(Gerard House)

A tablet used as a herbal laxative and astringent remedy to relieve the symptoms of constipation (particularly constipation which is aggravating piles).

Dose: 1-2 tablets at night.
Side effects:
Caution: pregnant women, nursing mothers, and patients who need laxatives regularly or repeatedly should consult a doctor before using this product.
Not to be used for: children under 12 years.
Not to be used with:

Contains: pilewort, senna, cranesbill, cascara.

Pilewort Ointment
(Potters)

An ointment used as a herbal remedy to relieve symptoms of discomfort from haemorrhoids (piles).

Dose: apply twice a day.
Side effects:
Caution:
Not to be used for: children.
Not to be used with:
Contains: pilewort.

Preparation H
(Whitehall)

An ointment and suppository used to relieve pain and itching from haemorrhoids (piles).

Dose: apply the ointment or insert 1 suppository into the rectum night and morning, and after each bowel movement.
Side effects:
Caution:
Not to be used for: children.
Not to be used with:
Contains: yeast cell extract, shark liver oil.

Rapolyte see Dioralyte Sachets
(Janssen)

Regulan
(Procter & Gamble)

Granules supplied in sachets and used as a bulking agent to treat constipation.

Dose: adults 1 sachet up to 3 times a day in water. (Children aged 6-12 years 2.5-5 ml up to 3 times a day in water.)
Side effects:
Caution: drink plenty of fluids. Do not take a dose immediately before going to bed.
Not to be used for: children under 6 years, or for patients suffering from blocked intestine, or who have difficulty swallowing.
Not to be used with:
Contains: ispaghula husk.

Reguletts
(Seton Healthcare)

A chewable tablet used as a strong laxative to treat occasional constipation.

Dose: 1 tablet at bedtime.
Side effects: skin rash, pink urine.
Caution: pregnant women, nursing mothers, and patients who need laxatives every day, or who have persistent abdominal pain should see a doctor before using this product.
Not to be used for: children under 12 years.
Not to be used with:
Contains: yellow phenolphthalein.

Regulose see **lactulose solution**
(Sandoz)

Rehidrat
(Searle Pharmaceuticals)

A powder supplied as sachets in various flavours, and used as a fluid and electrolyte replacement to treat diarrhoea.

Dose: adults and older children should drink the fluid freely. Bottle-fed babies should have the volume of their feeds substituted by the product. Breastfed babies should be given the product after a feed.
Side effects:
Caution: dissolve as directed before use. Consult a doctor before using for infants, or if diarrhoea persists for more than 24 hours.
Not to be used for:
Not to be used with:
Contains: sodium chloride, potassium chloride, sodium bicarbonate, citric acid, glucose, fructose, sucrose.

Relaxyl
(Whitehall)

A capsule used as an anti-spasmodic treatment for the pain and discomfort due to muscle spasm of irritable bowel syndrome.

Dose: adults 1-2 capsules up to 3 times a day.
Side effects: allergy.
Caution: pregnant women, nursing mothers, and patients experiencing bleeding from the back passage should consult a doctor.
Not to be used for: children under 12 years or for patients with obstruction in the bowel.
Not to be used with:
Contains: alverine citrate.

Safeway Health Salts see **Andrews Liver Salts**
(Safeway)

Senlax
(Intercare)

A chocolate tablet used as a stimulant laxative to treat constipation.

Dose: adults 1 tablet (children over 6 years ½ tablet) at bedtime.
Side effects:
Caution: pregnant women are advised to consult a doctor before using this product.
Not to be used for: children under 6 years, or for patients with severe abdominal pain, or who require laxatives regularly.
Not to be used with:
Contains: senna.

---

senna tablets

A tablet used as a stimulant laxative to treat occasional constipation.

Dose: adults 2 tablets at bedtime; children 6-12 years half adult dose.
Side effects:
Caution: pregnant women are advised to consult a doctor before using this product.
Not to be used for: children under 6 years, or for patients with severe abdominal pain or who require laxatives regularly.
Not to be used with:
Contains: sennosides.

Senokot
(Reckitt & Colman)

A tablet, syrup, or granule used as a stimulant laxative to treat constipation.

Dose: adults 2 tablets, 10 ml syrup, or 5 ml granules at bedtime;

children over 6 years half adult dose of syrup or granules in the morning.
Side effects:
Caution:
Not to be used for: children under 6 years.
Not to be used with:
Contains: senna.

Spanish Tummy Mixture
(Potters)

A mixture used as a herbal astringent remedy to relieve symptoms of non-persistent diarrhoea.

Dose: 5 ml every hour.
Side effects:
Caution:
Not to be used for: children.
Not to be used with:
Contains: blackberry root, catechu.

Spasmonal see **Relaxyl**
(Norgine)

Sure-lax
(English Grains Healthcare)

A chewable tablet used as a stimulant laxative to treat constipation.

Dose: adults 1 tablet chewed at bedtime. (Children over 8 years, half adult dose.)
Side effects: skin rash, pink urine.
Caution: pregnant women, nursing mothers, and patients who need laxatives every day or who have persistent abdominal pain should see a doctor before using this product.

Not to be used for: children under 8 years.
Not to be used with:
Contains: yellow phenolphthalein.

Trifyba
(Sanofi Winthrop)

A powder used as a bulking agent to treat constipation, diverticular disease, irritable colon, haemorrhoids, and fissures.

Dose: adults 1 sachet 2-3 times a day; children ½-1 sachet once or twice a day.
Side effects:
Caution: adequate fluids must be taken. Do not take a dose immediately before going to bed.
Not to be used for: patients suffering from blocked intestine.
Not to be used with:
Contains: concentrated extract of wheat husk.

Unichem Children's Diarrhoea Mixture
(Unichem)

A liquid used as an adsorbent treatment for upset stomach and diarrhoea.

Dose: 5-10 ml (according to age).
Side effects:
Caution: this product is not a substitute for oral rehydration therapy. Drink plenty of fluids during treatment. See note at start of chapter concerning the use of adsorbent medications.
Not to be used for: children with blocked intestines or for more than 3 days.
Not to be used with:
Contains: light kaolin.

Bladder and other urinary tract disorders

The most common urinary tract disorder is cystitis, an inflammation of the bladder, often due to infection. The symptoms of this can be particularly distressing, as the need to pass urine is frequent, and the action is usually painful. Fortunately, some preparations are available over the counter to relieve the symptoms in women, although medical advice should always be sought for men and children, because the condition is not common in these patients and needs further investigation. Women may be treated with citrates, which render the urine alkaline, helping to reduce the bacteria present and relieve the burning sensations. Herbal treatments generally contain urinary antiseptics to combat infection and diuretics to increase fluid output. Drinking plenty of fluids will also help to flush infections out of the urinary tract. If these measures fail to relieve the problem after 48 hours, however, a doctor should be consulted because more severe infections may require antibiotic treatment on prescription.

Prostate problems are common in older men, and these should always be treated by a doctor. There are, however, some herbal remedies available over the counter, which may help to relieve the symptoms temporarily, (for example, while awaiting surgery) if no medication has been prescribed by your doctor.

Diuretics are products which remove water from the body. Women may suffer from water retention before a period, and products specifically for premenstrual use are listed in the 'Women's disorders' section. The use of diuretics for other purposes should be strictly in accordance with a doctor's recommendation, and persistent water retention or swelling of the legs or ankles, particularly in elderly patients, should never be treated with over-the-counter remedies.

More serious urinary tract disorders, such as kidney infections, require urgent referral to a doctor. Similarly, any bleeding in the urine should also be reported without delay.

Antiglan
(Potters)

A tablet used as a herbal remedy to relieve mild bladder discomfort in elderly men. (May be of help in patients with enlarged prostate glands who are awaiting surgery.)

Dose: elderly males only, 2-3 tablets 3 times a day.
Side effects:
Caution: a doctor should be consulted in all cases of prostate disease.
Not to be used for: children, women, or younger men.
Not to be used with:
Contains: kava, saw palmetto, horsetail, hydrangea.

Antitis
(Potters)

A tablet used as a herbal diuretic and antiseptic treatment to relieve symptoms of cystitis.

Dose: 2 tablets 3 times a day for a maximum of 10 days.
Side effects:
Caution: fluid intake should be increased while taking this preparation.
Not to be used for: children.
Not to be used with:
Contains: buchu, clivers, couchgrass, horsetail, shepherd's purse, uva ursi.

Aqua-ban see entry in 'Women's disorders' section
(Thompson Medical)

Aqualette
(Kallo Foods)

A tablet used as a herbal diuretic to help promote normal water balance (for example, before a period, or when on a low-calorie diet).

Dose: 2-3 tablets 3 times a day.
Side effects:
Caution:
Not to be used for: children under 16 years, pregnant women, nursing mothers.
Not to be used with:
Contains: extracts of horsetail, dandelion root.

Boots Herbal Water Relief Tablets
(Boots)

A tablet used as a herbal diuretic to remove excess water from the body.

Dose: 2 tablets 3 times a day before food.
Side effects: allergy.
Caution:
Not to be used for: children under 12 years, pregnant women, nursing mothers.
Not to be used with:
Contains: uva ursi, clivers, burdock root.

Buchu Compound
(Gerard House)

A tablet used as a herbal diuretic, astringent, antiseptic, and calming remedy to aid normal urinary flow and regulate fluid balance.

Dose: 2 tablets 3 times a day.
Side effects:
Caution: pregnant women and nursing mothers should consult

a doctor before using this product.
Not to be used for: children.
Not to be used with:
Contains: dandelion root, buchu, uva ursi, clivers.

Cascade see entry in 'Women's disorders' section
(Lane)

Cymalon
(Sterling Health)

Granules supplied in sachets and used to make the urine alkaline and relieve symptoms of cystitis in women.

Dose: 1 sachet dissolved in water 3 times a day for 2 days. (If symptoms persist after 48 hours, consult a doctor.)
Side effects:
Caution: pregnant women, nursing mothers, and patients suffering from heart disease, kidney disease, high blood pressure, diabetes, or requiring a low-salt diet should consult a doctor before using this product.
Not to be used for: children and men.
Not to be used with: some antibiotics or tablets coated to protect the stomach.
Contains: sodium citrate, citric acid, sodium carbonate, sodium bicarbonate.

Cystemme see Cymalon
(Abbott)

Cystoleve
(Seton Healthcare)

Granules supplied in sachets and used to make the urine alkaline and relieve symptoms of cystitis in women.

Dose: 1 sachet dissolved in water 3 times a day for 2 days. (If symptoms persist after 48 hours, consult a doctor.)
Side effects:
Caution: pregnant women, nursing mothers, and patients suffering from heart disease, kidney disease, high blood pressure, diabetes, or requiring a low-salt diet should consult a doctor before using this product.
Not to be used for: children and men.
Not to be used with: some antibiotics or tablets coated to protect the stomach.
Contains: sodium citrate.

Cystopurin
(Roche Consumer Health)

Granules supplied in sachets and used to make the urine alkaline and relieve symptoms of cystitis in women.

Dose: 1 sachet dissolved in water 3 times a day for 2 days. (If symptoms persist after 48 hours, consult a doctor.)
Side effects: raised potassium levels, increased output of urine.
Caution: pregnant women, men, children, and patients suffering from heart or kidney disease should consult a doctor before using this product.
Not to be used for: children under 6 years.
Not to be used with: some diuretics, some antihypertensives.
Contains: potassium citrate.

De Witt's Kidney and Bladder Pills
(E. C. De Witt)

A tablet used as a diuretic to promote normal urinary elimination.

Dose: adults 1-2 pills before each meal and 2 at bedtime; children over 12 years 1 pill twice a day. (Maximum suggested use 5 days.)

Side effects:
Caution: pregnant women and nursing mothers should consult a doctor before using this product.
Not to be used for: children under 12 years.
Not to be used with:
Contains: uva ursi, buchu.

Diuretabs
(Potters)

A tablet used as a herbal diuretic, astringent, and soothing remedy to balance body fluids.

Dose: 2 tablets 3 times a day.
Side effects:
Caution: elderly patients should not use this product for more than 1 month. Patients taking other medication should consult a doctor before using this product.
Not to be used for: children, or for serious fluid-retention problems.
Not to be used with:
Contains: buchu leaf, juniper berry oil, parsley piert, uva ursi.

Effercitrate
(Typharm)

A white effervescent tablet used as an alkalizing agent to treat cystitis.

Dose: adults and children over 6 years 2 tablets dissolved in water up to 3 times a day after meals; children 1-6 years half adult dose.
Side effects: raised potassium levels, stomach irritation, increased urine output.
Caution: children under 12 years and adult males should consult a doctor if affected by cystitis. Pregnant women and

patients suffering from high blood pressure, heart disease, or kidney disorder should see a doctor before using this product.
Not to be used for: infants under 1 year or for patients suffering from ulcerated or blocked small bowel.
Not to be used with: some diuretics.
Contains: citric acid, potassium bicarbonate.

Heath & Heather Water Relief Tablets see entry in 'Women's disorders' section
(Ferrosan Healthcare)

Helonias Compound
(Gerard House)

A tablet used as a herbal diuretic and uterine tonic to help maintain normal fluid balance. (May be useful in relieving bloating in women.)

Dose: 1 tablet 3 times a day.
Side effects:
Caution:
Not to be used for: children, elderly patients, pregnant women, and nursing mothers.
Not to be used with:
Contains: unicorn root, parsley, black cohosh, raspberry leaf.

Kas-Bah Herb
(Potters)

A herb mixture used as a soothing, diuretic, astringent, and urinary antiseptic to relieve the symptoms of urinary or bladder discomfort and associated backache.

Dose: 15 ml (about 6 g) infused in 1 pint of boiling water and taken daily in portions when cool enough. (Strain before pouring.)

Side effects: harmless discoloration of urine or stools.
Caution:
Not to be used for: children, pregnant women, nursing mothers, or patients with intestinal disorders.
Not to be used with:
Contains: buchu, clivers, couchgrass, horsetail, uva ursi, senna leaf.

---

potassium citrate mixture

A mixture used to make the urine alkaline and relieve the symptoms of cystitis in women.

Dose: 10 ml 3 times a day, well diluted in water, for a maximum of 2 days.
Side effects: raised potassium levels, increased output of urine.
Caution: pregnant women, elderly women, and patients suffering from kidney or heart disease should consult a doctor before using this product.
Not to be used for: children or men.
Not to be used with: some diuretics, some antihypertensives.
Contains: potassium citrate.

Prostabrit*
(Britannia Health)

A capsule used as a food supplement, and thought to assist in the maintenance of a healthy prostate gland in men.

Dose: 2 capsules daily for at least 3 months.
Side effects:
Caution: a doctor should be consulted in all cases of prostate disease.
Not to be used for:
Not to be used with:
Contains: rye plant extracts.

Protat
(Potters)

A liquid used as a sedative and soothing herbal remedy for the short-term relief of symptoms of bladder discomfort, particularly in elderly men.

Dose: 5 ml 3 times a day.
Side effects: possible drowsiness.
Caution: a doctor should be consulted in all cases of prostate disease.
Not to be used for: children.
Not to be used with: other sedating medicines, alcohol.
Contains: cornsilk, kava.

Sabalin
(Kallo Foods)

A tablet used as a herbal remedy to relieve urinary discomfort and improve the flow of urine in men.

Dose: 2 tablets 3 times a day.
Side effects:
Caution: for short-term use only. A doctor should be consulted in all cases of prostate disease.
Not to be used for: women or children.
Not to be used with:
Contains: saw palmetto.

---

saw palmetto*
(Licensed product available from Kallo Foods – see Sabalin)

A herbal remedy believed to be of help in relieving the symptoms of prostatic enlargement in men. It may also help to restore lost weight, and is traditionally reputed to be aphrodisiac.

Dose: as specified for each individual product.
Side effects:
Caution: a doctor should be consulted in all cases of prostate disease.
Not to be used for: children.
Not to be used with:
Contains: saw palmetto.

Uvacin see entry in 'Women's disorders' section
(Kallo Foods)

Waterlex
(Gerard House)

A tablet used as a herbal diuretic and urinary antiseptic to assist normal urinary flow.

Dose: 1-2 tablets 3 times a day.
Side effects:
Caution: pregnant women and nursing mothers should consult a doctor before using this product.
Not to be used for: children under 12 years.
Not to be used with:
Contains: dandelion, horsetail, uva ursi.

Anti-worm preparations

Intestinal worms are normally present with abdominal pain, weight loss, and the passage of worms through the anus, although some infestations can be silent, with only anal itching (particularly at night) as a symptom. Once worms are detected, it is advisable to treat all family members, to prevent recurrence of the problem. Scrupulous attention to personal hygiene (hand washing and nail scrubbing) will also help to prevent the spread of worms. A bath first thing in the morning is also helpful because this removes eggs laid around the anus overnight. There are several medications available over the counter to treat these infestations.

De Witt's Worm Syrup
(E. C. De Witt)

A liquid used as an anti-worm treatment for threadworm and roundworm.

Dose: to treat threadworm: adults 15 ml daily, children 5-10 ml daily (according to age) for 7 days. To treat roundworm: adults 30 ml, children 10-25 ml (according to age) for one single dose only.
Side effects: rash, wheezing, upset stomach, dizziness, headache, aching muscles.
Caution: pregnant women and patients already taking medication should consult a doctor before using this product.
Not to be used for: children under 2 years, or for patients suffering from epilepsy.
Not to be used with: sedatives, antidepressants.
Contains: piperazine citrate.

Ovex
(Janssen)

A tablet used as an anti-worm treatment for threadworm.

Dose: 1 tablet only. (This may be repeated after 2 weeks if re-infestation occurs.)
Side effects:
Caution: treat all family members at the same time. Patients receiving other medication should consult a doctor or pharmacist before using this product.
Not to be used for: children under 2 years, pregnant women, or nursing mothers.
Not to be used with:
Contains: mebendazole.

Pripsen Mebendazole see Ovex
(Seton Healthcare)

Pripsen Powder
(Seton Healthcare)

A sachet used to treat threadworm and roundworm.

Dose: adults and children over 6 years 1 sachet (children 1-6 years ⅔ sachet) in milk or water. Repeat the dose after 14 days.
Side effects: rash, wheezing, upset stomach, dizziness, weakness, aching muscles.
Caution: pregnant women and patients already taking medication should consult a doctor before using this product.
Not to be used for: patients suffering from epilepsy.
Not to be used with: sedatives, antidepressants.
Contains: piperazine phosphate, senna.

Pripsen Worm Elixir
(Seton Healthcare)

A liquid used as an anti-worm treatment for threadworm and roundworm.

Dose: to treat threadworm: adults 15ml daily, children 5-10ml daily (according to age) for 7 days. To treat roundworm: adults 30 ml, children 10-25 ml (according to age) for one single dose only (repeated after 14 days).
Side effects: rash, wheezing, upset stomach, dizziness, headache, aching muscles.
Caution: pregnant women and patients already taking medication should consult a doctor before using this product.
Not to be used for: children under 1 year, or for patients suffering from epilepsy.
Not to be used with: sedatives, antidepressants.
Contains: piperazine citrate.

Stomach preparations

The main complaints affecting the upper gastro-intestinal system are pain, indigestion, acid reflux, distension, and wind. Loss of appetite can be treated with tonics (see 'Tonics'). Persistent vomiting may be due to acid reflux or gastro-enteritis. If vomiting does not settle in 24 hours, medical advice should be sought. (There are no specific over-the-counter remedies for vomiting, although rehydration products are useful in preventing dehydration.) Upper abdominal pain can also be due to gall bladder disease, which requires medical assistance.

The majority of products in this sections are antacids, which act directly to neutralize the acid in the stomach. Magnesium-containing antacids are usually laxative in nature, while aluminium- and sodium-containing preparations may constipate. The simplest of antacids (alkalis) is sodium bicarbonate, but care should be taken to avoid mineral overload. Sodium should be avoided in those with heart conditions or high blood pressure because it can lead to heart failure. Magnesium and aluminium should be used carefully in those with kidney disorders, and a combination of alkalis and milk can lead to excess calcium deposits in the kidney. Antacids should not be taken at the same time of day as iron because the absorption of the iron may be reduced by some antacids. Care should be taken not to overdose on antacid preparations.

Unlike most other conditions in pregnancy, heartburn and indigestion may be safely treated using some of the products listed below, once the twelfth week of pregnancy is passed. (Sodium and calcium products are marketed for use in pregnancy, but calcium is the drug of choice, because increasing sodium intake carries a small risk of increasing the blood pressure, which may be a problem to some pregnant women.)

Antacids will affect many other common medicines, and should not be taken at the same time of day as some antibiotics (commonly the tetracyclines), phenytoin (a common anti-epilepsy drug), some drugs used for mental illness, or aspirin. Sodium will affect lithium therapy, and magnesium trisilicate affects iron products. All antacids may affect the enteric coating found on products designed to protect the stomach, and should not be taken with such tablets. Check with a pharmacist if you wish to take an antacid with other medication.

The histamine H_2-receptor antagonists work by reducing the acid produced, but there are many restrictions with their use. They are not suitable for repeated or regular use, or for treating ulcers or hiatus hernia, (except when supplied on prescription), and should not be used as a substitute for regular prescription medication. Patients already taking other medicines, or who have a history of stomach ulcers should see a doctor before self-medicating, and patients who are middle-aged or older with symptoms of excess acid for the first time should also seek medical advice before using H_2-receptor antagonists. Any weight loss or difficulty swallowing should also be taken seriously and reported to a doctor, as should persistent stomach pain.

Persistent indigestion may mean that an ulcer is present and that medical evaluation is necessary. There are no preparations available over the counter to treat ulcers.

Travel sickness will respond to antihistamines, such as promethazine and cinnarizine, or to hyoscine, although all of these products have side effects that may impair driving performance, so drivers who need such medicines should beware. (Non-medicinal treatments, such as Sea-band, may be more suitable.)

Acidosis
(Potters)

A tablet used as a herbal acid-reducing, astringent, and absorbing remedy to treat the symptoms of stomach acid, indigestion, and heartburn.

Dose: 2 tablets 3 times a day after meals. (At least 10 days treatment is advised for full effect.)
Side effects:
Caution:
Not to be used for: children.
Not to be used with: any other medications.
Contains: meadowsweet, vegetable charcoal, rhubarb.

Actal
(Sterling Health)

A tablet used as an antacid to treat indigestion, heartburn, and stomach upset.

Dose: 2 tablets when needed (up to 8 times a day).
Side effects: few; sodium overload is possible.
Caution:
Not to be used for: children under 12 years.
Not to be used with: some antibiotics, iron, tablets coated to protect the stomach.
Contains: alexitol sodium.

Actonorm Gel
(Wallace)

A liquid used as an antacid to treat indigestion and wind.

Dose: 5-20 ml after meals.
Side effects: few; occasionally constipation or diarrhoea.

Caution:
Not to be used for: children.
Not to be used with: some antibiotics, iron, tablets coated to protect the stomach, homeopathic remedies.
Contains: aluminium hydroxide, magnesium hydroxide, activated dimethicone, peppermint oil.

Actonorm Powder
(Wallace)

A powder used as an antacid and anti-spasmodic treatment for excess acid, wind, indigestion, and discomfort due to over-indulgence.

Dose: 5 ml in water or milk 3 times a day.
Side effects: dry mouth, changes in vision, dry and flushed skin, abnormal heart rhythm, difficulty passing water, confusion, rash, fever.
Caution: children, the elderly, pregnant women, nursing mothers, and patients with difficulty passing water, prostate problems, heart or intestinal disease should consult a doctor before using this product.
Not to be used for: patients with glaucoma.
Not to be used with: some antibiotics, tablets coated to protect the stomach, antidepressants, MAOIs, glyceryl trinitrate, iron, homeopathic remedies.
Contains: atropine sulphate, aluminium hydroxide, calcium carbonate, magnesium trisilicate, magnesium carbonate, sodium bicarbonate, peppermint oil.

Algicon
(Rhone-Poulenc Rorer Family Health)

A tablet and suspension used as an antacid to treat excess acid and heartburn.

Dose: 1-2 tablets or 10-20 ml of suspension 4 times a day after meals and at night.

Side effects: few; constipation or diarrhoea.

Caution: patients suffering from diabetes should consult a doctor or dietician because of sucrose content of tablets.

Not to be used for: children, or in patients suffering from severe debilitation.

Not to be used with: some antibiotics, iron, tablets coated to protect the stomach.

Contains: magnesium alginate, aluminium hydroxide, magnesium carbonate, potassium bicarbonate.

Alka-Seltzer
(Warner Wellcome Consumer Healthcare)

An effervescent tablet used as an analgesic and antacid to treat headache and upset stomach, (for example, due to overindulgence in food or drink, migraine, period pain).

Dose: 2 tablets in water every 4 hours (up to 4 times a day) for up to 3 days.

Side effects: irritation of stomach and intestines.

Caution: pregnant women and patients with asthma or stomach disorder should consult a doctor before using this product.

Not to be used for: children under 12 years, nursing mothers, or patients with stomach ulcers, blood-clotting disorder, or allergy to aspirin.

Not to be used with: anticoagulants, some anti-epileptic drugs, some antibiotics, tablets coated to protect the stomach, iron.

Contains: aspirin, citric acid, sodium bicarbonate.

Altacite
(Roussel)

Tablets and suspension used as an antacid to treat indigestion.

Dose: adults 2 tablets or 10 ml suspension between meals and at bedtime; children 6-12 years half the adult dose.
Side effects:
Caution: chew or crush tablets before swallowing.
Not to be used for: children under 6 years.
Not to be used with: some antibiotics, tablets which are coated to protect the stomach, iron.
Contains: hydrotalcite.

Altacite Plus
(Hoechst Roussel)

A tablet and liquid used as an antacid and anti-wind preparation to treat wind and indigestion.

Dose: adults 10 ml liquid or 1-2 tablets between meals and at bedtime; children 8-12 years half adult dose.
Side effects: few; occasional diarrhoea and constipation.
Caution: chew or crush tablets before swallowing.
Not to be used for: children under 8 years.
Not to be used with: some antibiotics, iron, tablets coated to protect the stomach.
Contains: hydrotalcite, dimethicone (co-simalcite).

Alu-Cap
(3M Healthcare)

A capsule used as an antacid to treat excess acid.

Dose: 1 capsule 4 times a day and at bedtime.
Side effects: few; occasional bowel disorder such as constipation.
Caution:
Not to be used for: children.
Not to be used with: some antibiotics, iron, tablets coated to protect the stomach.

Contains: aluminium hydroxide gel.

Aludrox
(Charwell Health Care)

A tablet and liquid used as an antacid to treat indigestion, heartburn, and excess acid.

Dose: 1-2 tablets or 5-10 ml liquid 4 times a day and at bedtime.
Side effects:
Caution:
Not to be used for: children under 12 years.
Not to be used with: some antibiotics, iron, tablets that are coated to protect the stomach.
Contains: aluminium hydroxide. (Tablets also contain magnesium carbonate and magnesium hydroxide.)

Andrews Antacid
(Sterling Health)

A tablet available in original or fruit flavours, used as an antacid to relieve indigestion, heartburn, and wind.

Dose: 1-2 tablets sucked or chewed when required.
(Maximum 12 tablets in 24 hours.)
Side effects:
Caution:
Not to be used for: children.
Not to be used with: some antibiotics, iron, tablets coated to protect the stomach.
Contains: calcium carbonate, heavy magnesium carbonate.

Andrews Liver Salts
(Sterling Health)

An effervescent powder used treat upset stomach, indigestion, and symptoms of overindulgence. (For use in treating constipation, see 'Bowel disorders' section.)

Dose: adults 1 teaspoonful or sachet in water up to 4 times a day; children over 3 years half the adult dose.
Side effects:
Caution:
Not to be used for: children under 3 years.
Not to be used with: some antibiotics, iron, tablets coated to protect the stomach.
Contains: sodium bicarbonate, citric acid, magnesium sulphate.

APP Stomach Tablets
(Chancellor)

A tablet used as an antacid and antispasmodic treatment for indigestion and excess acid.

Dose: 1 tablet (chewed) 3-4 times a day.
Side effects: dry mouth, changes in vision, dry and flushed skin, abnormal heart rhythm, difficulty passing water, confusion, rash, fever.
Caution: the elderly, pregnant women, nursing mothers, and patients with difficulty passing water, prostate problems, heart or intestinal disease should consult a doctor before using this product.
Not to be used for: children under 12 years, and patients with glaucoma or myasthenia gravis.
Not to be used with: some antibiotics, iron, tablets coated to protect the stomach, antidepressants, MAOIs, glyceryl trinitrate.
Contains: calcium carbonate, aluminium hydroxide, magnesium carbonate, bismuth carbonate, homatropine methylbromide.

Asilone
(Seton Healthcare)

A liquid, suspension, or tablet used as an antacid, anti-wind preparation to treat indigestion, wind, excess acid, and heartburn.

Dose: 5-10 ml liquid/suspension or 1-2 tablets before meals and at bedtime.
Side effects: few; occasionally constipation.
Caution: tablets must be sucked or chewed.
Not to be used for: children under 12 years, women in the first 3 months of pregnancy, or severely debilitated patients.
Not to be used with: some antibiotics, warfarin, digoxin, iron, tablets coated to protect the stomach.
Contains: activated dimethicone, aluminium hydroxide. (The suspension and liquid also contain magnesium oxide.)

Atkinson & Barker's Infant Gripe Mixture
(Torbet Laboratories)

A liquid used as an antacid and aromatic carminative to treat wind pain in infants.

Dose: 2.5-10 ml (according to age).
Side effects:
Caution:
Not to be used for:
Not to be used with: some antibiotics, iron, tablets coated to protect the stomach.
Contains: sodium bicarbonate, dill oil, caraway oil.

Avomine
(Rhone-Poulenc Rorer Family Health)

A white, scored tablet used as an antihistamine treatment for travel sickness.

Dose: adults 1 tablet at bedtime before long journeys or 1-2 hours before short journeys. (Repeat the dose daily for long journeys.) Children 5-10 years half adult dose.

Side effects: drowsiness, blurred vision, dry mouth, difficulty passing water, stomach upset, cramp, muscle twitch, dizziness, sensitivity to sunlight.

Caution: pregnant women, nursing mothers, and patients suffering from asthma, bronchitis, glaucoma, epilepsy, heart disease, bladder problems, or otherwise being treated by a doctor should seek medical advice before using this product.

Not to be used for: children under 5 years.

Not to be used with: alcohol, other sedating medicines, MAOIs, pregnancy tests, allergy tests.

Contains: promethazine theoclate.

Barum Antacid Tablets see **Rap-eze**
(Wrafton Laboratories)

Bellocarb
(Sinclair Pharmaceuticals)

A tablet used as an antacid and anti-spasm treatment for bowel spasm and indigestion.

Dose: 1-2 tablets 4 times a day.

Side effects: dry mouth, changes in vision, dry and flushed skin, abnormal heart rhythm, difficulty passing water, confusion, rash, fever.

Caution: children, the elderly, pregnant women, nursing mothers, and patients with difficulty passing water, prostate problems, heart or intestinal disease should consult a doctor before using this product.

Not to be used for: patients suffereing from glaucoma.

Not to be used with: some antibiotics, iron, tablets coated to protect the stomach, antidepressants, MAOIs glyceryl trinitrate.

Contains: belladonna, magnesium trisilicate, magnesium carbonate.

Bio-Strath Artichoke Formula
(Cedar Health)

A liquid used as a herbal digestive remedy to relieve the symptoms of indigestion after eating fatty foods.

Dose: 20 drops (0.6 ml) in a little water 3 times a day before meals, or as directed by a doctor.
Side effects:
Caution:
Not to be used for: children.
Not to be used with: homeopathic remedies.
Contains: yeast, artichoke, thistle seed, peppermint.

Bio-Strath Liquorice Formula
(Cedar Health)

A liquid used as a herbal remedy to aid digestion.

Dose: 20 drops (0.6 ml) in a little water 3 times a day, or as directed by a doctor.
Side effects: high doses may cause sodium retention, potassium loss, water retention, high blood pressure, headache, and shortness of breath.
Caution:
Not to be used for: children.
Not to be used with:
Contains: yeast, liquorice root, camomile, gentian.

Biobalm Powder
(Lane)

A powder used as a herbal soothing remedy to relieve

symptoms of indigestion, wind, and stomach upset.

Dose: adults 1-2 level teaspoonsful (mixed into fluid, as directed) up to 4 times a day; children aged 5-12 years half the adult dose.
Side effects:
Caution:
Not to be used for: children under 5 years.
Not to be used with:
Contains: slippery elm bark, marshmallow root, Irish moss, camomile.

Birley's Antacid Powder
(Torbet Laboratories)

A powder used as an antacid to treat indigestion, excess acid, heartburn, and wind.

Dose: adults 5 ml in water after each meal, or twice a day; children ¼-1 adult dose, according to age.
Side effects:
Caution:
Not to be used for:
Not to be used with: some antibiotics, iron, tablets coated to protect the stomach.
Contains: aluminium hydroxide, magnesium trisilicate, magnesium carbonate.

Bismag
(Whitehall)

A tablet used as an antacid to treat indigestion, wind, and acid.

Dose: 2-4 tablets with water after meals, repeated after 15 minutes if needed and at bedtime.
Side effects:

Caution:
Not to be used for: children.
Not to be used with: some antibiotics, iron, tablets coated to protect the stomach.
Contains: sodium bicarbonate, heavy magnesium carbonate, light magnesium carbonate.

Bisodol
(Whitehall)

A tablet and sugar-free powder used as an antacid to treat indigestion, heartburn, wind, and acid.

Dose: 1-2 tablets sucked or chewed, (or 5 ml powder in water), after meals if required.
Side effects:
Caution:
Not to be used for: children.
Not to be used with: some antibiotics, iron, tablets coated to protect the stomach.
Contains: light magnesium carbonate, sodium bicarbonate. (Tablets also contain calcium carbonate, powder also contains heavy magnesium carbonate.)

Bisodol Extra
(Whitehall)

A tablet used as an antacid and anti-wind preparation to treat heartburn, acidity, and wind.

Dose: 1-2 sucked or chewed when required.
Side effects:
Caution:
Not to be used for:
Not to be used with: some antibiotics, iron, tablets coated to protect the stomach.

Contains: calcium carbonate, magnesium carbonate, sodium bicarbonate, simethicone.

Bisodol Heartburn
(Whitehall)

A tablet used as an antacid and reflux suppressant to treat heartburn (including heartburn of pregnancy).

Dose: adults 1-2 tablets chewed when required (children 6-12 years 1 tablet after meals and at bedtime).
Side effects:
Caution: patients taking other medications should see a doctor before using this product.
Not to be used for: children under 6 years, or for women during the first 3 months of pregnancy.
Not to be used with: some antibiotics, iron, tablets coated to protect the stomach.
Contains: sodium bicarbonate, magaldrate, alginic acid.

Boots Antacid Tablets see Rap-eze
(Boots)

Boots Children's Gripe Mixture
(Boots)

A sugar-free mixture used as an antacid to treat wind and gripe pains in infants.

Dose: 5-10 ml (according to age) before or after each feed (up to 6 times a day).
Side effects: allergy.
Caution:
Not to be used for: babies under 1 month or children over 1 year.
Not to be used with: some antibiotics, iron.

Contains: sodium bicarbonate.

Boots Cream of Magnesia see magnesium hydroxide mixture
(Boots)

Boots Cream of Magnesia Tablets
(Boots)

A tablet used to treat acid indigestion, heartburn, and wind.

Dose: adults 2 tablets after meals, at bedtime, and when required. (Children aged 5-12 years half the adult dose.)
Side effects:
Caution:
Not to be used for:
Not to be used with: some antibiotics, iron, tablets coated to protect the stomach.
Contains: magnesium hydroxide.

Boots Double Action Indigestion Remedies
(Boots)

A liquid or tablet used as an antacid, anti-wind preparation to treat painful wind, indigestion, heartburn, and excess acid.

Dose: adults 1-2 tablets or 10 ml liquid after meals, at bedtime, or when required. (Children 5-12 years half the adult dose.)
Side effects:
Caution:
Not to be used for: children under 5 years.
Not to be used with: some antibiotics, iron, tablets coated to protect the stomach.
Contains: aluminium hydroxide, magnesium hydroxide,

polymethylsiloxane.

Boots Health Salts
(Boots)

An effervescent powder used as an antacid to treat upset stomach, heartburn, and indigestion. (For use as a laxative see entry in 'Bowel disorders' section.)

Dose: 1 teaspoonful in water every 3-4 hours, for a maximum of 5 days.
Side effects:
Caution:
Not to be used for: children under 12 years.
Not to be used with: some antibiotics, iron, tablets coated to protect the stomach.
Contains: sucrose, sodium bicarbonate, magnesium sulphate, citric acid, tartaric acid, sodium chloride.

Boots Herbal Indigestion Tablets
(Boots)

A tablet used as a herbal remedy to relieve symptoms of indigestion and wind.

Dose: 2 tablets 3 times a day before food.
Side effects:
Caution:
Not to be used for: children under 12 years, pregnant women, and nursing mothers.
Not to be used with:
Contains: parsley root, centaury, marshmallow root.

Boots Indigestion Tablets
(Boots)

A tablet used as an antacid to relieve excess acid, indigestion, heartburn, and wind.

Dose: adults 1-2 tablets after meals, at bedtime, or when required. (Children under 12 years, half the adult dose.)
Side effects:
Caution: chew or suck before swallowing.
Not to be used for:
Not to be used with: some antibiotics, iron, tablets coated to protect the stomach.
Contains: calcium carbonate, magnesium trisilicate, magnesium carbonate, sodium bicarbonate.

Boots Travel Band* see Sea-Band*
(Boots)

Boots Travel Calm
(Boots)

A tablet used as an anti-spasm treatment to prevent travel sickness.

Dose: ¼-1 tablet (according to age) 20 minutes before journey. Repeat every 6-8 hours. (Maximum of 3 doses in 24 hours.)
Side effects: drowsiness, dry mouth, dizziness, blurred vision, difficulty passing water.
Caution: patients suffering from heart or circulatory disorder, having difficulty passing water, or taking any other medication should consult a doctor before using this product.
Not to be used for: children under 3 years, pregnant women, nursing mothers, and patients suffering from glaucoma.
Not to be used with: alcohol, antidepressants, MAOIs, other

sedating medicines.
Contains: hyoscine hydrobromide.

Buscopan
(Windsor Healthcare)

A tablet used as an anti-spasm treatment for stomach cramps and period pain.

Dose: adults 2 tablets 4 times a day. (Children aged 6-12 years 1 tablet 3 times a day.)
Side effects: dry mouth, blurred vision, palpitations.
Caution: patients over 65 and those suffering from heart conditions should consult a doctor before using this product.
Not to be used for: children under 6 years or for patients suffering from glaucoma.
Not to be used with: antidepressants, MAOIs, glyceryl trinitrate, alcohol, sedating medicines.
Contains: hyoscine butylbromide.

Cantassium Herbal Travel Sickness Tablets
(Cantassium)

A tablet used as a herbal remedy for travel sickness.

Dose: adults 3 tablets (children aged 6-12 years 1-2 tablets) half-an-hour before journey.
Side effects:
Caution:
Not to be used for: children under 6 years.
Not to be used with:
Contains: ginger.

Carbellon
(Torbet)

A black tablet used as an anti-wind, antacid preparation to treat excess acid, indigestion, and wind.

Dose: adults 2-4 tablets 3 times a day; children 1½-2 tablets 3 times a day.
Side effects:
Caution:
Not to be used for: children under 1 year.
Not to be used with: antibiotics, iron, tablets coated to protect the stomach, homeopathic remedies.
Contains: magnesium hydroxide, charcoal, peppermint oil.

Carminative Tea
(Weleda)

A tea used as a herbal calming and anti-spasm remedy to relieve wind.

Dose: adults use 5 ml tea added to 200 ml boiling water and allowed to simmer for 1 minute. Filter before drinking. Use this dose twice a day if required. (Children use half adult dose.)
Side effects:
Caution: prepare freshly for each dose. Pregnant women should consult a doctor before using this product.
Not to be used for:
Not to be used with:
Contains: aniseed, fennel, caraway, yarrow, matricaria.

---

charcoal tablets
(licensed preparations available from Lanes, Potters)

A tablet used as an absorbing treatment to relieve symptoms of wind, indigestion, heartburn, and diarrhoea.

Dose: as specified for each individual product.
Side effects: black-coloured stools.
Caution:
Not to be used for:
Not to be used with: any other medication.
Contains: charcoal.

De Witt's Antacid
(E. C. De Witt)

A tablet and powder used as an antacid to treat upset stomach, indigestion, excess acid, and wind. (The powder is also adsorbent.)

Dose: 1-2 tablets (or 5 ml powder in water) at first sign of discomfort. (If using powder, repeat the dose after 10 minutes if necessary.)
Side effects:
Caution: for powder, see note concerning use of adsorbent medications at start of 'Bowel disorders' section.
Not to be used for: children.
Not to be used with: some antibiotics, iron, tablets coated to protect the stomach, homeopathic remedies.
Contains: magnesium trisilicate, magnesium carbonate, calcium carbonate, peppermint oil. (The powder also contains light kaolin.)

Dentinox Colic Drops
(Dendron)

A liquid used as an anti-wind preparation to treat wind and griping pains in infants (from birth onwards).

Dose: 2.5 ml with or after each feed (up to 6 times a day).
Side effects:
Caution:

Not to be used for:
Not to be used with:
Contains: simethicone.

Digest
(Lane)

A tablet used as a herbal calming and anti-wind preparation to relieve indigestion and wind.

Dose: 2 tablets 3 times a day before meals.
Side effects:
Caution:
Not to be used for: children under 12 years, pregnant women, or nursing mothers.
Not to be used with:
Contains: parsley, centaury, marshmallow root.

Dijex
(Seton Healthcare)

A liquid or tablet used as an antacid to treat indigestion.

Dose: adults 1-2 tablets (chewed) or 5-10 ml liquid 3 times a day and at bedtime. (Children over 5-6 years half adult dose.) Tablets may be used every 2-4 hours if needed.
Side effects:
Caution:
Not to be used for: children under 5 years (tablets) or under 6 years (liquid).
Not to be used with: some antibiotics, iron, tablets coated to protect the stomach.
Contains: aluminium hydroxide. (Tablets also contain magnesium carbonate and liquid also contains magnesium hydroxide.)

Diovol
(Pharmax)

A white suspension used as an antacid and anti-wind preparation to treat wind and acidity.
Dose: 5-10 ml 3 times a day.
Side effects: few; occasionally constipation.
Caution:
Not to be used for: children.
Not to be used with: some antibiotics, iron, tablets coated to protect the stomach.
Contains: aluminium hydroxide, magnesium hydroxide, dimethicone.

Dramamine
(Searle)

A tablet used as an antihistamine to prevent travel sickness.

Dose: adults 1-2 tablets (children ¼-1 tablet according to age) 2-3 times a day. (Take the first dose 30 minutes before journey starts.)
Side effects: drowsiness
Caution: pregnant women should consult a doctor before using this product.
Not to be used for: children under 1 year.
Not to be used with: alcohol, MAOIs, other sedating medicines.
Contains: dimenhydrinate.

Enos
(SmithKline Beecham Consumer)

An effervescent powder available in two flavours (original or lemon) and used as an antacid to relieve stomach upsets, heartburn, wind, nausea, and acid indigestion.

Dose: 1 sachet or 1 teaspoonful every 2-3 hours if needed. (Maximum of 6 doses in 24 hours.)
Side effects:
Caution:
Not to be used for: children under 12 years.
Not to be used with: some antibiotics, iron, tablets coated to protect the stomach.
Contains: sodium bicarbonate, citric acid, sodium carbonate.

Fenulin
(Gerard House)

A tablet used as a herbal soothing remedy to treat digestive upsets.

Dose: 2 tablets 3 times a day after meals.
Side effects:
Caution:
Not to be used for: children under 12 years, pregnant women, or nursing mothers.
Not to be used with:
Contains: fenugreek, slippery elm, golden seal.

Gastrocote
(Boehringer Mannheim)

A tablet and liquid used as an antacid and reflux suppressant to treat heartburn, including heartburn associated with pregnancy or hiatus hernia.
Dose: adults and children over 6 years 1-2 tablets (chewed) or 5-15 ml liquid 4 times a day.
Side effects:
Caution: diabetics and patients requiring a low salt or low phosphate diet should consult a doctor before using this product.
Not to be used for: children under 6 years.

Not to be used with: some antibiotics, iron, tablets coated to protect the stomach.
Contains: aluminium hydroxide, magnesium trisilicate, sodium bicarbonate. (Tablets also contains alginic acid. Liquid also contains sodium alginate.)

Gastron
(Sanofi-Winthrop)

A tablet used as an antacid and reflux suppressant to treat reflux symptoms.

Dose: 1-2 tablets 3 times a day and 2 at bedtime.
Side effects: few; occasionally constipation.
Caution: pregnant women and patients suffering from high blood pressure or heart disease should consult a doctor before using this product.
Not to be used for: children.
Not to be used with: some antibiotics, iron, tablets coated to protect the stomach.
Contains: alginic acid, aluminium hydroxide, magnesium trisilicate, sodium bicarbonate.

Gaviscon
(Reckitt & Colman)

A tablet (available in two strengths) and liquid used as an antacid and reflux suppressant to treat reflux, heartburn, and acid indigestion. (Suitable for the treatment of pregnant women.)
Dose: adults 1-2 tablets (chewed) or 10-20 ml liquid after meals and at night. (Children aged 6-12 years 5 ml liquid after meals and at night.)
Side effects: few; occasionally constipation.
Caution: pregnant women and patients requiring a low-salt diet should consult their doctor before using this product.
Not to be used for: children under 6 years (liquid) or under 12

years (tablets).
Not to be used with: some antibiotics, iron, tablets coated to protect the stomach.
Contains: sodium bicarbonate. (Liquid also contains sodium alginate and calcium carbonate. Tablets also contain alginic acid, aluminium hydroxide, and magnesium trisilicate.)

G. B. Tablets
(Potters)

A tablet used as a herbal remedy to increase bile flow and relieve the symptoms of upper abdominal discomfort after meals.

Dose: 2 tablets 3 times a day for a 10-day course.
Side effects:
Caution:
Not to be used for: children.
Not to be used with:
Contains: black root, wahoo, kava, burdock.

Gelusil
(Warner Wellcome Consumer Healthcare)

A tablet used as an antacid to treat indigestion and heartburn.

Dose: adults 1-2 tablets after meals; children over 6 years half adult dose.
Side effects: few; occasionally constipation.
Caution:
Not to be used for: children under 6 years.
Not to be used with: some antibiotics, iron, tablets coated to protect the stomach.
Contains: magnesium trisilicate, aluminium hydroxide.

Ginger Tablets
(Gerard House)

A tablet used as a calming herbal remedy to treat nausea.

Dose: 1 tablet 3 times a day.
Side effects:
Caution: pregnant women and nursing mothers should consult a doctor before using this product.
Not to be used for: children.
Not to be used with:
Contains: ginger.

Golden Seal Compound
(Gerard House)

A tablet used as a herbal soothing and astringent remedy to stimulate the digestive organs and relieve indigestion, heartburn, wind, nausea, and stomach irritation.

Dose: 2 tablets 3 times a day between meals.
Side effects:
Caution:
Not to be used for: children under 12 years, pregnant women, and nursing mothers.
Not to be used with:
Contains: marshmallow root, cranesbill, golden seal, dandelion root.

Heath and Heather Indigestion and Flatulence Tablets
(Ferrosan Healthcare)

A tablet used as a herbal remedy to relieve the symptoms of indigestion and wind.

Dose: 2 tablets 3 times a day after meals.

Side effects:
Caution: pregnant women should consult a doctor before using this medicine.
Not to be used for: children.
Not to be used with: homeopathic remedies.
Contains: peppermint oil, fennel oil, capsicum oleoresin.

Indian Brandee
(Potters)

A liquid used as a herbal warming remedy to relieve the symptoms of digestive discomfort.

Dose: 5 ml in or with a little water. Repeat once or twice if needed.
Side effects:
Caution:
Not to be used for: children or pregnant women.
Not to be used with:
Contains: capsicum tincture, strong ginger tincture, compound rhubarb tincture.

Indigestion Mixture
(Potters)

A mixture used as a herbal antacid and digestive remedy to treat the symptoms of indigestion, heartburn, and wind.

Dose: 5 ml 3-4 times a day after meals.
Side effects:
Caution:
Not to be used for: children, pregnant women, or nursing mothers.
Not to be used with:
Contains: meadowsweet, concentrated compound gentian infusion, wahoo.

Infacol
(Pharmax)

A sugar-free liquid, supplied with a measuring dropper, and used as an anti-wind preparation to treat griping pain and colic in infants (from birth onwards).

Dose: 0.5-1.0 ml before each feed.
Side effects:
Caution:
Not to be used for:
Not to be used with:
Contains: simethicone.

Jaap's Health Salt
(Askit Laboratories)

An effervescent powder used as an antacid and laxative to treat indigestion, heartburn, and constipation.

Dose: 5-10 ml in water in the morning, or during the day if needed.
Side effects:
Caution:
Not to be used for:
Not to be used with: some antibiotics, iron, tablets coated to protect the stomach.
Contains: sodium potassium tartrate, acid tartrate, sodium hydrogen carbonate, sucrose, dextrose.

Joy-Rides
(Stafford-Miller)

A chewable tablet used as an anti-spasm treatment to prevent travel sickness.

Dose: adults 2 tablets, children ½-2 tablets (according to age). Repeat the dose after 6 hours if needed. (Maximum of 2 doses in 24 hours.)
Side effects: drowsiness.
Caution: children under 3 years and patients suffering from glaucoma must be seen by a doctor before taking this product.
Not to be used for:
Not to be used with: alcohol, other sedating medicines.
Contains: hyoscine hydrobromide.

Kolanticon
(Marion Merrell Dow)

A gel used as an antacid, anti-spasm preparation to treat the symptoms of indigestion.

Dose: 10-20 ml every 4 hours.
Side effects: blurred vision, confusion, dry mouth, dry and flushed skin, abnormal heart rhythm, difficulty passing water, rash.
Caution: the elderly, pregnant women, nursing mothers, and patients with difficulty passing water or suffering from heart conditions should consult a doctor before using this product.
Not to be used for: children or for patients suffering from glaucoma, inflammatory bowel disease, intestinal obstruction, or enlarged prostate.
Not to be used with: some antibiotics, iron, tablets coated to protect the stomach, MAOIs, antidepressants, glyceryl trinitrate.
Contains: aluminium hydroxide, magnesium oxide, dicyclomine hydrochloride, simethicone.

Kwells
(Roche Consumer Health)

A tablet available in standard or junior strengths, and used as an anti-spasm product to treat and prevent travel sickness.

Dose: standard tablets: adults 1 tablet every 6 hours (maximum 3 in 24 hours); children aged 7-12 years half the adult dose. Junior tablets: for ages 8-12 years 1-2 tablets every 6 hours (maximum 3-6 in 24 hours), for ages 3-7 years, ½-1 tablet every 6 hours (maximum 1½-3 in 24 hours).
Side effects: drowsiness, dry mouth, blurred vision, difficulty passing water.
Caution: children under 3 years, elderly patients, and patients with heart or circulation disease, glaucoma, blocked intestines, or difficulty passing water should see a doctor before using this product. Junior-strength tablets should be used for children aged 3-7 years.
Not to be used for: patients suffering from glaucoma.
Not to be used with: alcohol, other sedating medicines.
Contains: hyoscine hydrobromide.

Maalox/Maalox TC
(Rhone-Poulenc Rorer)

A tablet (Maalox TC) and a liquid (available as Maalox and higher-strength Maalox TC) used as an antacid to treat indigestion, heartburn, and acidity.

Dose: 1-2 tablets or 5-10 ml liquid 3 times a day after meals and at bedtime.
Side effects: constipation, diarrhoea.
Caution:
Not to be used for: children under 14 years, women in the first 3 months of pregnancy, nursing mothers, or for severely debilitated patients, or those with severe stomach pains or possible bowel obstruction.
Not to be used with: some antibiotics, iron, tablets coated to protect the stomach.
Contains: aluminium hydroxide, magnesium hydroxide.

Maalox Plus
(Rhone-Poulenc Rorer)

A liquid and tablet used as an antacid and anti-wind preparation to treat indigestion, heartburn, and wind.

Dose: 1-2 tablets (chewed) or 5-10 ml liquid 4 times a day after meals and at bedtime. (Reduced doses of liquid may be used for children.)
Side effects: constipation, diarrhoea.
Caution: pregnant women and patients receiving medical treatment should consult a doctor before using this product.
Not to be used for: children under 5 years, women in the first 3 months of pregnancy, nursing mothers, or for patients who are severely debilitated or who have severe stomach pains or possible bowel obstruction.
Not to be used with: some antibiotics, iron, tablets coated to protect the stomach.
Contains: aluminium hydroxide, simethicone, magnesium hydroxide.

Maclean
(SmithKline Beecham Consumer)

A tablet used as an antacid to treat indigestion, excess acid, nausea, heartburn, and wind.

Dose: 1-2 tablets sucked or chewed when needed. (Maximum 16 tablets in 24 hours.)
Side effects:
Caution:
Not to be used for: children under 12 years.
Not to be used with: some antibiotics, iron, tablets coated to protect the stomach.
Contains: calcium carbonate, magnesium carbonate, aluminium hydroxide.

Magnatol
(Sterling Health)

A liquid used as an antacid to treat the symptoms of heartburn.

Dose: 20 ml up to 4 times a day.
Side effects:
Caution:
Not to be used for: children.
Not to be used with: some antibiotics, iron, tablets coated to protect the stomach.
Contains: heavy magnesium carbonate, potassium bicarbonate, alexitol sodium, xanthan gum.

---

magnesium trisilicate mixture BP

A suspension used as an antacid to treat acidity and indigestion.

Dose: adults 10 ml 3 times a day in water.
Side effects: diarrhoea.
Caution: children should be seen by a doctor before using this product.
Not to be used for:
Not to be used with: some antibiotics, iron, tablets coated to protect the stomach.
Contains: magnesium trisilicate.

---

magnesium trisilicate powder compound BP

A powder used as an antacid to treat acidity and indigestion.

Dose: 1-5 g powder taken in liquid when required.
Side effects: diarrhoea.
Caution: children should be seen by a doctor before using this product.
Not to be used for:

Not to be used with: some antibiotics, iron, tablets coated to protect the stomach.
Contains: magnesium trisilicate, chalk, heavy magnesium carbonate, sodium bicarbonate.

magnesium trisilicate tablets compound BP

A tablet used as an antacid to treat acidity and indigestion.

Dose: 1-2 tablets chewed when required.
Side effects: diarrhoea.
Caution: children should be seen by a doctor before using this product.
Not to be used for:
Not to be used with: some antibiotics, iron, tablets coated to protect the stomach.
Contains: magnesium trisilicate, aluminium hydroxide.

Melissa Comp. see entry in 'Bowel disorders' section (Weleda)

Milk of Magnesia
(Sterling Health)

A liquid or tablet used as an antacid to treat indigestion, upset stomach, wind, heartburn and excess acid. (For use as a laxative see 'Bowel disorders' section.)

Dose: adults 2-4 tablets or 5-10 ml liquid when required; (maximum of 16 tablets or 60 ml liquid in 24 hours). Children aged 6-12 years half adult dose. Children aged 3-6 years half adult dose of liquid only.
Side effects:
Caution: children under 3 years should be seen by a doctor before using this product.
Not to be used for:

Not to be used with: some antibiotics, iron, or tablets coated to protect the stomach.
Contains: magnesium hydroxide.

Moorland
(Crookes Healthcare)

A tablet used as an antacid to treat indigestion, heartburn, and wind.

Dose: 2 tablets dissolved in the mouth after meals and at bedtime.
Side effects:
Caution:
Not to be used for: children under 6 years.
Not to be used with: some antibiotics, iron, tablets coated to protect the stomach.
Contains: bismuth aluminate, magnesium trisilicate, aluminium hydroxide, magnesium carbonate, light kaolin, calcium carbonate.

Mucogel
(Pharmax)

A liquid used as an antacid to treat heartburn and indigestion.

Dose: 10-20 ml 3 times a day and at bedtime.
Side effects:
Caution:
Not to be used for: children under 12 years.
Not to be used with: some antibiotics, iron, tablets coated to protect the stomach.
Contains: aluminium hydroxide, magnesium hydroxide.

Natraleze
(English Grains Healthcare)

A tablet used as a herbal remedy to treat the symptoms of heartburn, indigestion, and trapped wind.

Dose: adults 2 tablets (children aged 7-12 years 1 tablet) after meals.
Side effects:
Caution:
Not to be used for: children under 7 years, or for pregnant women.
Not to be used with:
Contains: slippery elm bark, meadow sweet, liquorice.

Neo Baby Mixture
(Neo Laboratories)

A mixture used as an antacid and aromatic carminative to treat wind indigestion, griping, and teething in babies.

Dose: 2.5-15 ml 3 times a day, according to age.
Side effects:
Caution:
Not to be used for:
Not to be used with: some antibiotics, iron.
Contains: sodium bicarbonate, dill oil, essence of ginger.

Nulacin
(Goldshield Healthcare)

A tablet used as an antacid to treat indigestion, excess acid, heartburn.

Dose: 1 tablet sucked slowly when required (up to 8 a day).
Side effects:

Caution:
Not to be used for: children, or for patients suffering from coeliac disease.
Not to be used with: some antibiotics, iron, tablets coated to protect the stomach, homeopathic remedies.
Contains: milk solids with dextrins and maltose, magnesium oxide, magnesium carbonate, magnesium trisilicate, calcium carbonate, peppermint oil.

Nurse Harvey's Gripe Mixture
(Harvey Scruton)

An alcohol-free mixture used as an antacid and aromatic carminative to treat wind, gripe pains, and stomach upsets in babies.

Dose: 5-10 ml, according to age, during or after feeds. (Maximum 6 doses in 24 hours.)
Side effects:
Caution:
Not to be used for: babies under 1 month.
Not to be used with: some antibiotics, iron.
Contains: sodium bicarbonate, dill oil, caraway oil.

Opas
(Rybar)

A tablet used as an antacid to treat acid indigestion, heartburn, and wind.

Dose: 1-2 tablets after each meal if needed.
Side effects:
Caution:
Not to be used for: children.
Not to be used with: some antibiotics, iron, tablets coated to protect the stomach.

Contains: sodium bicarbonate, calcium carbonate, heavy magnesium carbonate, magnesium trisilicate.

Papaya Plus
(Gerard House)

A tablet used as a herbal absorbing and soothing remedy to relieve the symptoms of indigestion, heartburn, excess acid, and wind.

Dose: 1 tablet before meals 3 times a day.
Side effects:
Caution: pregnant women and nursing mothers should consult a doctor before using this product.
Not to be used for: children.
Not to be used with: any other medication.
Contains: charcoal, papain, slippery elm, golden seal.

Pepcid-AC
(Centra Healthcare)

A tablet used as a histamine H_2-receptor antagonist to treat symptoms of heartburn, indigestion, and excess acid.
(Doctors may prescribe this medication for different disorders. Self-medication should be limited to the conditions and doses stated.)

Dose: 1 tablet (one hour before eating). Repeat if the symptoms return. (Maximum 2 tablets in 24 hours). Maximum period of treatment : 2 weeks.
Side effects: headache, dizziness, dry mouth, nausea, vomiting, abdominal bloating and discomfort, constipation, diarrhoea, loss of appetite, tiredness, jaundice, breast swelling and tenderness, itching, rash, allergic reaction.
Caution: patients suffering from any other illness, taking any other medicines, regularly being seen by a doctor or with a

history of stomach ulcer should consult their doctor before using this product.

Not to be used for: children under 16 years, pregnant women, nursing mothers, patients with unintended weight loss, difficulty swallowing or persistent stomach pain, patients middle aged or older with new or changed symptoms.

Not to be used with: see caution above.

Contains: famotidine.

---

peppermint*

Peppermint in various forms is used to calm the stomach, and is particularly effective in the form of peppermint water (available from pharmacies) in treating wind, especially after surgery. Peppermint oil can be useful in relieving colic and bloating associated with irritable bowel syndrome, but it must be taken in the form of specially designed capsules, which release the contents in the bowel, and not higher up in the digestive tract. (See 'Mintec', 'Colpermin'.) The pure oil is irritant to the mouth and oesophagus, and should not be swallowed in any other form. It is also useful as an aromatic decongestant when inhaled, for relieving nasal congestion. (See 'Respiratory conditions – inhaled remedies'.)

Dose: as specified for each individual product.

Side effects: the oil is irritant to the mouth and throat.

Caution:

Not to be used for:

Not to be used with: homeopathic remedies.

Contains: peppermint.

Pepto-Bismol see entry in 'Bowel disorders' section
(Procter & Gamble)

Phenergan see entry in 'Allergic disorders' section
(M & B)

Prefil
(Norgine)

Granules used as a bulking agent to control the appetite.

Dose: 1-2 sachets swallowed with water ½-1 hour before eating.
Side effects:
Caution: take with plenty of water. Children should be seen by a doctor before using this product.
Not to be used for: patients suffering from blocked intestine.
Not to be used with:
Contains: sterculia.

Q-Mazine see entry in 'Allergic disorders' section
(Seton Healthcare)

Rap-eze
(Roche Consumer Health)

A tablet used as an antacid to treat indigestion, wind, heartburn, and excess acid. Suitable for the treatment of indigestion in pregnancy.

Dose: 2 tablets to be chewed or sucked when required. (Maximum 16 tablets in 24 hours.)
Side effects:
Caution:
Not to be used for: children under 12 years.
Not to be used with: some antibiotics, iron, tablets coated to protect the stomach.
Contains: calcium carbonate.

Remegel
(Warner Wellcome Consumer Healthcare)

A chewy square used as an antacid to treat excess acid, heartburn, and indigestion.

Dose: 2 squares to be chewed every hour. (Maximum of 12 in 24 hours.)
Side effects:
Caution:
Not to be used for: children under 12 years.
Not to be used with: some antibiotics, iron, tablets coated to protect the stomach.
Contains: calcium carbonate.

Rennie
(Roche Consumer Health)

A tablet used as an antacid to treat indigestion, heartburn, excess acid, and wind.

Dose: adults 2 tablets (children aged 6-12 years 1 tablet) sucked or chewed when necessary. (Maximum 16 in 24 hours for adults, 8 in 24 hours for children.)
Side effects:
Caution:
Not to be used for: children under 6 years.
Not to be used with: some antibiotics, iron, tablets coated to protect the stomach.
Contains: calcium carbonate, magnesium carbonate.

Rennie Gold
(Roche Consumer Health)

A tablet used as an antacid to treat indigestion, acidity, heartburn, wind.

Dose: 2 tablets sucked or chewed when needed. (Maximum

of 14 in 24 hours.)
Side effects:
Caution:
Not to be used for: children under 12 years.
Not to be used with: some antibiotics, iron, tablets coated to protect the stomach.
Contains: calcium carbonate.

Rennie Rap-eze see **Rap-eze**
(Roche Consumer Health)

Resolve
(SmithKline Beecham Consumer Healthcare)

A powder supplied in sachets, used as an analgesic and antacid to treat headache and settle stomach.

Dose: 1 sachet in water every 4 hours (up to 4 times a day).
Side effects:
Caution:
Not to be used for: children under 16 years.
Not to be used with: some antibiotics, iron, tablets coated to protect the stomach, other medicines containing paracetamol.
Contains: paracetamol, sodium bicarbonate, citric acid, potassium bicarbonate, sodium carbonate, vitamin C.

Safeway Health Salt see **Andrews Liver Salts**
(Safeway)

Sea-Band*
(Sea-Band)

An elasticated wrist band which provides pressure to relieve travel sickness without medication.

Sea-Legs
(Seton Healthcare)

A tablet used as an antihistamine to prevent travel sickness.

Dose: adults 2 tablets (children ½-1 tablet according to age) taken 1 hour before journey or the previous night. (Effects last for 24 hours.)
Side effects: drowsiness.
Caution: pregnant women should consult a doctor before taking this product.
Not to be used for: children under 2 years.
Not to be used with: other sedating medicines, alcohol, antidepressants.
Contains: meclozine hydrochloride.

Setlers
(SmithKline Beecham)

A tablet available as original Setlers or flavoured Setlers 'Tums', used as an antacid to treat acid and nervous indigestion, wind, heartburn, and discomfort after eating.

Dose: 1-2 sucked or chewed when required, (up to 8 times a day).
Side effects:
Caution:
Not to be used for: children under 12 years.
Not to be used with: some antibiotics, iron, tablets coated to protect the stomach.
Contains: calcium carbonate.

---

slippery elm tablets
(licensed product available from Gerard House.)

A tablet used as a herbal soothing remedy to aid digestion and relieve the symptoms of stomach disorders.

Dose: as specified for each individual product.
Side effects:
Caution: pregnant women should consult a doctor before using this product.
Not to be used for: children under 12 years.
Not to be used with:
Contains: slippery elm bark.

Slippery Elm Stomach Tablets
(Potters)

A tablet used as a soothing herbal remedy to relieve the symptoms of indigestion, heartburn, and wind.

Dose: 1-2 tablets chewed after each meal, up to 5 times a day.
Side effects:
Caution: pregnant women should consult a doctor before using this product.
Not to be used for: children.
Not to be used with: homeopathic remedies.
Contains: slippery elm bark, cinnamon oil, clove oil, peppermint oil.

---

soda mint tablets BP

A tablet used as an antacid to treat indigestion and excess acid.

Dose: 2-6 to be sucked when required after meals and at bedtime.
Side effects: belching.
Caution: avoid prolonged use. Pregnant women, elderly patients, and patients with heart disease or on a sodium-restricted diet should consult a doctor before using this product.

Not to be used for:
Not to be used with: some antibiotics, iron, tablets coated to protect the stomach.
Contains: sodium bicarbonate.

---

sodium bicarbonate compound tablets BP see **soda mint tablets BP**

Stomach Mixture
(Potters)

A mixture used as a traditional remedy to treat the symptoms of stomach upset and stomach ache.

Dose: 5 ml 3 times a day.
Side effects:
Caution:
Not to be used for: children or pregnant women.
Not to be used with:
Contains: dandelion root, gentian, compound rhubarb tincture, bismuth ammonium citrate.

Stugeron
(Janssen)

A tablet used as an antihistamine treatment to prevent travel sickness.

Dose: adults 2 tablets 2 hours before the journey, then 1 tablet every 8 hours. Children 5-12 years half adult dose.
Side effects: drowsiness.
Caution:
Not to be used for: children under 5 years.
Not to be used with: MAOIs, alcohol, other sedating medicines.

Contains: cinnarizine.

Tagamet-100
(SmithKline Beecham Consumer)

A tablet used as a histamine H_2-receptor antagonist to relieve symptoms of heartburn, excess acid, and indigestion. (Doctors may prescribe this medication for different disorders. Self-medication should be limited to the conditions and doses stated.)

Dose: 2 tablets when symptoms appear. 2 more tablets may be taken after a further hour if needed. (Maximum of 4 in 4 hours, and 8 in 24 hours.) For heartburn at night, take 1 tablet an hour before bedtime. Maximum treatment period: 2 weeks.
Side effects: diarrhoea, tiredness, dizziness, headache, rash, confusion, heart and blood disorders, fever, joint or muscular pain, allergic reaction, kidney liver or pancreas disorder.
Caution: side effects are more likely in the elderly. Patients with a past history of stomach ulcer should consult a doctor before using this product. Consult a doctor or pharmacist if taking any other medicines (prescribed or purchased).
Not to be used for: children under 16 years, pregnant women, nursing mothers, patients suffering from any other illness or being seen regularly by a doctor, patients middle aged or older with new or changed symptoms, patients with unintended weight loss.
Not to be used with: see caution above. Anticoagulants, phenytoin, and theophylline.
Contains: cimetidine.

Tagamet Dual Action
(SmithKline Beecham)

A liquid used as a histamine H_2-receptor antagonist and reflux suppressant to treat symptoms of heartburn associated with acid reflux. (Doctors may prescribe Tagamet for different disorders. Self-medication should be limited to the conditions and doses stated.)

Dose: 10 ml at onset of symptoms, followed by a further 10 ml after 1 hour if symptoms have not improved. (Maximum of 20 ml in 4 hours or 40 ml in 24 hours.) Maximum treatment period: 2 weeks.

Side effects: diarrhoea, tiredness, dizziness, headache, rash, confusion, heart and blood disorders, fever, joint or muscular pain, allergic reaction, kidney, liver, or pancreas disorder.

Caution: side effects are more likely in the elderly. Patients with a past history of stomach ulcer should consult a doctor before using this product. Patients on a sodium-restricted diet should be aware of the sodium content of this product. Consult a doctor or pharmacist if taking any other medicines (prescribed or purchased).

Not to be used for: children under 16 years, pregnant women, nursing mothers, patients suffering from any other illness or being seen regularly by a doctor, patients middle aged or older with new or changed symptoms, patients with unintended weight loss.

Not to be used with: see caution above. Anticoagulants, phenytoin, and theophylline.

Contains: cimetidine, sodium alginate.

Topal
(Novex Pharma)

A tablet used as an antacid to treat heartburn.

Dose: adults 1-3 tablets 4 times a day after meals and at bedtime; children half adult dose.

Side effects:

Caution:

Not to be used for: infants, or for severely debilitated patients, or those on low-phosphorus diets or with high blood magnesium levels.

Not to be used with: some antibiotics, iron, tablets coated to

protect the stomach.
Contains: aluminium hydroxide, magnesium carbonate, alginic acid.

Tums see **Setlers**
(SmithKline Beecham Consumer)

Unigest
(Unigreg)

A tablet used as an antacid, anti-wind preparation to treat indigestion, heartburn, and wind.

Dose: 1-2 tablets sucked or chewed after meals and at bedtime.
Side effects:
Caution:
Not to be used for: children under 12 years.
Not to be used with: some antibiotics, iron, tablets coated to protect the stomach.
Contains: aluminium hydroxide gel, dimethicone.

Windcheaters
(Napp Consumer Products)

A capsule used as an anti-wind preparation to treat wind pains, bloating, and other symptoms of intestinal gas.

Dose: 1-2 capsules 3-4 times a day.
Side effects:
Caution:
Not to be used for: children.
Not to be used with:
Contains: simethicone.

Woodward's Gripe Water
(LRC Products)

A sugar-free and alcohol-free mixture used as an antacid and aromatic carminative to treat wind and gripe pains in babies.

Dose: 5-10 ml according to age before or after each feed. (Maximum of 6 doses in 24 hours.)
Side effects:
Caution:
Not to be used for: babies under 1 month.
Not to be used with: some antibiotics, iron.
Contains: sodium bicarbonate, dill oil.

Zantac-75
(Glaxo)

A tablet used as a histamine H_2-receptor antagonist to relieve heartburn and indigestion. (Doctors may prescribe this medication for different disorders. Self-medication should be limited to the conditions and doses stated.)

Dose: 1 tablet. Repeat if the symptoms return. (Maximum 4 tablets in 24 hours.) Maximum treatment period : 2 weeks.
Side effects: headaches, dizziness, diarrhoea, nausea, aches and pains, jaundice, blood disorder, rash, allergic reaction.
Caution: patients with a past history of stomach ulcer should consult a doctor before using this product. Consult a doctor or pharmacist if taking any other medicines (prescribed or purchased).
Not to be used for: children under 16 years, pregnant women, nursing mothers, patients suffering from any other illness or being seen regularly by a doctor, patients middle aged or older with new or changed symptoms, patients with unintended weight loss.
Not to be used with: see caution above.
Contains: ranitidine.

Respiratory conditions

1   Cough and cold remedies

Most upper respiratory conditions are caused by virus infections and allergies such as hayfever. The common cold will not respond to antibiotics unless there is added bacterial infection. Symptomatic treatment with many of the preparations listed below will benefit many cold sufferers. Pollution and cigarette smoking will exacerbate upper respiratory symptoms.

Antihistamines are anti-allergic preparations used to treat allergies, and are dealt with in a separate section (see 'Allergic disorders'), but they also dry up the nasal passages, so they are included in combination with some other drugs in numerous cold treatments.

Other ingredients in cold remedies include sympathomimetic decongestants, which open the airways and reduce congestion, but these can cause an increase in blood pressure, and should be avoided by patients with heart disease, high blood pressure, overactive thyroid, or diabetes. These products may also affect a significant number of other medicines, and care should be taken before adding a sympathomimetic decongestant to other medication already taken.

When treating coughs, care should be taken to differentiate between dry, unproductive coughs and those where congestion is a feature. Dry coughs may be treated with suppressants, although these are not recommended under the age of 1 year. Alternatively, soothing agents, such as glycerin or syrup, may be used. Chesty, congestive coughs require the use of an expectorant to clear the phlegm. Never treat a chesty cough with a suppressant, as congestion will remain in the lungs and may precipitate a chest infection.

Coughing of blood should be reported to a doctor.

Painkillers, such as aspirin and paracetamol, are also commonly found in cold remedies, to relieve pain and discomfort, and to reduce fever. Care should be taken not to exceed the total daily dose for any ingredient when more than one product is used to treat symptoms. (Ask a pharmacist for advice on mixing remedies.)

Actifed
(Warner Wellcome Consumer Healthcare)

A tablet or liquid used as a sympathomimetic decongestant and antihistamine treatment for nasal congestion due to colds, influenza, or hayfever.

Dose: adults 1 tablet or 10 ml syrup (children aged 6-12 years 5 ml syrup, children aged 2-5 years 2.5 ml syrup) 4 times a day.
Side effects: drowsiness, rapid or abnormal heart rate, dry mouth, excitement, anxiety, shaking hands.
Caution: pregnant women, asthmatics, and patients taking other medication should consult a doctor before using this product.
Not to be used for: children under 12 years (tablets) or children under 2 years (syrup), or for patients with high blood pressure, overactive thyroid, heart disease, diabetes.
Not to be used with: MAOIs, tricyclic antidepressants, beta-blockers, antihypertensives, other sedating medicines, alcohol.
Contains: triprolidine hydrochloride, pseudoephedrine hydrochloride.

Actifed Compound
(Warner Wellcome Consumer Healthcare)

A linctus used as an antihistamine opiate cough suppressant and sympathomimetic decongestant to treat dry cough and nasal congestion.

Dose: adults 10 ml (children aged 6-12 years 5 ml, children aged 2-5 years 2.5 ml) 4 times a day.
Side effects: drowsiness, rapid or abnormal heart rate. dry mouth, anxiety, shaking hands.
Caution: pregnant women, asthmatics, and patients taking other medication should consult a doctor before taking this product.

Not to be used for: children under 2 years, or for patients with high blood pressure, thyroid disease, heart disease, or diabetes.
Not to be used with: alcohol, other sedating medicines, MAOIs, betablockers, antihypertensives, tricyclic antidepressants.
Contains: triprolidine hydrochloride, pseudoephedrine hydrochloride, dextromethorphan hydrobromide.

Actifed Expectorant
(Warner Wellcome Consumer Healthcare)

A liquid used as an antihistamine, sympathomimetic decongestant and expectorant treatment for chesty coughs and nasal congestion.

Dose: adults 10 ml (children aged 6-12 years 5 ml, children aged 2-5 years 2.5 ml) 4 times a day.
Side effects: drowsiness, rapid or abnormal heart rate, dry mouth, excitement, anxiety, shaking hands.
Caution: pregnant women, asthmatics and patients receiving other medication should consult a doctor before using this product.
Not to be used for: children under 2 years, or for patients with high blood pressure, overactive thyroid, heart disease, diabetes.
Not to be used with: MAOIs, tricyclic antidepressants, beta-blockers, antihypertensives, other sedating medicines, alcohol.
Contains: triprolidine hydrochloride, pseudoephedrine hydrochloride, guaiphenesin.

Actifed Junior Cough Relief
(Warner Wellcome Consumer Healthcare)

A liquid used as an antihistamine and opiate cough suppressant to treat dry coughs in children.

Dose: 2.5-10 ml (according to age) 3-4 times a day.

Side effects: drowsiness, constipation, dependence.
Caution: asthmatics should consult a doctor or pharmacist before using this product.
Not to be used for: children under 1 year.
Not to be used with: MAOIs, other sedating medicines.
Contains: triprolidine hydrochloride, dextromethorphan hydrobromide.

Allens Chesty Cough
(Allens & Co.)

A mixture used as an expectorant and aromatic decongestant to treat chesty coughs.

Dose: adults 10 ml up to 4 times a day; children aged 7-14 years half the adult dose.
Side effects:
Caution: patients with heart disease should consult a doctor before using this product.
Not to be used for: children under 7 years.
Not to be used with:
Contains: ammonium chloride, tolu tincture, squill tincture, menthol, liquid extract of horehound.

Allens Dry Cough
(Allens & Co.)

A liquid used as an antiseptic, expectorant, and aromatic decongestant to relieve dry tickly coughs.

Dose: adults 10 ml up to 4 times a day; children aged 7-14 years half the adult dose.
Side effects:
Caution:
Not to be used for: children under 7 years.
Not to be used with:

Contains: benzoin tincture, ipecacuanha tincture, capsicum tincture, cetylpyridinium chloride.

Antibron
(Potters)

A tablet used as an expectorant, soothing, anti-spasm, and sedative herbal remedy to treat coughs.

Dose: adults 2 tablets (children over 7 years 1 tablet) 3 times a day.
Side effects:
Caution: do not exceed the stated dose – lobelia may cause nausea and vomiting in high doses.
Not to be used for: children under 7 years.
Not to be used with:
Contains: lobelia, wild lettuce, coltsfoot, euphorbia, pleurisy root, senega.

Antifect
(Potters)

A tablet used as an expectorant and anti-infective herbal remedy to treat symptoms of catarrh, rhinitis, and nasal congestion.

Dose: adults 2 tablets (children over 8 years 1 tablet) 3 times a day.
Side effects:
Caution:
Not to be used for: children under 8 years.
Not to be used with:
Contains: garlic, echinacea.

Balm of Gilead
(Potters)

A liquid used as a herbal expectorant to relieve the symptoms of coughs.

Dose: adults 10 ml (children over 5 years 5 ml) 3-4 times a day. (May be diluted with water if required.)
Side effects:
Caution: do not exceed the stated dose – high doses of lobelia may cause nausea and vomiting. Patients with heart disease should consult a doctor before using this product.
Not to be used for: children under 5 years, or for pregnant women or nursing mothers.
Not to be used with:
Contains: squill, lobelia, balm of Gilead, lungwort.

Barum Cold Relief Capsules
(Wrafton Laboratories)

A capsule used as an analgesic, stimulant, and sympathomimetic decongestant treatment for fever, pain, and blocked nose associated with colds and influenza.

Dose: adults 2 capsules (children aged 6-12 years 1 capsule) every 3-4 hours. (Maximum of 12 in 24 hours for adults or 6 in 24 hours for children.)
Side effects: rapid or abnormal heart rate, dry mouth, excitement, anxiety, shaking hands.
Caution: pregnant women, asthmatics, and patients taking other medication should consult a doctor before using this product.
Not to be used for: children under 6 years, or for patients with high blood pressure, overactive thyroid, heart disease, diabetes.
Not to be used with: MAOIs, tricyclic antidepressants, beta-blockers, antihypertensives, other medicines containing paracetamol, excess tea and coffee.

Contains: paracetamol, caffeine, phenylephrine hydrochloride.

Beechams All-In-One Cold & Flu Remedy
(SmithKline Beecham Consumer)

A liquid used as an analgesic, expectorant, and sympathomimetic decongestant treatment for pain, fever, nasal congestion, and chesty cough.

Dose: adults 20 ml (children aged 6-12 years 10 ml) up to 4 times a day.
Side effects: rapid or abnormal heart rate, dry mouth, excitement, anxiety, shaking hands.
Caution: asthmatics should consult a doctor or pharmacist before using this product, because prescribed medication may be affected.
Not to be used for: children under 6 years, or patients with high blood pressure, overactive thyroid, heart disease, diabetes.
Not to be used with: MAOIs, tricyclic antidepressants, beta-blockers, antihypertensives, other medicines containing paracetamol.
Contains: paracetamol, guaiphenesin, phenylephrine hydrochloride.

Beechams Coughcaps see Contac Coughcaps
(SmithKline Beecham Consumer)

Beechams Hot Blackcurrant see Lemsip
(SmithKline Beecham Healthcare)

Beechams Hot Lemon see Lemsip
(SmithKline Beecham Healthcare)

Beechams Hot Lemon and Honey see **Lemsip**
(SmithKline Beecham Healthcare)

Beechams Powders see entry in 'Simple pain killers' section
(SmithKline Beecham Healthcare)

Beechams Powders Capsules
(SmithKline Beecham Healthcare)

A capsule used as an analgesic, stimulant, and sympathomimetic decongestant treatment for fever, pain, and blocked nose associated with colds and influenza.

Dose: 2 capsules every 3-4 hours, up to a maximum of 12 in 24 hours. (Children aged 6-12 years, half the adult dose.)
Side effects: rapid or abnormal heart rate, dry mouth, excitement, anxiety, shaking hands.
Caution: pregnant women, asthmatics, and patients taking other medication should consult a doctor before using this product.
Not to be used for: children under 6 years, or for patients with high blood pressure, overactive thyroid, heart disease, diabetes.
Not to be used with: MAOIs, tricyclic antidepressants, beta-blockers, antihypertensives, other medicines containing paracetamol, excess tea or coffee.
Contains: paracetamol, caffeine, phenylephrine hydrochloride.

Benylin Chesty Cough Original
(Warner Wellcome Consumer Healthcare)

A syrup used as an antihistamine, aromatic decongestant and expectorant treat chesty cough and nasal congestion.

Dose: adults 10 ml (children 6-12 years 5 ml) 4 times a day.
Side effects: drowsiness.

Caution: pregnant women should consult a doctor before using this product.
Not to be used for: children under 6 years.
Not to be used with: other sedating medicines, alcohol.
Contains: diphenhydramine hydrochloride, ammonium chloride, menthol.

Benylin 4-Flu
(Warner Wellcome)

A tablet and liquid used as a decongestant, antihistamine, and analgesic treatment for the relief of fevers, aches, and pains of influenza.

Dose: adults 2 tablets or 20 ml liquid 4 times a day; children aged 6-12 years half adult dose.
Side effects: drowsiness, rapid or abnormal heart rate, dry mouth, excitement, anxiety, shaking hands.
Caution: asthmatics should consult a doctor or pharmacist before using this product, as prescribed medication may be affected. Pregnant women and patients suffering from enlarged prostate or glaucoma should also take advice before using this product.
Not to be used for: children under 6 years, patients with high blood pressure, overactive thyroid, heart disease, diabetes.
Not to be used with: MAOIs, tricyclic antidepressants, beta-blockers, antihypertensives, alcohol, other sedating medicines, other preparations containing paracetamol.
Contains: diphenhydramine hydrochloride, paracetamol, pseudoephedrine hydrochloride.

Benylin Chesty Cough Non-Drowsy
(Warner Wellcome Consumer Healthcare)

A mixture used as an expectorant and aromatic decongestant to treat chesty coughs.

Dose: adults 10 ml 4 times a day; children aged 6-12 years half the adult dose.
Side effects:
Caution: pregnant women should consult a doctor before using this product.
Not to be used for: children under 6 years.
Not to be used with:
Contains: guaiphenesin, menthol.

Benylin Children's Cough Mixture
(Warner Wellcome Consumer Healthcare)

A liquid available in normal or sugar-free varieties, and used as an antihistamine and aromatic decongestant treatment for children's coughs.

Dose: children aged 1-5 years 5 ml (aged 6-12 years 10 ml) 4 times a day.
Side effects: drowsiness.
Caution:
Not to be used for: children under 1 year.
Not to be used with: other sedating medicines, alcohol.
Contains: diphenhydramine hydrochloride, menthol.

Benylin Cough and Congestion
(Warner Wellcome Consumer Healthcare)

A liquid used as a sympathomimetic and aromatic decongestant, antihistamine and opiate cough suppressant, used to treat dry coughs and nasal congestion due to colds.

Dose: adults 10 ml (children aged 6-12 years 5 ml) 4 times a day.
Side effects: drowsiness, rapid or abnormal heart rate, dry mouth, excitement, anxiety, shaking hands, constipation, dependence.

Caution: pregnant women and asthmatics should consult a doctor or pharmacist before using this product.
Not to be used for: children under 6 years, patients with high blood pressure, overactive thyroid, heart disease, diabetes.
Not to be used with: MAOIs, tricyclic antidepressants, beta-blockers, antihypertensives, other sedating medicines, alcohol.
Contains: diphenhydramine hydrochloride, dextromethorphan hydrobromide, pseudoephedrine hydrochloride, menthol.

Benylin Day and Night
(Warner Wellcome Consumer Healthcare)

A yellow daytime tablet containing an analgesic and sympathomimetic decongestant, and a blue night-time tablet containing an analgesic and antihistamine, used to treat the symptoms of colds and influenza.

Dose: 1 yellow tablet 3 times a day and 1 blue tablet at night.
Side effects: rapid or abnormal heart rate, dry mouth, excitement, anxiety, shaking hands (from yellow tablets), drowsiness (from blue tablets).
Caution: asthmatics should consult a doctor or pharmacist before using this product, because prescribed medication may be affected.
Not to be used for: children under 12 years, or for patients with high blood pressure, overactive thyroid, heart disease, diabetes.
Not to be used with: MAOIs, tricyclic antidepressants, beta-blockers, antihypertensives, alcohol, other sedating medicines, other medicines containing paracetamol.
Contains: paracetamol. (Yellow tablets also contain phenylpropanolamine hydrochloride, blue tablets also contain diphenhydramine hydrochloride.)

Benylin Dry Cough Non-Drowsy
(Warner Wellcome Consumer Healthcare)

A liquid used as an opiate cough suppressant to treat dry coughs.

Dose: adults 10 ml (children aged 6-12 years 5 ml) 4 times a day.
Side effects: constipation, dependence.
Caution: asthmatics should consult a doctor or pharmacist before using this product.
Not to be used for: children under 6 years.
Not to be used with: MAOIs.
Contains: dextromethorphan hydrobromide.

Benylin Dry Cough Original
(Warner Wellcome Consumer Healthcare)

A mixture used as an antihistamine, aromatic decongestant and opiate cough suppressant to treat dry coughs.

Dose: adults 10 ml (children aged 6-12 years 5 ml) 4 times a day.
Side effects: drowsiness, constipation, dependence.
Caution: pregnant women and asthmatics should consult a doctor before using this product.
Not to be used for: children under 6 years.
Not to be used with: MAOIs, other sedating medicines, alcohol.
Contains: diphenhydramine hydrochloride, dextromethorphan hydrobromide, menthol.

Benylin With Codeine
(Warner Wellcome Consumer Healthcare)

A liquid used as an antihistamine, aromatic decongestant and opiate cough suppressant to treat persistent dry coughs.

Dose: adults 10 ml (children aged 6-12 years 5 ml) 4 times a day.
Side effects: drowsiness, constipation, dependence.
Caution: asthmatics should consult a doctor or pharmacist before using this product.
Not to be used for: children under 6 years.
Not to be used with: MAOIs, other sedating medicines, alcohol.
Contains: codeine phosphate, menthol, diphenhydramine hydrochloride.

Bio-Strath Thyme Formula
(Cedar Health)

A liquid used as a herbal antiseptic remedy to give temporary relief from cough symptoms.

Dose: 20 drops (0.6 ml) in a little water 3 times a day before meals, or as directed by a doctor.
Side effects:
Caution:
Not to be used for: children or pregnant women.
Not to be used with:
Contains: yeast, thyme, primula root.

Boots Bronchial Cough Mixture
(Boots)

An expectorant liquid used to treat chesty coughs and colds on the chest.

Dose: adults 10 ml (children 5-12 years 5 ml) up to 3-4 times a day. (The dose to be taken in water.)
Side effects:

Caution:
Not to be used for: children under 5 years.
Not to be used with:
Contains: ammonium chloride, ammonium carbonate, guaiphenesin.

Boots Catarrh Cough Syrup see **Famel Original**
(Boots)

Boots Children's Chesty Cough Syrup
(Boots)

A sugar-free medicine used as an expectorant to treat chesty coughs.

Dose: 5-10 ml up to 4 times a day (according to age).
Side effects:
Caution: rarely stomach upset.
Not to be used for: children under 1 year, pregnant women, and nursing mothers.
Not to be used with:
Contains: guaiphenesin.

Boots Children's Cold Relief
(Boots)

A sachet used to make a sugar-free hot drink containing an analgesic to treat pain and fever due to colds and influenza, and as a source of extra vitamin C.

Dose: 1 sachet in hot water every 4 hours (up to 4 times a day).
Side effects: allergy, skin rash.
Caution: pregnant women and nursing mothers should consult a doctor before using this product.
Not to be used for: children under 3 years.

Not to be used with: other medicines containing paracetamol.
Contains: paracetamol, vitamin C.

Boots Children's Cough and Cold Syrup
(Boots)

A sugar-free liquid used as a sympathomimetic decongestant and expectorant to treat chesty coughs and nasal congestion.

Dose: 2.5-10 ml every 4 hours (up to 4 times a day) according to age.
Side effects: rapid or abnormal heart rate, dry mouth, excitement, anxiety, shaking hands, headache, stomach upset, dizziness.
Caution: asthmatics or children taking heart drugs or any other medication should be seen by a doctor before using this product.
Not to be used for: children under 6 months, pregnant women, nursing mothers, and patients with high blood pressure, overactive thyroid, heart disease, circulation problems or diabetes.
Not to be used with: MAOIs, tricyclic antidepressants, beta-blockers, antihypertensives.
Contains: ephedrine hydrochloride, ipecacuanha.

Boots Children's Decongestant Syrup
(Boots)

A sugar-free liquid used as a sympathomimetic decongestant and antihistamine treatment for stuffy blocked-up noses and symptoms of colds and influenza.

Dose: 2.5-10 ml up to 4 times a day (according to age).
Side effects: rapid or abnormal heart rate, dry mouth, excitement, anxiety, shaking hands, drowsiness, upset stomach, headache or blurred vision.
Caution: asthmatics and children already taking heart drugs,

antidepressants, or other medicines should consult a doctor before using this product.

Not to be used for: children under 1 year, pregnant women, nursing mothers, or patients with high blood pressure, overactive thyroid, heart disease, circulation problems, or diabetes.

Not to be used with: MAOIs, tricyclic antidepressants, beta-blockers, antihypertensives, other sedating medicines, alcohol.

Contains: diphenhydramine hydrochloride, pseudoephedrine hydrochloride.

Boots Children's Dry Cough Syrup
(Boots)

A sugar-free liquid used as an antihistamine and opiate cough suppressant to treat dry, tickly, unproductive coughs.

Dose: 5-10 ml every 4 hours (up to 4 times a day) according to age.

Side effects: constipation, dependence, drowsiness, upset stomach, dry mouth, mood changes.

Caution: asthmatics or children taking any other medicines should be seen by a doctor before using this product.

Not to be used for: children under 1 year, pregnant women, or nursing mothers.

Not to be used with: MAOIs, other sedating medicines.

Contains: diphenhydramine hydrochloride, pholcodine.

Boots Cold and Influenza Mixture
(Boots)

A liquid used as an expectorant to treat chesty coughs associated with colds and influenza.

Dose: adults 10 ml (children aged 5-12 years 5 ml) every 2 hours when required.

Side effects:

Caution:
Not to be used for: children under 5 years, or patients suffering from heart disease.
Not to be used with:
Contains: squill vinegar, ammonium acetate.

Boots Cold and Flu Caplets
(Boots)

A caplet used as a sympathomimetic decongestant, analgesic, and stimulant to relieve colds, influenza, and blocked-up nose, and to provide extra vitamin C.

Dose: adults 2 tablets (repeated to a maximum of 8 in 24 hours); children aged 5-12 years 1 tablet (up to a maximum of 4 in 24 hours).
Side effects: rapid or abnormal heart rate, dry mouth, excitement, anxiety, shaking hands.
Caution: asthmatics should consult a doctor or pharmacist before using this product, because prescribed medication may be affected.
Not to be used for: children under 5 years, or patients with high blood pressure, overactive thyroid, heart disease, diabetes.
Not to be used with: MAOIs, tricyclic antidepressants, beta-blockers, antihypertensives, other medicines containing paracetamol, excess tea or coffee.
Contains: paracetamol, vitamin C, caffeine, phenylephrine hydrochloride.

Boots Day Cold Comfort
(Boots)

A capsule or liquid used as an analgesic, sympathomimetic decongestant and opiate cough suppressant to treat headache, runny nose, sore throat, tickly cough, fever, and pain associated with colds and influenza.

Dose: adults 2 capsules or 30 ml liquid every 4 hours (up to 4 times a day). Children aged 6-12 years half the adult dose.
Side effects: rapid or abnormal heart rate, dry mouth, excitement, anxiety, shaking hands, constipation, dependence.
Caution: asthmatics or patients already receiving medical advice or treatment should consult a doctor before using this product.
Not to be used for: children under 6 years or patients with high blood pressure, overactive thyroid, heart disease, diabetes.
Not to be used with: MAOIs, tricyclic antidepressants, beta-blockers, antihypertensives, other medicines containing paracetamol.
Contains: pholcodine, pseudoephedrine hydrochloride, paracetamol.

Boots Decongestant Tablets see **Sudafed**
(Boots)

Boots Glycerin and Blackcurrant Linctus
(Boots)

A soothing linctus used to treat tickly coughs and sore throats.

Dose: 5-10 ml 3-4 times a day (according to age).
Side effects:
Caution:
Not to be used for: children under 1 year.
Not to be used with:
Contains: glycerin.

Boots Herbal Catarrh Tablets
(Boots)

A tablet used as a herbal remedy to relieve symptoms of catarrh and blocked sinuses.

Dose: adults 2 tablets (children aged 5-12 years 1 tablet) 3 times a day before food.
Side effects:
Caution:
Not to be used for: children under 5 years, pregnant women, and nursing mothers.
Not to be used with:
Contains: marshmallow root, echinacea, elderflower.

Boots Herbal Cold Relief Tablets
(Boots)

A tablet used as a herbal remedy to relieve symptoms of colds and catarrh.

Dose: adults 1 tablet 3 times a day; children aged 5-12 years 1 tablet at night.
Side effects:
Caution: pregnant women and nursing mothers should consult a doctor before using this product.
Not to be used for: children under 5 years.
Not to be used with:
Contains: marshmallow root, parsley root, garlic oil.

Boots Hot Blackcurrant Cold Relief
(Boots)

A hot blackcurrant drink used as an analgesic to treat pain and fever associated with colds and influenza.

Dose: 1 sachet in freshly boiled hot water every 4 hours when required (up to 4 times a day).
Side effects: rarely drowsiness, confusion, allergy, rash, temperature or blood changes.
Caution: pregnant women, nursing mothers, and patients receiving medical treatment should see a doctor before using this product.

Not to be used for: children under 12 years, or for alcoholics.
Not to be used with: other medicines containing paracetamol, or drugs used to treat high cholesterol.
Contains: paracetamol, vitamin C.

Boots Hot Blackcurrant Cold Relief with Decongestant
(Boots)

A powder to make a hot blackcurrant drink, and used as an analgesic and sympathomimetic decongestant treatment for pain, fever, and blocked nose associated with colds and influenza.

Dose: 1 sachet in hot water every 4 hours. (Maximum 4 in 24 hours.)
Side effects: rapid or abnormal heart rate, dry mouth, excitement, anxiety, shaking hands.
Caution: pregnant women, asthmatics and patients taking other medication should consult a doctor before using this product.
Not to be used for: children under 12 years, or patients with high blood pressure, overactive thyroid, heart disease, diabetes.
Not to be used with: MAOIs, tricyclic antidepressants, beta-blockers, antihypertensives, other medicines containing paracetamol.
Contains: paracetamol, phenylephrine hydrochloride, vitamin C.

Boots Hot Lemon Cold Relief
(Boots).

A hot lemon drink used as an analgesic to treat pain and fever associated with colds and influenza.

Dose: 1 sachet in freshly boiled hot water every 4 hours when required (up to 4 times a day).
Side effects: rarely drowsiness, confusion, allergy, rash, temperature, or blood changes.

Caution: pregnant women, nursing mothers, and patients receiving medical treatment should see a doctor before using this product.
Not to be used for: children under 12 years, or for alcoholics.
Not to be used with: other medicines containing paracetamol, or drugs used to treat high cholesterol.
Contains: paracetamol, vitamin C.

Boots Hot Lemon Cold Relief with Decongestant see **Lemsip**
(Boots)

Boots Hot Lemon Flu Relief
(Boots)

A hot lemon drink used as an analgesic to treat pain and fever associated with colds and influenza.

Dose: 1 sachet in freshly boiled hot water every 4 hours when required (up to 4 times a day).
Side effects: rarely drowsiness, confusion, allergy, rash, temperature or blood changes.
Caution: pregnant women, nursing mothers and patients receiving medical treatment should see a doctor before using this product.
Not to be used for: children under 12 years, or for alcoholics.
Not to be used with: other medicines containing paracetamol, or drugs used to treat high cholesterol.
Contains: paracetamol, vitamin C.

Boots Night Cold Comfort
(Boots)

A capsule or liquid used as an analgesic, sympathomimetic decongestant, antihistamine and opiate cough suppressant to treat headache, runny nose, sore throat, tickly cough, pain, and fever associated with colds and influenza at night-time.

Dose: 2 capsules or 30 ml liquid at night.
Side effects: rapid or abnormal heart rate, dry mouth, excitement, anxiety, shaking hands, constipation, dependence, drowsiness.
Caution: asthmatics or patients already receiving medical advice or treatment should consult a doctor before using this product.
Not to be used for: children under 12 years or patients with high blood pressure, overactive thyroid, heart disease, diabetes.
Not to be used with: MAOIs, tricyclic antidepressants, beta-blockers, antihypertensives, other medicines containing paracetamol, other sedating medicines, alcohol.
Contains: pholcodine, pseudoephedrine hydrochloride, paracetamol, diphenhydramine hydrochloride. (Liquid also contains alcohol.)

Boots Nirolex (Linctus)
(Boots)

A sympathomimetic and aromatic decongestant and expectorant liquid used to treat chesty cough.

Dose: adults 10 ml (children aged 5-12 years 5 ml) every 4 hours (up to 4 times a day).
Side effects: rapid or abnormal heart rate, dry mouth, excitement, anxiety, shaking hands.
Caution: asthmatics should consult a doctor or pharmacist before using this product, because prescribed medication may be affected.
Not to be used for: children under 5 years, patients with high blood pressure, overactive thyroid, heart disease, diabetes.
Not to be used with: MAOIs, tricyclic antidepressants, beta-blockers, antihypertensives.
Contains: guaiphenesin, ephedrine, levomenthol, sucrose, glycerol.

Boots Nirolex Lozenges
(Boots)

A lozenge used as an opiate cough suppressant to treat dry tickly coughs.

Dose: 1 sucked when required (maximum for adults 10 in 24 hours). Children aged 6-12 years maximum 2 in 4 hours or 7 in 24 hours.
Side effects: constipation, dependence.
Caution: asthmatics should consult a doctor or pharmacist before using this product.
Not to be used for: children under 6 years.
Not to be used with: MAOIs.
Contains: dextromethorphan hydrochloride.

Boots Prolonged Release Cold Capsules
(Boots)

A long-acting capsule used as a sympathomimetic decongestant and antihistamine treatment for congestion.

Dose: 1 capsule every 12 hours.
Side effects: rapid or abnormal heart rate, dry mouth, excitement, anxiety, shaking hands, drowsiness.
Caution: pregnant women, nursing mothers, asthmatics, and patients already receiving medical advice or treatment should consult a doctor or pharmacist before using this product
Not to be used for: children under 12 years, and for patients with high blood pressure, overactive thyroid, heart disease, diabetes.
Not to be used with: MAOIs, tricyclic antidepressants, beta-blockers, antihypertensives, other sedating medicines, alcohol.
Contains: phenylpropanolamine hydrochloride, diphenylpyraline hydrochloride.

Boots Tusana Cough Syrup see **Benylin Non-Drowsy Dry Cough**
(Boots)

Bronalin Decongestant see **Sudafed Elixir**
(Seton Healthcare)

Bronalin Dry Cough Elixir
(Seton Healthcare)

An elixir used as a sympathomimetic decongestant and opiate cough suppressant to treat dry coughs and colds.

Dose: adults 5-10 ml (children aged 6-12 years 2.5 ml) 4 times a day.
Side effects: rapid or abnormal heart rate, dry mouth, excitement, anxiety, shaking hands, constipation, dependence.
Caution: asthmatics should consult a doctor or pharmacist before using this product.
Not to be used for: children under 6 years, or for patients with high blood pressure, overactive thyroid, heart disease, diabetes.
Not to be used with: MAOIs, tricyclic antidepressants, beta-blockers, antihypertensives.
Contains: dextromethorphan hydrobromide, pseudoephedrine hydrochloride, alcohol.

Bronalin Expectorant Linctus
(Seton Healthcare)

A linctus used as an antihistamine and expectorant treatment for chesty coughs and colds.

Dose: adults 5-10 ml (children aged 6-12 years 5 ml) up to 4 times a day.
Side effects: drowsiness.
Caution:

Not to be used for: children under 6 years.
Not to be used with: other sedating medicines, alcohol.
Contains: ammonium chloride, sodium citrate, diphenhydramine hydrochloride.

Bronalin Junior Linctus
(Seton Healthcare)

A linctus used as an antihistamine treatment for coughs and colds in children.

Dose: 5-10 ml (according to age) 3 times a day.
Side effects: drowsiness.
Caution:
Not to be used for: children under 1 year.
Not to be used with: other sedating medicines, alcohol.
Contains: sodium citrate, diphenhydramine hydrochloride.

Buttercup Syrup (Traditional)
(Charwell Health Care)

A syrup used as an expectorant to treat coughs, colds, sore throats, and hoarseness.

Dose: adults 10 ml (children over 2 years 5 ml) 3 times a day and at bedtime.
Side effects:
Caution: patients with heart disease should consult a doctor before using this product.
Not to be used for: children under 2 years.
Not to be used with:
Contains: squill liquid extract, capsicum tincture.

Buttercup Syrup (Blackcurrant/Honey & Lemon)
(Charwell Health Care)

A syrup used as an expectorant, soothing, and aromatic decongestant treatment for chesty or dry coughs, and to soothe sore throats and ease congestion.

Dose: adults 10 ml (children 5 ml) every 2-3 hours.
Side effects:
Caution:
Not to be used for:
Not to be used with:
Contains: menthol, glucose, ipecacuanha. (Honey and Lemon product also contains purified honey.)

Cabdrivers Cough Linctus
(Seven Seas)

A liquid available as standard or sugar-free versions, used as an expectorant, opiate cough suppressant and aromatic decongestant to treat bronchial coughs.

Dose: 5 ml every 4 hours.
Side effects: constipation, dependence.
Caution: asthmatics should consult a doctor or pharmacist before using this product.
Not to be used for: children.
Not to be used with: MAOIs.
Contains: dextromethorphan hydrobromide, pumilio pine oil, menthol, eucalyptus oil, terpin hydrate.

Catarrh-eeze
(English Grains)

A tablet used as a herbal remedy to relieve the symptoms of catarrh.

Dose: adults 2 tablets (children aged 5-12 years 1 tablet) 3 times a day.
Side effects:
Caution:
Not to be used for: children under 5 years, pregnant women, or nursing mothers.
Not to be used with:
Contains: horehound, yarrow, inula.

Catarrh Mixture
(Potters)

A sugar-free liquid used as a herbal remedy to relieve the symptoms of nasal catarrh and catarrh of the throat.

Dose: adults 5 ml 3 times a day; children over 7 years 5 ml twice a day.
Side effects:
Caution:
Not to be used for: children under 7 years.
Not to be used with:
Contains: boneset, blue flag, burdock root, hyssop, capsicum.

Catarrh-Ex see Lemsip Capsules
(Thompson Medical)

Chest Mixture
(Potters)

A liquid used as a herbal expectorant and soothing remedy to relieve the symptoms of coughs and catarrh of the upper respiratory tract.

Dose: 5 ml every 3 hours.
Side effects:
Caution: do not exceed the stated dose. (Lobelia may cause

nausea and vomiting in high doses.) Patients with heart disease should consult a doctor before using this product.
Not to be used for: children or pregnant women.
Not to be used with:
Contains: horehound, pleurisy root, senega, lobelia, squill.

Co-op Bronchial Mixture
(Co-op)

A mixture used as an expectorant to treat the symptoms of coughs and colds.

Dose: 5 ml in warm water 2-3 times a day.
Side effects:
Caution:
Not to be used for: children under 3 years.
Not to be used with: homeopathic remedies.
Contains: acetic acid, anise oil, peppermint oil, capsicum oleoresin.

Co-op Dry Tickly Cough Linctus
(Co-op)

A soothing linctus used to treat dry tickly coughs and sore throats.

Dose: 10 ml 3-4 times a day; children aged 5-12 years, half adult dose.
Side effects:
Caution:
Not to be used for: children under 5 years.
Not to be used with:
Contains: sugar syrup, glycerin, citric acid, ipecacuanha, lemon oil.

Co-op Hot Lemon Cold & Flu Relief see **Lemplus Powders**
(Co-op)

---

codeine linctus

A linctus available as standard (BP) formula, and as a paediatric
(children's) formula, used as an opiate cough suppressant to
treat dry coughs. Sugar-free versions are also available.

Dose: adults 5-10 ml of standard formula 3-4 times a day;
children aged 5-12 years 2.5-5 ml of standard formula 3-4 times
a day; children aged 1-5 years 5 ml of paediatric formula 3-4
times a day.
Side effects: constipation, dependence.
Caution: asthmatics should consult a doctor or pharmacist
before using this product.
Not to be used for: children under 1 year.
Not to be used with: MAOIs.
Contains: codeine phosphate.

Cold-eeze
(English Grains)

A tablet used as a herbal remedy to relieve the symptoms of
colds.

Dose: 2 tablets 3 times a day.
Side effects:
Caution: do not chew the tablets.
Not to be used for: children, pregnant women, or nursing
mothers.
Not to be used with:
Contains: garlic, echinacea.

373

Cold Relief Capsules see **Lemsip Capsules**
(Sussex Pharmaceuticals)

Coldrex Tablets
(Sterling Health)

A tablet used as a sympathomimetic decongestant, analgesic, stimulant, expectorant, and vitamin C supplement to treat the symptoms of colds and influenza.

Dose: adults 2 tablets (children aged 6-12 years 1 tablet) up to 4 times a day.
Side effects: rapid or abnormal heart rate, dry mouth, excitement, anxiety, shaking hands.
Caution: asthmatics should consult a doctor or pharmacist before using this product, because prescribed medication may be affected.
Not to be used for: children under 6 years, patients with high blood pressure, overactive thyroid, heart disease, diabetes.
Not to be used with: MAOIs, tricyclic antidepressants, beta-blockers, antihypertensives, excess tea or coffee, other medicines containing paracetamol.
Contains: paracetamol, caffeine, vitamin C, phenylephrine hydrochloride, terpin hydrate.

---

comfrey* see entry in 'Skin disorders' section

Contac Coughcaps
(SmithKline Beecham Consumer)

A long-acting capsule used as an opiate cough suppressant to treat dry coughs.

Dose: 1 capsule twice a day (with at least 8 hours between doses).
Side effects: constipation, dependence.

Caution: asthmatics should consult a doctor or pharmacist before using this product.
Not to be used for: children under 12 years.
Not to be used with: MAOIs.
Contains: dextromethorphan hydrobromide.

Contac-400
(SmithKline Beecham)

A long-acting capsule used as an antihistamine and sympathomimetic decongestant treatment for nasal congestion in colds, sinusitis, and hayfever.

Dose: 1 capsule twice a day.
Side effects: rapid or abnormal heart rate, dry mouth, excitement, anxiety, shaking hands, drowsiness.
Caution: do not chew or crush the capsules. Asthmatics or patients already receiving medical attention should consult a doctor before using this product.
Not to be used for: children under 12 years, or patients with high blood pressure, overactive thyroid, heart disease, diabetes.
Not to be used with: MAOIs, tricyclic antidepressants, beta-blockers, antihypertensives, alcohol, other sedating medicines.
Contains: phenylpropanolamine hydrochloride, chlorpheniramine maleate.

Copholco
(Roche Consumer Health)

A linctus used as an opiate cough suppressant, expectorant, and aromatic decongestant to treat unproductive, tickly coughs.

Dose: adults 10 ml (children over 8 years 5 ml) 4-5 times a day.
Side effects: constipation, dependence.
Caution: asthmatics should consult a doctor or pharmacist

before using this product.
Not to be used for: children under 8 years.
Not to be used with: MAOIs.
Contains: pholcodine, menthol, cineole, terpin hydrate.

Copholcoids
(Roche Consumer Health)

A pastille used as an opiate cough suppressant and expectorant to treat tickly coughs.

Dose: adults 1-2 pastilles sucked 3-4 times a day; children over 5 years 1 pastille sucked 3 times a day.
Side effects: constipation, dependence.
Caution: asthmatics should consult a doctor or pharmacist before using this product.
Not to be used for: children under 5 years.
Not to be used with: MAOIs.
Contains: pholcodine, menthol, cineole, terpin hydrate.

Cough Drops
(Weleda)

A liquid used as a herbal remedy to relieve irritating coughs.

Dose: 10-20 drops every 2 hours, taken in warm water.
Side effects:
Caution:
Not to be used for: children, pregnant women, or nursing mothers.
Not to be used with: homeopathic remedies.
Contains: angelica root, cinnamon, clove, coriander, lemon oil, lemon balm leaf, nutmeg, aqua cherry laurel.

Cough-eeze
(English Grains)

A tablet used as a herbal expectorant remedy to relieve chesty coughs.

Dose: adults 2 tablets (children aged 8-12 years 1 tablet) 3 times a day.
Side effects:
Caution:
Not to be used for: children under 8 years, pregnant women, or nursing mothers.
Not to be used with:
Contains: ipecacuanha, horehound, inula.

Covonia
(Thornton & Ross)

A bronchial balsam liquid containing an opiate cough suppressant and aromatic decongestant, used to treat dry coughs.

Dose: adults 10 ml (children 6-12 years 5 ml) every 4 hours.
Side effects: constipation, dependence.
Caution: asthmatics should consult a doctor or pharmacist before using this product. Elderly patients may need reduced doses.
Not to be used for: children under 6 years.
Not to be used with: MAOIs.
Contains: dextromethorphan hydrobromide, menthol.

Covonia For Children
(Thornton & Ross)

A sugar-free linctus used as an opiate cough suppressant to treat dry coughs in children.

Dose: 5-10 ml (according to age) every 4-6 hours when required.
Side effects: constipation, dependence.
Caution: asthmatics should consult a doctor or pharmacist before using this product.
Not to be used for: children under 2 years.
Not to be used with: MAOIs.
Contains: dextromethorphan hydrobromide.

Day Nurse
(SmithKline Beecham Consumer)

A liquid, capsule, and sachet (used to make a hot drink), used as an analgesic, sympathomimetic decongestant, and opiate cough suppressant to treat pain, fever, dry cough, nasal congestion, and sore throat due to colds and influenza.

Dose: adults 20 ml liquid, 2 capsules, or 1 sachet (children aged 6-12 years 10 ml liquid or 1 capsule) up to 4 times a day. (Reduce doses to 3 times a day if 'Night Nurse' also being used.)
Side effects: rapid or abnormal heart rate, dry mouth, excitement, anxiety, shaking hands, constipation, dependence.
Caution: children under 6 years (liquid and capsules) or children under 12 years (sachets), pregnant women, asthmatics and patients already taking other medication or under medical supervision should consult a doctor before using this product.
Not to be used for: patients with high blood pressure, overactive thyroid, heart disease, diabetes.
Not to be used with: MAOIs, tricyclic antidepressants, beta-blockers, antihypertensives, other cough or cold remedies, other medication containing paracetamol.
Contains: paracetamol, phenylpropanolamine hydrochloride, dextromethorphan hydrobromide. (Hot drink also contains vitamin C.)

Dimotane Co
(Whitehall)

A sugar-free liquid, available in adult or children's strengths, and used as an antihistamine, sympathomimetic decongestant and opiate cough suppressant to treat dry, irritating coughs and nasal congestion.

Dose: adults 10 ml (adult strength) 3 times a day; children 2.5-7.5 ml (adult strength) or 5-15 ml (children's strength) 3 times a day.
Side effects: drowsiness, rapid or abnormal heart rate, dry mouth, excitement, anxiety, shaking hands, constipation, dependence.
Caution: asthmatics or patients taking other medications or receiving medical treatment should consult a doctor before using this product.
Not to be used for: children under 2 years, or for patients with high blood pressure, overactive thyroid, heart disease, diabetes.
Not to be used with: MAOIs, tricyclic antidepressants, beta-blockers, antihypertensives, other sedating medicines, alcohol.
Contains: brompheniramine maleate, pseudoephedrine hydrochloride, codeine phosphate.

Dimotane Expectorant
(Whitehall Laboratories)

A liquid used as an antihistamine, expectorant, and sympathomimetic treatment for chesty cough and congestion.

Dose: adults 5-10 ml (children 2.5-5 ml according to age) 3 times a day.
Side effects: anxiety, hands shaking, rapid or abnormal heart rate, dry mouth, drowsiness.
Caution: asthmatics should consult a doctor or pharmacist before using this product, as prescribed medication may be affected.

Not to be used for: children under 2 years or for patients suffering from overactive thyroid, heart disease, high blood pressure, or diabetes.
Not to be used with: MAOIs, tricyclic antidepressants, alcohol, other sedating medicines, beta-blockers, antihypertensives.
Contains: brompheniramine maleate, guaiphenesin, pseudoephedrine hydrochloride.

Dimotapp
(Whitehall Laboratories)

A long-acting tablet and sugar-free elixir (available in adult and children's strengths) used as an antihistamine and sympathomimetic decongestant treatment for colds, nasal congestion, and hayfever.

Dose: adults 1-2 tablets night and morning or 5-10 ml adult elixir 3 times a day; children 2.5-5 ml adult elixir or 5-10 ml children's elixir 3 times a day, according to age.
Side effects: drowsiness, rapid or abnormal heart rate, dry mouth, excitement, anxiety, shaking hands.
Caution: asthmatics and patients taking other medicines or receiving medical treatment should consult a doctor before using this product.
Not to be used for: children under 2 years or patients suffering from high blood pressure, heart disease, overactive thyroid gland, or diabetes.
Not to be used with: MAOIs, tricyclic antidepressants, alcohol, beta-blockers, antihypertensives, and other sedating medicines.
Contains: brompheniramine maleate, phenylephrine hydrochloride, phenylpropanolamine hydrochloride.

Do-do Expectorant
(Zyma Healthcare)

An expectorant linctus, used to treat and loosen bronchial catarrh and ease coughing.

Dose: adults 5-10 ml every 2-4 hours. (Children aged 6-12 years 5-10 ml every 4 hours.)
Side effects:
Caution: children under 6 years should see a doctor before using this product.
Not to be used for:
Not to be used with:
Contains: guaiphenesin.

Do-do Tablets see entry in 'Respiratory conditions – bronchodilators' section
(Zyma Healthcare)

Dolvan
(Norma Chemicals)

A tablet used as a sympathomimetic decongestant, analgesic, antihistamine, and stimulant treatment for the symptoms of colds, influenza, and nasal congestion with allergy.

Dose: 1-2 tablets 3 times a day. (Elderly patients 1 tablet 3 times a day.)
Side effects: drowsiness, rapid or abnormal heart rate, dry mouth, excitement, anxiety, shaking hands.
Caution: asthmatics should consult a doctor or pharmacist before using this product, because prescribed medication may be affected.
Not to be used for: patients with high blood pressure, overactive thyroid, heart disease, diabetes.
Not to be used with: MAOIs, tricyclic antidepressants, beta-blockers, antihypertensives, other medicines containing paracetamol, excess tea or coffee, other sedating medicines, alcohol.
Contains: diphenhydramine hydrochloride, ephedrine hydrochloride, paracetamol, caffeine.

Dristan Tablets
(Whitehall Laboratories)

A tablet used as an analgesic, sympathomimetic decongestant, antihistamine, and stimulant treatment for pain and nasal congestion associated with colds and influenza.

Dose: 2 tablets up to 4 times a day.
Side effects: drowsiness, irritation of stomach and intestines, rapid or abnormal heart rate, dry mouth, excitement, anxiety, shaking hands.
Caution: pregnant women and patients with asthma or indigestion should consult a doctor before using this product.
Not to be used for: children under 12 years, nursing mothers, or patients with stomach ulcers, blood-clotting disorder, high blood pressure, overactive thyroid, heart disease, diabetes, or allergy to aspirin.
Not to be used with: anticoagulants, some anti-epileptic drugs, MAOIs, tricyclic antidepressants, beta-blockers, antihypertensives, other sedating medicines, alcohol, excess tea or coffee.
Contains: aspirin, chlorpheniramine maleate, phenylephrine hydrochloride, caffeine.

Ecdylin
(E. C. De Witt)

A syrup used as an expectorant and antihistamine treatment for chesty coughs.

Dose: adults 5-10 ml every 2-3 hours; children 2.5-5 ml every 3-4 hours.
Side effects: drowsiness.
Caution:
Not to be used for:
Not to be used with: other sedating medicines, alcohol.
Contains: ammonium chloride, diphenhydramine

hydrochloride.

echinacea* see entry in 'Skin disorders' section

Echinacea and Garlic
(Gerard House)

A tablet used as a herbal remedy to relieve symptoms of colds and influenza.

Dose: 1-2 tablets 3 times a day.
Side effects:
Caution: pregnant women and nursing mothers should consult a doctor before using this product.
Not to be used for: children.
Not to be used with:
Contains: echinacea root, garlic powder.

Elderflower and Peppermint with Composition Essence
(Potters)

A liquid used as a herbal expectorant, stimulant, and anti-infection treatment to relieve the symptoms of colds, chills, and sore throats.

Dose: adults 10 ml (children over 5 years 5 ml) in a-third of a cupful of warm water 3 times a day.
Side effects:
Caution: do not exceed the stated dose. (May cause nausea and vomiting in high doses.)
Not to be used for: children under 5 years.
Not to be used with: homeopathic remedies.
Contains: bayberry bark, hemlock spruce, elderflowers, peppermint oil.

Eldermint Life Drops
(Potters)

A liquid used as a herbal remedy to relieve the symptoms of influenza, colds, fever, and sore throat.

Dose: adults 11 drops every hour. (Children over 7 years 11 drops every 2 hours.) Take the dose in warm water.
Side effects:
Caution:
Not to be used for: children under 7 years.
Not to be used with: homeopathic remedies.
Contains: capsicum, elder flowers, peppermint oil.

Ernest Jackson's Catarrh Pastilles
(Ernest Jackson)

A pastille used as an aromatic decongestant to treat catarrh.

Dose: 1 pastille dissolved in the mouth when required.
Side effects: (rarely allergy).
Caution:
Not to be used for:
Not to be used with:
Contains: menthol, creosote, abietis pine oil, sylvestris pine oil.

Ernest Jackson's Children's Cough Pastilles
(Ernest Jackson)

A pastille used as an expectorant to treat coughs in children.

Dose: 1 pastille sucked slowly when required. (Maximum of 8 in 24 hours for children aged 3-5 years, 10 in 24 hours for children aged 6-8 years, and 12 in 24 hours for children over 8 years.)

Side effects:
Caution: patients with heart disease should consult a doctor before using this product.
Not to be used for: children under 3 years.
Not to be used with:
Contains: honey, citric acid, ipecacuanha, squill.

Ernest Jackson's Cough Pastilles
(Ernest Jackson)

A pastille used as an aromatic decongestant to treat coughs.

Dose: suck 1 when required.
Side effects:
Caution:
Not to be used for:
Not to be used with:
Contains: menthol, eucalyptus oil.

Ernest Jackson's Night Cough Pastilles
(Ernest Jackson)

A pastille used as an opiate cough suppressant to treat dry coughs.

Dose: up to 4 sucked every 2 hours. (Maximum 15 in 24 hours.)
Side effects: constipation, dependence.
Caution: asthmatics should consult a doctor or pharmacist before using this product.
Not to be used for: children.
Not to be used with: MAOIs.
Contains: codeine phosphate, wild cherry bark.

ES Bronchial Mixture
(Torbet Laboratories)

A mixture used as an expectorant to treat coughs, colds, and catarrh.

Dose: 10 ml in water 3 times a day.
Side effects:
Caution: patients with heart disease should consult a doctor before using this product.
Not to be used for: children.
Not to be used with:
Contains: squill, ipecacuanha, senna, ammonium bicarbonate.

Eskornade
(Goldshield Healthcare)

A syrup and long-acting capsule used as a sympathomimetic decongestant and antihistamine treatment to relieve nasal congestion due to colds, influenza, and allergies.

Dose: adults 1 capsule every 12 hours, or 10 ml syrup up to 4 times a day; children 2.5-5 ml syrup (according to age) up to 4 times a day.
Side effects: drowsiness, rapid or abnormal heart rate, dry mouth, excitement, anxiety, shaking hands.
Caution: pregnant women, asthmatics, and patients suffering from glaucoma or prostate problems, or anyone already receiving medical treatment should consult a doctor before using this product.
Not to be used for: children under 12 years (capsules) or under 2 years (syrup), or for patients with high blood pressure, overactive thyroid, heart disease, diabetes.
Not to be used with: MAOIs, tricyclic antidepressants, beta-blockers, antihypertensives, alcohol, other sedating medicines.
Contains: phenylpropanolamine hydrochloride, diphenylpyraline hydrochloride.

Expulin Children's Cough Linctus
(Monmouth)

A sugar-free linctus used as an antihistamine and opiate cough suppressant to treat dry coughs and relieve nasal itch and sneezing.

Dose: children aged 1-5 years 5-10 ml (aged 6-12 years 10 ml) 2-3 times a day.

Side effects: constipation, dependence, nausea, drowsiness.

Caution: asthmatics and patients with other breathing disorders should consult a doctor before using this product.

Not to be used for: children under 1 year or pregnant women.

Not to be used with: MAOIs, alcohol, other sedating medicines.

Contains: pholcodine, chlorpheniramine maleate.

Expulin Cough Linctus
(Monmouth)

A sugar-free linctus used as an antihistamine, opiate cough suppressant and sympathomimetic treatment for dry cough and nasal congestion associated with colds and influenza.

Dose: adults 10 ml (children 2-6 years 2.5-5 ml, 6-12 years 5-10 ml) 4 times a day.

Side effects: constipation, drowsiness, reduced reactions, anxiety, hands shaking, irregular or rapid heart rate, dry mouth, excitement, rarely skin eruptions, dependence.

Caution: patients suffering from prostate or bladder problems should consult a doctor before using this product.

Not to be used for: children under 2 years, pregnant women, nursing mothers, asthmatics, or for patients suffering from high blood pressure, heart or thyroid disorders.

Not to be used with: MAOIs, alcohol, tricyclic antidepressants, beta-blockers, antihypertensives, other sedating medicines.

Contains: pholcodine, pseudoephedrine hydrochloride,

chlorpheniramine maleate.

Expulin Decongestant Linctus
(Monmouth)

A sugar-free linctus used as a sympathomimetic decongestant and antihistamine treatment for nasal congestion due to colds, influenza, and hayfever in children.

Dose: children aged 3-12 months 2.5-5 ml twice a day; aged 1-5 years 5-10 ml (aged 6-12 years 10-15 ml) 3 times a day.
Side effects: drowsiness, rapid or abnormal heart rate, dry mouth, excitement, anxiety, shaking hands.
Caution: asthmatics should consult a doctor or pharmacist before using this product, because prescribed medication may be affected.
Not to be used for: patients with high blood pressure, overactive thyroid, heart disease, diabetes.
Not to be used with: MAOIs, tricyclic antidepressants, beta-blockers, antihypertensives, alcohol, other sedating medicines.
Contains: ephedrine, chlorpheniramine maleate.

Expulin Dry Cough Linctus see pholcodine linctus strong BP
(Monmouth)

Famel Catarrh and Throat Pastilles
(Seton Healthcare)

A pastille used as an aromatic decongestant and expectorant to treat sore throat, cough, and catarrh.

Dose: 1 pastille sucked when required.
Side effects:
Caution:
Not to be used for:

Not to be used with:
Contains: menthol, creosote.

Famel Expectorant
(Seton Healthcare)

A liquid used as an expectorant to treat chesty coughs and catarrh.

Dose: adults 20 ml (children 5-10 ml) every 2-4 hours when required.
Side effects:
Caution:
Not to be used for: children under 1 year.
Not to be used with:
Contains: guaiphenesin.

Famel Honey and Lemon Pastilles
(Seton Healthcare)

A pastille used as an expectorant to treat chesty coughs, catarrh, and sore throats.

Dose: adults and children over 10 years 1 pastille sucked every hour if required; children aged 5-10 years 1 pastille sucked every 2 hours if required.
Side effects:
Caution:
Not to be used for: children under 5 years.
Not to be used with:
Contains: guaiphenesin.

Famel Linctus see **pholcodine linctus**
(Seton Healthcare)

Famel Original
(Seton Healthcare)

A liquid used as an opiate cough suppressant to treat dry coughs.

Dose: 10-15 ml 3 times a day for a maximum of 7 days.
Side effects: constipation, dependence, drowsiness.
Caution: asthmatics should consult a doctor or pharmacist before using this product.
Not to be used for: children under 12 years.
Not to be used with: MAOIs.
Contains: creosote, codeine phosphate.

Fedril Expectorant
(Pinewood Healthcare)

A sugar-free liquid used as an antihistamine, expectorant, and aromatic decongestant to treat chesty coughs.

Dose: adults 5-10 ml (children 2.5-5 ml) 3-4 times a day.
Side effects: drowsiness.
Caution:
Not to be used for: children under 2 years.
Not to be used with: other sedating medicines, alcohol.
Contains: diphenhydramine hydrochloride, ammonium chloride, menthol.

Fedril Paediatric see Benylin Children's Cough
(Pinewood Healthcare)

Fedril Tickly Cough
(Pinewood Healthcare)

A liquid used as an antiseptic, expectorant, and soothing treatment for tickly coughs.

Dose: adults 15 ml (children 5-10 ml) every 2-3 hours.
Side effects:
Caution:
Not to be used for:
Not to be used with:
Contains: cetylpyridinium chloride, ipecacuanha, lemon oil, honey, ammonium chloride, glycerin, citric acid.

Fennings Little Healers
(Waterhouse)

A tablet used as an expectorant to assist in treating coughs and catarrh.

Dose: adults 2 tablets (children over 5 years 1 tablet) 3 times a day.
Side effects:
Caution: pregnant women should consult a doctor before using this product.
Not to be used for:
Not to be used with:
Contains: ipecacuanha.

Flucaps
(Ernest Jackson)

A capsule used as an opiate analgesic to relieve the symptoms of colds and influenza.

Dose: 1 capsule 3 times a day and 2 at bedtime.
Side effects: constipation, dependence.
Caution: asthmatics should consult a doctor or pharmacist before using this product.
Not to be used for: children under 12 years.
Not to be used with: MAOIs, other medicines containing paracetamol.

Contains: paracetamol, codeine phosphate.

___

Flurex Cold/Flu Capsules with Cough Suppressant
(Seton Healthcare)

A capsule used as a sympathomimetic decongestant, analgesic, and opiate cough suppressant to treat the symptoms of colds and influenza.

Dose: adults 2 capsules (children aged 6-12 years 1 capsule) every 4 hours.
Side effects: rapid or abnormal heart rate, dry mouth, excitement, anxiety, shaking hands, constipation, dependence.
Caution: asthmatics should consult a doctor before using this product.
Not to be used for: children under 6 years, or for patients with high blood pressure, overactive thyroid, heart disease, diabetes.
Not to be used with: MAOIs, tricyclic antidepressants, beta-blockers, antihypertensives, other medicines containing paracetamol.
Contains: paracetamol, phenylephrine hydrochloride, dextromethorphan hydrobromide.

___

Flurex Tablets
(Seton Healthcare)

A tablet used as a sympathomimetic decongestant, analgesic, and stimulant to relieve the symptoms of colds, influenza, and catarrh.

Dose: adults 2 capsules (children aged 6-12 years 1 capsule) up to 4 times a day.
Side effects: rapid or abnormal heart rate, dry mouth, excitement, anxiety, shaking hands.
Caution: asthmatics should consult a doctor or pharmacist before using this product, because prescribed medication may

be affected.
Not to be used for: children under 6 years, or for patients with high blood pressure, overactive thyroid, heart disease, diabetes.
Not to be used with: MAOIs, tricyclic antidepressants, beta-blockers, antihypertensives, other medicines containing paracetamol, excess tea or coffee.
Contains: paracetamol, caffeine, phenylephrine hydrochloride.

Franolyn for Dry Coughs
(Centra Healthcare)

A liquid used as an opiate cough suppressant to treat dry coughs.

Dose: adults 10 ml (children aged 7-12 years 5 ml) up to 4 times a day.
Side effects: constipation, dependence.
Caution: asthmatics should consult a doctor or pharmacist before using this product.
Not to be used for: children under 7 years.
Not to be used with: MAOIs.
Contains: dextromethorphan hydrobromide.

Galcodine see **codeine linctus (sugar-free)**
(Galen)

Galenphol Adult Linctus
(Galen)

A sugar-free linctus used as an opiate cough suppressant to treat dry cough.

Dose: adults 10-15 ml 3-4 times a day; children 6-12 years 5-10 ml 4 times a day.
Side effects: constipation, dependence.
Caution: asthmatics should consult a doctor or pharmacist

before using this product.
Not to be used for: children under 6 years.
Not to be used with: MAOIs.
Contains: pholcodine.

Galenphol Paediatric
(Galen)

A sugar-free linctus used as an opiate cough suppressant to treat dry coughs in children.

Dose: children aged 1-5 years 5-10 ml (children aged 3-12 months 2.5 ml) 3 times a day.
Side effects: constipation, dependence.
Caution: asthmatics should consult a doctor or pharmacist before using this product. Children under 1 year should be seen by a doctor before being treated.
Not to be used for:
Not to be used with: MAOIs.
Contains: pholcodine.

Galloways
(Charwell Health Care)

A mixture used as an expectorant to treat cough and hoarseness.

Dose: adults and children over 10 years 10 ml 3-4 times a day; children under 10 years half the adult dose.
Side effects:
Caution: patients with heart disease should consult a doctor before using this product.
Not to be used for:
Not to be used with:
Contains: ipecacuanha liquid extract, squill vinegar.

Galpseud
(Galen)

A tablet and sugar-free elixir, used as a sympathomimetic decongestant to relieve nasal and sinus congestion.

Dose: adults 1 tablet or 10 ml elixir 3 times a day; children 2.5-5 ml elixir (according to age) 3-4 times a day.
Side effects: rapid or abnormal heart rate, dry mouth, excitement, anxiety, shaking hands.
Caution: pregnant women, asthmatics, and patients taking prescribed medication should consult a doctor before using this product.
Not to be used for: patients with high blood pressure, overactive thyroid, heart disease, diabetes.
Not to be used with: MAOIs, tricyclic antidepressants, beta-blockers, antihypertensives.
Contains: pseudoephedrine hydrochloride.

---

garlic preparations see entry in 'Miscellaneous' section

Garlic Perles
(Gerard House)

A capsule used as a herbal remedy to treat the symptoms of coughs, colds, and catarrh.

Dose: 1 capsules 3 times a day or 2-3 capsules at night.
Side effects:
Caution: pregnant women should consult a doctor before using this product.
Not to be used for: children.
Not to be used with:
Contains: garlic.

Garlic Tablets
(Potters)

A tablet used as a herbal remedy to treat the symptoms of colds and to give temporary relief from rhinitis and catarrh.

Dose: adults 2 tablets 3 times a day; children over 8 years 1 tablet 3-4 times a day.
Side effects:
Caution:
Not to be used for:
Not to be used with:
Contains: garlic.

Garlodex
(Lane)

A tablet used as a herbal antibacterial, anti-inflammatory, and expectorant remedy to treat the symptoms of colds and catarrh.

Dose: adults 1 tablet 3 times a day; children aged 5-12 years 1 tablet at bedtime.
Side effects:
Caution:
Not to be used for: children under 5 years, pregnant women, or nursing mothers.
Not to be used with:
Contains: garlic oil, marshmallow, parsley.

Gee's linctus

A linctus or pastille used as an expectorant and opiate cough suppressant to treat coughs.

Dose: 5 ml linctus 3-4 times a day or 1 pastille every 2 hours.
Side effects: constipation, dependence.

Caution: asthmatics and patients suffering from heart disease should consult a doctor before using this product.
Not to be used for: children under 12 years.
Not to be used with: MAOIs.
Contains: camphorated opium tincture, squill oxymel. (The linctus also contains tolu syrup.)

---

glycerin BP

A liquid used to soothe dry coughs and irritated throats. (For use as a skin emollient see 'Skin disorders' section.)

Dose: 2.5-10 ml, according to age, mixed with water four times a day.
Side effects:
Caution:
Not to be used for:
Not to be used with:
Contains: glycerin.

---

glycerin, lemon, and honey linctus

A soothing linctus used to treat tickly coughs and sore throats.

Dose: 2.5-10 ml 3-4 times a day (according to age).
Side effects:
Caution:
Not to be used for: (see individual brand product labels for guidance).
Not to be used with:
Contains: glycerin, lemon oil, honey.

---

glycerin, lemon, and honey linctus with ipecacuanha

An expectorant linctus used to treat tickly coughs and sore throats.

Dose: 2.5-10 ml 3-4 times a day (according to age).
Side effects:
Caution:
Not to be used for: (see individual brand product labels for guidance).
Not to be used with:
Contains: glycerin, lemon oil, honey, ipecacuanha.

Heath & Heather Balm of Gilead Cough Pastilles
(Ferrosan Healthcare)

A herbal pastille used as an expectorant to relieve the symptoms of coughs and catarrh.

Dose: dissolve 1 pastille in the mouth when required. (Maximum of 12 in 24 hours.)
Side effects: nausea and vomiting in high doses.
Caution: patients with heart disease should consult a doctor before using this product.
Not to be used for: children, pregnant women, or nursing mothers.
Not to be used with: homeopathic remedies.
Contains: balm of Gilead buds, squill, lobelia.

Heath & Heather Catarrh Tablets
(Ferrosan Healthcare)

A herbal remedy used to relieve the symptoms of coughs and catarrh.

Dose: 1 tablet 3 times a day.
Side effects:
Caution: pregnant women and patients with heart disease should consult a doctor before using this product.
Not to be used for: children.
Not to be used with:

Contains: white horehound, squill.

Hedex Headcold
(Sterling Health)

A powder or tablet used as a sympathomimetic decongestant and analgesic treatment for sinus pain and symptoms of influenza.

Dose: 1 sachet (in hot water) or 2 tablets every 4 hours when required. (Maximum of 4 sachets or 8 tablets in 24 hours.)
Side effects: rapid or abnormal heart rate, dry mouth, excitement, anxiety, shaking hands.
Caution: asthmatics should consult a doctor or pharmacist before using this product, because prescribed medication may be affected. Pregnant women and patients taking prescribed medicines should also consult a doctor.
Not to be used for: children under 12 years, patients with high blood pressure, overactive thyroid, heart disease, diabetes.
Not to be used with: MAOIs, tricyclic antidepressants, beta-blockers, antihypertensives, other medicines containing paracetamol. (Tablets also not to be used with excess tea or coffee.)
Contains: paracetamol, phenylephrine hydrochloride, vitamin C, (tablets also contain caffeine).

Herb and Honey Cough Elixir
(Weleda)

An elixir used as a herbal soothing remedy for relief of dry and irritating cough symptoms.

Dose: adults 10 ml (children over 6 years 5 ml) in water every 3-4 hours, up to 4 times a day.
Side effects:
Caution:

Not to be used for: children under 6 years, diabetics, or pregnant women.
Not to be used with:
Contains: marshmallow, elder flowers, horehound, Iceland moss, thyme, aniseed.

Herbelix
(Lane)

A liquid used as a herbal expectorant to relieve symptoms of catarrh and congestion.

Dose: adults and children over 14 years 5 ml at bedtime; children aged 7-14 years half the adult dose.
Side effects:
Caution:
Not to be used for: children under 7 years, pregnant women, or nursing mothers.
Not to be used with:
Contains: lobelia, tolu solution, sodium bicarbonate.

Hill's Balsam Adult Expectorant
(Windsor Healthcare)

A mixture used as an expectorant to treat chesty coughs.

Dose: 5-10 ml every 2-4 hours. (Maximum 60 ml in 24 hours.)
Side effects:
Caution: pregnant women, nursing mothers, and patients taking other medication should consult a doctor before using this product.
Not to be used for: children under 12 years.
Not to be used with:
Contains: guaiphenesin.

Hill's Balsam Adult Suppressant see **pholcodine linctus strong BP**
(Windsor Healthcare)

Hill's Balsam Children's Mixture for Chesty Coughs
(Windsor Healthcare)

A mixture used as an expectorant to treat chesty coughs.

Dose: 2.5-5 ml 3 times a day and at bedtime (according to age).
Side effects:
Caution:
Not to be used for:
Not to be used with:
Contains: citric acid, ipecacuanha liquid extract.

Hill's Balsam Flu Strength Hot Lemon Powders see **Lemplus Powders**
(Windsor Healthcare)

Hill's Balsam Menthol and Eucalyptus Pastilles
(Windsor Healthcare)

A pastille used as an aromatic decongestant to treat colds and blocked noses.

Dose: 1 pastille sucked when required.
Side effects:
Caution:
Not to be used for: children.
Not to be used with:
Contains: menthol, eucalyptus oil.

Hill's Balsam Pastilles for Chesty Coughs
(Windsor Healthcare)

A pastille used as an expectorant and aromatic decongestant to treat coughs, colds, and catarrh.

Dose: 1 pastille sucked when required.
Side effects:
Caution:
Not to be used for: children under 12 years.
Not to be used with: homeopathic remedies.
Contains: ipecacuanha liquid extract, compound benzoin tincture, capsicum oleoresin, peppermint oil, tincture of lobelia, menthol.

Höfels Garlic with Parsley
(Seven Seas)

Capsules of garlic with parsley (to mask the taste and odour of garlic), used as a herbal remedy to relieve catarrh, rhinitis, and cold symptoms.

Dose: 1 each day.
Side effects:
Caution: do not chew or swallow with hot liquids.
Not to be used for: children under 7 years.
Not to be used with:
Contains: garlic, parsley.

Höfels One-a-day Garlic Pearles
(Seven Seas)

Capsules of garlic used as a herbal remedy to relieve catarrh, rhinitis, and cold symptoms.

Dose: 1 capsule daily.

Side effects:
Caution: do not chew or swallow with hot liquids.
Not to be used for: children under 7 years.
Not to be used with:
Contains: garlic.

Höfels Original Garlic Pearles
(Seven Seas)

Capsules of garlic used as a herbal remedy to relieve catarrh, rhinitis, and cold symptoms.

Dose: adults 3 capsules (children aged 7-12 years 2 capsules) daily.
Side effects:
Caution: do not chew or swallow with hot liquids.
Not to be used for: children under 7 years.
Not to be used with:
Contains: garlic.

Honey and Molasses Cough Mixture
(Lane)

A liquid used as a herbal expectorant to relieve coughs, colds, hoarseness, sore throats, and catarrh.

Dose: adults 5 ml (children aged 7-14 years 2.5 ml) 3 times a day. Children aged 2-7 years may use 2.5 ml once a day.
Side effects:
Caution: pregnant women should consult a doctor before using this medicine.
Not to be used for: children under 2 years, women in the early stages of pregnancy, nursing mothers, or patients with heart or kidney disorders.
Not to be used with: digoxin, some beta-blockers.
Contains: ipecacuanha, squill, white horehound.

Horehound and Aniseed Cough Mixture
(Potters)

A mixture used as a herbal remedy to relieve the symptoms of coughs.

Dose: adults 10 ml (children over 5 years 5 ml) 3 times a day.
Side effects:
Caution: do not exceed the stated dose.
Not to be used for: children under 5 years, pregnant women, or nursing mothers.
Not to be used with:
Contains: lobelia, pleurisy root, elecampane, horehound, skunk cabbage.

Hot Lemon Cold Relief Powders see Lemplus Powders
(Sussex Pharmaceuticals)

Jackson's All Fours
(Waterhouse)

A syrup used as an expectorant to treat the symptoms of chesty coughs.

Dose: 10-20 ml at bedtime or at 4-hourly intervals.
Side effects:
Caution:
Not to be used for: children under 12 years.
Not to be used with:
Contains: guaiphenesin.

Jackson's Febrifuge
(Waterhouse)

A liquid used as an analgesic to relieve the symptoms of influenza, sore throat, colds, and muscular pain.

Dose: 5-10 ml in water every 6 hours or 3 times a day. (Elderly patients should use only 5 ml.)
Side effects: irritation of stomach and intestines.
Caution: patients with asthma or indigestion should consult a doctor before using this product.
Not to be used for: children under 12 years, pregnant women, nursing mothers, or patients with stomach ulcers, blood-clotting disorder, or allergy to aspirin.
Not to be used with: anticoagulants, some anti-epileptic drugs.
Contains: sodium salicylate.

JW Glycerin Lemon and Honey see **glycerin, lemon, and honey linctus**
(Waterhouse)

Lemplus Capsules see **Lemsip Capsules**
(Adcock Ingram)

Lemplus Powders
(Adcock Ingram)

A hot lemon drink used as an analgesic to treat pain and fever associated with colds and influenza.

Dose: 1 sachet in freshly boiled hot water up to 4 times a day.
Side effects:
Caution: pregnant women, nursing mothers, and patients receiving medical treatment should see a doctor before using this product.
Not to be used for: children under 12 years.
Not to be used with: other medicines containing paracetamol.
Contains: paracetamol, vitamin C.

Lemsip
(Reckitt & Colman)

A powder available to make the original hot lemon drink, hot lemon drink with added menthol, or cool lemon drink, and used as an analgesic and sympathomimetic decongestant treatment for pain, fever, and blocked nose associated with colds and influenza.

Dose: 1 sachet in hot water every 4 hours. (Maximum 4 in 24 hours.)
Side effects: rapid or abnormal heart rate, dry mouth, excitement, anxiety, shaking hands.
Caution: pregnant women, asthmatics and patients taking other medication should consult a doctor before using this product.
Not to be used for: children under 12 years, or patients with high blood pressure, overactive thyroid, heart disease, diabetes.
Not to be used with: MAOIs, tricyclic antidepressants, beta-blockers, antihypertensives, other medicines containing paracetamol.
Contains: paracetamol, phenylephrine hydrochloride, vitamin C.

Lemsip Capsules
(Reckitt & Colman)

A capsule used as an analgesic, stimulant, and sympathomimetic decongestant treatment for fever, pain, and blocked nose associated with colds and influenza.

Dose: 1-2 capsules every 4 hours. (Maximum of 8 in 24 hours.)
Side effects: rapid or abnormal heart rate, dry mouth, excitement, anxiety, shaking hands.
Caution: pregnant women, asthmatics, and patients taking other medication should consult a doctor before using this product.
Not to be used for: children under 12 years, or patients with

high blood pressure, overactive thyroid, heart disease, diabetes.
Not to be used with: MAOIs, tricyclic antidepressants, beta-blockers, antihypertensives, other medicines containing paracetamol, excess tea or coffee.
Contains: paracetamol, caffeine, phenylephrine hydrochloride.

Lemsip Chesty Cough
(Reckitt & Colman)

A liquid used as an expectorant to treat chesty coughs and to soothe the throat.

Dose: adults 10-20 ml (children 5-10 ml according to age) 3-4 times a day.
Side effects:
Caution:
Not to be used for: children under 2 years.
Not to be used with:
Contains: guaiphenesin.

Lemsip Dry Tickly Cough
(Reckitt & Colman)

A liquid used as a soothing treatment for dry tickly coughs.

Dose: adults 10 ml (children under 12 years 5 ml) 3-4 times a day.
Side effects:
Caution:
Not to be used for:
Not to be used with:
Contains: honey, lemon oil, glycerol, citric acid, syrup.

Lemsip Flu Strength Sachets
(Reckitt & Colman)

A sachet used as an analgesic and sympathomimetic decongestant to treat the symptoms of influenza and heavy colds.

Dose: 1 sachet in hot water up to three times a day.
Side effects: rapid or abnormal heart rate, dry mouth, excitement, anxiety, shaking hands.
Caution: asthmatics and patients with glaucoma should consult a doctor before using this product.
Not to be used for: children under 12 years, patients with high blood pressure, overactive thyroid, heart disease, diabetes.
Not to be used with: MAOIs, tricyclic antidepressants, beta-blockers, antihypertensives, other medicines containing paracetamol.
Contains: paracetamol, pseudoephedrine hydrochloride, vitamin C.

Lemsip Flu Strength Night-time
(Reckitt & Colman)

A liquid used as an analgesic, sympathomimetic decongestant, antihistamine, and opiate cough suppressant to treat fever, pain, dry cough, and nasal congestion at night-time, due to colds and influenza.

Dose: 30 ml at night.
Side effects: drowsiness, rapid or abnormal heart rate, dry mouth, excitement, anxiety, shaking hands, constipation, dependence, blurred vision, upset stomach.
Caution: asthmatics and patients already taking other medication should consult a doctor before using this product.
Not to be used for: children under 13 years, pregnant women, or patients with high blood pressure, overactive thyroid, heart disease, diabetes. Not to be used for prolonged periods.

Not to be used with: MAOIs, tricyclic antidepressants, beta-blockers, antihypertensives, other cough or cold remedies, other medication containing paracetamol, other sedating medicines, alcohol.

Contains: paracetamol, phenylpropanolamine hydrochloride, dextromethorphan hydrobromide, chlorpheniramine maleate, alcohol.

Life Drops
(Potters)

A liquid used as a herbal remedy to relieve the discomfort of colds, influenza, chills, and sore throat.

Dose: adults 11 drops (0.2 ml) in 1-2 tablespoonsful of warm water every hour when required; children over 7 years adult dose every 2 hours when required.
Side effects:
Caution:
Not to be used for: children under 7 years.
Not to be used with: homeopathic remedies.
Contains: capsicum, elderflower, peppermint oil.

Lightning Cough Remedy
(Potters)

A liquid used as a traditional remedy to treat the symptoms of coughs.

Dose: adults 10 ml 3-4 times a day; children aged 5 years and over, 5 ml every 5-6 hours.
Side effects:
Caution:
Not to be used for: children under 5 years.
Not to be used with:
Contains: liquorice, anise oil.

Liqufruta Blackcurrant
(Charwell Health Care)

A liquid used as an expectorant and aromatic decongestant to treat dry or chesty coughs, congestion, and sore throats.

Dose: adults 10 ml (children 5 ml) every 2-3 hours.
Side effects:
Caution:
Not to be used for:
Not to be used with:
Contains: menthol, liquid glucose, ipecacuanha.

Liqufruta Garlic
(Charwell Health Care)

A mixture used as an expectorant to treat chesty coughs, hoarseness, and sore throat.

Dose: adults 10-15 ml, children aged 3-12 years 10 ml, children aged 1-2 years 5 ml – all three times a day and at bedtime.
Side effects:
Caution:
Not to be used for:
Not to be used with:
Contains: guaiphenesin.

Lobelia Compound
(Gerard House)

A tablet used as a herbal expectorant, anti-spasmodic, and respiratory stimulant remedy to treat the symptoms of coughs, colds, and catarrh.

Dose: 1 tablet 3 times a day.
Side effects:

Caution: pregnant women and patients with heart disease should consult a doctor before using this product. Do not exceed the stated dose. (Large doses of lobelia may cause nausea and vomiting.)
Not to be used for: children under 12 years.
Not to be used with:
Contains: lobelia, gum ammoniacum, squill.

Lockets
(Mars)

A medicated lozenge with a liquid centre, available in three flavours, and used as an aromatic decongestant to clear the nose and soothe the throat.

Dose: suck one when required. Maximum in 24 hours: adults 3 packs, young children 1 pack, older children 2 packs.
Side effects:
Caution:
Not to be used for:
Not to be used with:
Contains: honey, menthol, eucalyptol.

Lusty's Garlic Perles
(Lane)

A capsule used as a herbal remedy to treat the symptoms of coughs, colds, rhinitis, and catarrh.

Dose: adults 1 capsule 3 times a day with meals or up to 3 at night; children aged 5-12 years 1 capsule twice a day with meals.
Side effects:
Caution:
Not to be used for:
Not to be used with:

Contains: garlic.

Meggezones
(Schering-Plough Consumer Health)

A pastille used as an aromatic decongestant to treat sore throats, coughs, catarrh, and nasal congestion.

Dose: 1 pastille sucked when required. (Maximum in 24 hours: 15 for adults, 10 for children aged 6-12 years, 5 for children under 6 years.)
Side effects: irritation, allergy.
Caution:
Not to be used for:
Not to be used with:
Contains: menthol.

Melo Glycerin Lemon and Honey with Ipecac see glycerin, lemon and honey with ipecacuanha
(Waterhouse)

Meltus Adult Expectorant
(Seton Healthcare)

A mixture used as an expectorant and antiseptic to treat chesty coughs and catarrh.

Dose: 5-10 ml every 3-4 hours.
Side effects:
Caution:
Not to be used for: children under 12 years.
Not to be used with:
Contains: guaiphenesin, cetylpyridinium chloride, sucrose, purified honey.

Meltus Baby Linctus
(Seton Healthcare)

A linctus used as an expectorant to relieve irritating coughs in young children.

Dose: 2.5-10 ml (according to age) every 2-3 hours as needed.
Side effects:
Caution:
Not to be used for: babies under 3 months.
Not to be used with:
Contains: dilute acetic acid.

Meltus Cough Control Capsules
(Seton Healthcare)

A chewable capsule used as an opiate cough suppressant to control dry coughs.

Dose: 1 capsule every 4 to 6 hours as required. (Maximum of 6 in 24 hours.)
Side effects: constipation, dependence, drowsiness, dizziness, stomach upset.
Caution: asthmatics should consult a doctor or pharmacist before using this product.
Not to be used for: children under 12 years, pregnant women, and nursing mothers.
Not to be used with: MAOIs, alcohol.
Contains: dextromethorphan hydrobromide.

Meltus Dry Cough Elixir
(Seton Healthcare)

An elixir used as a sympathomimetic decongestant and opiate cough suppressant to treat dry coughs and catarrh.

Dose: 5 ml 4 times a day.

Side effects: rapid or abnormal heart rate, dry mouth, excitement, anxiety, shaking hands, constipation, dependence.

Caution: asthmatics should consult a doctor or pharmacist before using this product.

Not to be used for: children under 12 years, or for patients with high blood pressure, overactive thyroid, heart disease, diabetes.

Not to be used with: MAOIs, tricyclic antidepressants, beta-blockers, antihypertensives.

Contains: dextromethorphan hydrobromide, pseudoephedrine hydrochloride.

Meltus Honey and Lemon
(Seton Healthcare)

A linctus used as an expectorant to treat chesty coughs and soothe the throat.

Dose: adults 10-20 ml (children aged 6-12 years 10 ml, aged 2-6 years 5 ml) 3-4 times a day.

Side effects:

Caution: children under 2 years should be seen by a doctor before using this medicine.

Not to be used for:

Not to be used with:

Contains: guaiphenesin.

Meltus Junior Dry Cough
(Seton Healthcare)

An elixir used as a sympathomimetic decongestant and opiate cough suppressant to treat dry coughs and congestion.

Dose: 5-10 ml (according to age) 4 times a day.

Side effects: rapid or abnormal heart rate, dry mouth,

excitement, anxiety, shaking hands, constipation, dependence.
Caution: asthmatics should consult a doctor or pharmacist before using this product.
Not to be used for: children under 2 years, or for patients with high blood pressure, overactive thyroid, heart disease, diabetes.
Not to be used with: MAOIs, tricyclic antidepressants, beta-blockers, antihypertensives.
Contains: dextromethorphan hydrobromide, pseudoephedrine hydrochloride.

Meltus Junior Expectorant
(Seton Healthcare)

A liquid used as an antiseptic, expectorant, and soothing treatment for chesty coughs, catarrh and sore throats.

Dose: 5-10 ml (according to age) 3-4 times a day.
Side effects:
Caution:
Not to be used for:
Not to be used with:
Contains: guaiphenesin, cetylpyridinium chloride, purified honey.

Mentholatum Antiseptic Lozenges
(Mentholatum)

A lozenge used as an aromatic decongestant and antiseptic treatment for nasal congestion, coughs, and sore throat.

Dose: dissolve 1 lozenge slowly in the mouth when required. (Maximum of 9 in 24 hours.)
Side effects:
Caution:
Not to be used for: children under 3 years.
Not to be used with:

Contains: amylmetacresol, menthol, eucalyptus oil.

Merothol
(Marion Merrell Dow)

A lozenge used as an antiseptic and aromatic decongestant to treat blocked noses and sore throats.

Dose: 1 lozenge sucked every 3 hours.
Side effects: rarely allergy or burning sensation in mouth.
Caution:
Not to be used for: children under 6 years.
Not to be used with:
Contains: cetylpyridinium chloride, menthol, eucalyptus oil.

Mu-Cron
(Zyma Healthcare)

A tablet used as an analgesic and sympathomimetic decongestant to treat nasal congestion, sinus pain, and fever due to colds and influenza.

Dose: 1 tablet up to 4 times a day.
Side effects: rapid or abnormal heart rate, dry mouth, excitement, anxiety, shaking hands.
Caution: pregnant women, asthmatics, diabetics, and patients with high blood pressure, glaucoma, prostate problems, angina, overactive thyroid, heart disease or a high fever should consult a doctor before using this product.
Not to be used for: children under 12, or for patients with high blood pressure.
Not to be used with: MAOIs, tricyclic antidepressants, beta-blockers, antihypertensives, other medicines containing paracetamol.
Contains: phenylpropanolamine hydrochloride, paracetamol.

Mu-Cron Junior
(Zyma Healthcare)

A liquid used as a sympathomimetic decongestant and expectorant to treat blocked noses and chesty coughs in children.

Dose: children aged 2-6 years 5 ml (aged 6-12 years 5-10 ml) up to 4 times a day.
Side effects: rapid or abnormal heart rate, dry mouth, excitement, anxiety, shaking hands.
Caution: asthmatics and children already taking other medication should consult a doctor or pharmacist before using this product.
Not to be used for: patients with high blood pressure, overactive thyroid, heart disease, diabetes.
Not to be used with: MAOIs, tricyclic antidepressants, beta-blockers, antihypertensives.
Contains: phenylpropanolamine hydrochloride, ipecacuanha.

Night Nurse
(SmithKline Beecham Consumer)

A liquid or capsule used as an analgesic, antihistamine, and opiate cough suppressant to treat sore throat, dry cough, congestion, pain, and fever due to colds and influenza.

Dose: adults 20 ml liquid or 2 capsules (children aged 6-12 years 10 ml liquid or 1 capsule) at night-time.
Side effects: constipation, dependence, drowsiness.
Caution: children under 6 years, pregnant women, asthmatics, and patients already taking other medication should consult a doctor before using this product.
Not to be used for:
Not to be used with: MAOIs, other sedating medicines, alcohol, or other medication containing paracetamol.
Contains: paracetamol, dextromethorphan hydrobromide,

promethazine hydrochloride.

Nurofen Cold and Flu
(Crookes Healthcare)

A tablet used as a non-steroidal anti-inflammatory and sympathomimetic decongestant treatment for pain, headache, fever, sore throat, blocked nose and sinuses.

Dose: 2 tablets initially, then 1 or 2 tablets every 4 hours if required. (Maximum of 6 tablets per day.)
Side effects: stomach discomfort, nausea, diarrhoea, stomach ulcers, rapid or abnormal heart rate, dry mouth, anxiety, excitement, shaking hands, rash, rarely blood disorders.
Caution: elderly patients may require reduced doses. Asthmatics, nursing mothers, and patients taking other medication should consult a doctor before taking this product.
Not to be used for: children under 12 years, pregnant women, patients with stomach ulcers or other stomach disorder, heart disease, asthma, allergy to aspirin or anti-inflammatory drugs, high blood pressure, overactive thyroid or diabetes.
Not to be used with: antihypertensives, MAOIs, tricyclic antidepressants, beta-blockers, some antibiotics.
Contains: ibuprofen, pseudoephedrine hydrochloride.

Nurse Sykes Balsam
(Waterhouse)

A liquid used as an expectorant to treat bronchial catarrh and cough.

Dose: 5-10 ml at bedtime or every 4 hours.
Side effects:
Caution:
Not to be used for: children.
Not to be used with:

Contains: guaiphenesin.

Olbas Pastilles
(Lane)

A pastille used as an aromatic decongestant to treat sore throats and catarrh.

Dose: 1 pastille sucked when required. (Maximum of 8 pastilles in 24 hours for adults, and 6 pastilles in 24 hours for children aged 7-12 years.)
Side effects:
Caution:
Not to be used for: children under 7 years.
Not to be used with: homeopathic remedies.
Contains: peppermint oil, eucalyptus oil, wintergreen oil, menthol, juniper berry oil, clove oil.

Owbridges Childrens Cough Medicine
(Chefaro)

A liquid used as an antihistamine, expectorant, and aromatic decongestant to treat cough and congestion.

Dose: 5-10 ml (according to age) every 3 hours.
Side effects: drowsiness.
Caution:
Not to be used for: children under 1 year.
Not to be used with: other sedating medicines, alcohol.
Contains: diphenhydramine hydrochloride, sodium citrate, menthol.

Owbridges for Chesty Coughs
(Chefaro)

A liquid used as an expectorant to treat chesty coughs.

Dose: adults 10-20 ml (children 6-12 years 5-10 ml) every 4 hours if required. Maximum in 24 hours 120 ml (adults) 60 ml (children).
Side effects:
Caution:
Not to be used for: children under 6 years.
Not to be used with:
Contains: guaiphenesin.

Owbridges for Dry, Tickly and Allergy Coughs
(Chefaro)

A liquid used as an opiate cough suppressant and soothing product for relief of dry or allergic coughs.

Dose: 5 ml 3 times a day.
Side effects: constipation, dependence.
Caution: asthmatics should consult a doctor or pharmacist before using this product.
Not to be used for: children under 12 years.
Not to be used with: MAOIs.
Contains: dextromethorphan hydrobromide, glycerin.

Pavacol-D
(Boehringer Ingelheim)

A sugar-free mixture containing an opiate cough suppressant used to treat dry, irritating coughs.
Dose: adults 5-10 ml up to 4 times a day (children 2.5-5 ml 3-5 times a day, according to age).
Side effects: constipation, dependence.
Caution: asthmatics should consult a doctor or pharmacist before using this product.
Not to be used for: children under 1 year.
Not to be used with: MAOIs.
Contains: pholcodine.

Peerless Composition Essence
(Potters)

A liquid used as a herbal astringent and analgesic remedy to relieve symptoms of colds and chills.

Dose: adults 5-10 ml (children over 8 years 5 ml) every 3 hours when necessary.
Side effects:
Caution:
Not to be used for: children under 8 years, pregnant women, or nursing mothers.
Not to be used with:
Contains: oak bark, hemlock spruce, poplar bark, prickly ash bark, bayberry bark.

Penetrol Lozenges
(Seton Healthcare)

A lozenge used as a sympathomimetic and aromatic decongestant to treat nasal congestion due to colds or hayfever.

Dose: initially suck one lozenge, followed immediately by another, then use 1 every 2-3 hours if needed. (Maximum of 8 in 24 hours.)
Side effects: rapid or abnormal heart rate, dry mouth, excitement, anxiety, shaking hands.
Caution: asthmatics should consult a doctor or pharmacist before using this product, because prescribed medication may be affected.
Not to be used for: children under 10 years, or for patients with high blood pressure, thyroid disease, heart disease, diabetes.
Not to be used with: MAOIs, tricyclic antidepressants, beta-blockers, antihypertensives.
Contains: menthol, ammonium chloride, phenylephrine hydrochloride, creosote.

Phensedyl Plus Linctus
(Rhone Poulenc Rorer Family Health)

A linctus used as an antihistamine, opiate cough suppressant and sympathomimetic decongestant treatment for dry coughs with congestion.

Dose: 5-10 ml 3-4 times a day.

Side effects: constipation, drowsiness, anxiety, shaking hands, irregular or rapid heart rate, dry mouth, excitement, dependence.

Caution: asthmatics should consult a doctor or pharmacist before using this product.

Not to be used for: children, or for patients suffering from heart disease, overactive thyroid, high blood pressure, or diabetes.

Not to be used with: MAOIs, alcohol, tricyclic antidepressants, other sedating medicines, beta-blockers, antihypertensives.

Contains: promethazine hydrochloride, pholcodine, psuedoephedrine hydrochloride.

---

pholcodine linctus BP

A linctus used as an opiate cough suppressant to treat dry coughs. (Some brands are sugar-free.)

Dose: adults 5-10 ml (children aged 5-12 years 2.5-5 ml) 3-4 times a day.

Side effects: constipation, dependence.

Caution: asthmatics should consult a doctor or pharmacist before using this product.

Not to be used for: children under 5 years.

Not to be used with: MAOIs.

Contains: pholcodine.

---

pholcodine linctus strong BP

A linctus used as an opiate cough suppressant to treat dry coughs. (Some brands are sugar-free.)

Dose: adults 5 ml 3-4 times a day.
Side effects: constipation, dependence.
Caution: asthmatics should consult a doctor or pharmacist before using this product.
Not to be used for: children under 12 years.
Not to be used with: MAOIs.
Contains: pholcodine.

---

pholcodine pastilles

A pastille used as an opiate cough suppressant to treat dry coughs.

Dose: up to 2 pastilles sucked every 4 hours.
Side effects: constipation, dependence.
Caution: asthmatics, pregnant women, and nursing mothers should consult a doctor or pharmacist before using this product.
Not to be used for: children under 12 years.
Not to be used with: MAOIs.
Contains: pholcodine.

Pholcomed Diabetic Forte see pholcodine linctus strong
(Medo)

Potter's Catarrh Pastilles
(Ernest Jackson)

A pastille used as an aromatic decongestant treatment for congestion.

Dose: 1 pastille sucked when required.

Side effects:
Caution:
Not to be used for: children.
Not to be used with:
Contains: menthol, pumilio pine oil, creosote, eucalyptus oil.

Potter's Traditional Cough Pastilles
(Ernest Jackson)

A sugar-free pastille used as an aromatic decongestant and expectorant to treat the symptoms of coughs, colds, and catarrh.

Dose: suck 1 pastille slowly when required.
Side effects:
Caution:
Not to be used for:
Not to be used with: homeopathic remedies.
Contains: liquorice extract, menthol, benzoin tincture, aniseed oil, clove oil, peppermint oil, capsicum.

Proctor's Pinelyptus Pastilles see entry in 'Diseases of the mouth and throat' section
(Ernest Jackson)

Pulmo Bailly
(Bengue & Co)

A liquid used as an expectorant and opiate cough suppressant to treat coughs associated with catarrh, colds, influenza, laryngitis, etc.

Dose: adults up to 10 ml (children aged 5-15 years 5 ml) 3 times a day in water, before food.
Side effects: drowsiness, constipation, dependence.
Caution: asthmatics or patients taking other medication should consult a doctor or pharmacist before using this product.

Not to be used for: children under 5 years, pregnant women, nursing mothers.
Not to be used with: MAOIs.
Contains: guaiacol, codeine.

Revitonil
(Kallo Foods)

A chewable tablet used as a herbal remedy to relieve the symptoms of colds and upper respiratory tract infections.

Dose: adults 2-3 tablets (children aged 10-15 years 2 tablets, children aged 6-10 years 1 tablet) 3 times a day.
Side effects: high doses may cause diarrhoea.
Caution: patients using other medicines should consult a doctor before using this product.
Not to be used for: children under 6 years, or for diabetics.
Not to be used with:
Contains: echinacea.

Ricola Original Herb Lozenges
(Cedar Health)

A lozenge used as an aromatic decongestant to relieve stuffy noses, sore throats, and coughs.

Dose: dissolve 1 lozenge in the mouth at regular intervals. (Maximum 24 lozenges in 24 hours for adults, 10 lozenges in 24 hours for children.)
Side effects:
Caution:
Not to be used for:
Not to be used with: homeopathic remedies.
Contains: menthol, peppermint oil.

Robitussin Chesty Cough
(Whitehall)

A liquid used as an expectorant to treat chesty coughs.

Dose: adults 10 ml (children 2.5-5 ml according to age) 4 times a day.
Side effects:
Caution:
Not to be used for: children under 1 year.
Not to be used with:
Contains: guaiphenesin.

Robitussin Chesty Cough and Congestion see Sudafed Expectorant
(Whitehall)

Robitussin Dry Cough see Benylin Dry Cough Non-Drowsy
(Whitehall)

Robitussin Junior
(Whitehall)

A liquid used as an opiate cough suppressant to treat dry coughs in children.

Dose: 5-10 ml (according to age) 3-4 times a day.
Side effects: constipation, dependence.
Caution: asthmatics should consult a doctor or pharmacist before using this product.
Not to be used for: children under 1 year.
Not to be used with: MAOIs.
Contains: dextromethorphan hydrobromide.

Safeway Adult Chesty Cough Linctus see **Meltus Adult Expectorant**
(Safeway)

Safeway Cold Relief Tablets see **Flurex Tablets**
(Safeway)

Safeway Dry Cough Elixir see **Bronalin Dry Cough Elixir**
(Safeway)

Safeway Expectorant Linctus see **Bronalin Expectorant Linctus**
(Safeway)

Safeway Family Cough Linctus see **Meltus Honey and Lemon**
(Safeway)

Safeway Real Lemon Cold Powders see **Lemsip**
(Safeway)

Secron
(E. C. De Witt)

A syrup used as a sympathomimetic decongestant and expectorant to treat nasal congestion associated with colds and chesty coughs in children.

Dose: 2.5-10 ml (according to age) 2-3 times a day.
Side effects: rapid or abnormal heart rate, dry mouth, excitement, anxiety, shaking hands.
Caution: asthmatics should consult a doctor or pharmacist

before using this product, because prescribed medication may be affected.

Not to be used for: children under 2 years, or for patients with high blood pressure, overactive thyroid, heart disease, diabetes.

Not to be used with: MAOIs, tricyclic antidepressants, beta-blockers, antihypertensives.

Contains: ephedrine hydrochloride, ipecacuanha.

Sinotar
(Lane)

A tablet used as an antiseptic, soothing, and expectorant herbal remedy to relieve the symptoms of sinusitis and catarrh.

Dose: adults 2 tablets (children aged 5-12 years 1 tablet) 3 times a day before meals.

Side effects:

Caution:

Not to be used for: children under 5 years, pregnant women, or nursing mothers.

Not to be used with:

Contains: elderflower, marshmallow root, echinacea.

Sinutab
(Warner Wellcome Consumer Healthcare)

A tablet used as an analgesic and sympathomimetic decongestant to treat nasal and sinus congestion, headache, and pain.

Dose: adults 2 tablets 3 times a day, (children aged 6-12 years, half the adult dose).

Side effects: rapid or abnormal heart rate, dry mouth, excitement, anxiety, shaking hands.

Caution: asthmatics, diabetics, and patients with angina, overactive thyroid, heart disease, or a high fever should consult a doctor before using this product.

Not to be used for: children under 6, pregnant women, or patients with high blood pressure.

Not to be used with: MAOIs, tricyclic antidepressants, beta-blockers, antihypertensives, other medicines containing paracetamol.

Contains: phenylpropanolamine hydrochloride, paracetamol.

Sinutab Night-time
(Warner Wellcome Consumer Healthcare)

A tablet used as an analgesic, antihistamine, and sympathomimetic decongestant to treat nasal and sinus congestion, headache, and pain at night.

Dose: 1 tablet at night.

Side effects: drowsiness, rapid or abnormal heart rate, dry mouth, excitement, anxiety, shaking hands.

Caution: asthmatics and patients taking prescribed medication should consult a doctor before using this product.

Not to be used for: children under 12 years, pregnant women, or patients with high blood pressure, thyroid disease, heart disease, diabetes.

Not to be used with: MAOIs, tricyclic antidepressants, beta-blockers, antihypertensives, other sedating medicines, alcohol, other medicines containing paracetamol.

Contains: phenylpropanolamine hydrochloride, paracetamol, phenyltoloxamine citrate.

squill linctus, opiate see Gee's linctus

Sudafed
(Warner Wellcome Consumer Healthcare)

A tablet and elixir used as a sympathomimetic decongestant to relieve nasal congestion.

Dose: adults 1 tablet or 10 ml elixir 4 times a day; children 2.5-5 ml elixir (according to age) 4 times a day.

Side effects: anxiety, rapid or abnormal heart rate, dry mouth, excitement, shaking hands.

Caution: pregnant women, asthmatics, and patients taking prescribed medication should consult a doctor before using this product.

Not to be used for: children under 2 years, or for patients suffering from high blood pressure, overactive thyroid, heart disease, or diabetes.

Not to be used with: MAOIs, tricyclic antidepressants, beta-blockers, antihypertensives.

Contains: pseudoephedrine hydrochloride.

Sudafed-Co
(Warner Wellcome Consumer Healthcare)

A tablet used as an analgesic, antihistamine, and sympathomimetic decongestant to treat nasal congestion, pain, and fever.

Dose: adults 1 tablet (children aged 6-12 years ½ tablet) 4 times a day.

Side effects: rapid or abnormal heart rate, dry mouth, excitement, anxiety, shaking hands.

Caution: asthmatics, diabetics and patients with angina, overactive thyroid, heart disease or a high fever should consult a doctor before using this product.

Not to be used for: children under 6 years, pregnant women, or patients with high blood pressure.

Not to be used with: MAOIs, tricyclic antidepressants, beta-blockers, antihypertensives, other medicines containing paracetamol.

Contains: pseudoephedrine hydrochloride, paracetamol.

Sudafed Expectorant
(Warner Wellcome Consumer Healthcare)

A liquid used as a sympathomimetic decongestant and expectorant treatment for chesty coughs, nasal congestion, and blocked sinuses.

Dose: adults 10 ml (children aged 6-12 years 5 ml, children aged 2-5 years 2.5 ml) 4 times a day.
Side effects: rapid or abnormal heart rate, dry mouth, excitement, anxiety, shaking hands.
Caution: pregnant women, asthmatics, and patients taking other medication should consult a doctor before using this product, because prescribed medication may be affected.
Not to be used for: children under 2 years, or patients with high blood pressure, overactive thyroid, heart disease, diabetes.
Not to be used with: MAOIs, tricyclic antidepressants, beta-blockers, antihypertensives.
Contains: pseudoephedrine hydrochloride, guaiphenesin.

Sudafed Linctus
(Warner Wellcome Consumer Healthcare)

A linctus used as a sympathomimetic decongestant and opiate cough suppressant to treat dry tickly coughs, blocked sinuses, and nasal congestion.

Dose: adults 10 ml (children aged 6-12 years 5 ml, children aged 2-5 years 2.5 ml) 4 times a day.
Side effects: rapid or abnormal heart rate, dry mouth, excitement, anxiety, shaking hands, constipation, dependence.
Caution: pregnant women, asthmatics and patients taking other medication should consult a doctor before using this product.
Not to be used for: children under 2 years, or patients with high blood pressure, overactive thyroid, heart disease, diabetes.
Not to be used with: MAOIs, tricyclic antidepressants, beta-blockers, antihypertensives.

Contains: dextromethorphan hydrobromide, pseudoephedrine hydrochloride.

Sudafed Plus
(Warner Wellcome Consumer Healthcare)

A tablet and syrup used as an antihistamine, sympathomimetic treatment for allergic rhinitis.

Dose: adults 1 tablet or 10 ml syrup 4 times a day; children 2.5-5 ml syrup (according to age) 4 times a day.
Side effects: drowsiness, rash, dry mouth, excitement, anxiety, rapid or abnormal heart rate, shaking hands.
Caution: asthmatics and patients with raised eye pressure or enlarged prostate should consult a doctor before using this product.
Not to be used for: children under 2 years, or for patients suffering from high blood pressure, heart disease, overactive thyroid, diabetes.
Not to be used with: MAOIs, alcohol, other sedating medicines, tricyclic antidepressants, beta-blockers, antihypertensives.
Contains: triprolidine hydrochloride, pseudoephedrine hydrochloride.

Tancolin
(Roche Consumer Healthcare)

A liquid used as an opiate cough suppressant to treat coughs associated with upper respiratory tract infection or inflammation in children.

Dose: 2.5-15 ml (according to age) up to 3 times a day.
Side effects: constipation, dependence.
Caution: asthmatics should consult a doctor or pharmacist before using this product.

Not to be used for: children under 6 months.
Not to be used with: MAOIs.
Contains: dextromethorphan hydrobromide, vitamin C.

Terpoin
(Hough, Hoseason)

An elixir used as an opiate cough suppressant to treat dry coughs.

Dose: 5 ml every 3 hours.
Side effects: constipation, dependence.
Caution: patients suffering from asthma should consult a doctor or pharmacist before using this product.
Not to be used for: children under 16 years.
Not to be used with: MAOIs.
Contains: codeine phosphate.

Throaties Catarrh Pastilles see **Ernest Jackson's Catarrh Pastilles**
(Ernest Jackson)

Throaties Family Cough Linctus
(Ernest Jackson)

A liquid used as an expectorant and soothing treatment for sore throats and tickly coughs.

Dose: adults 10 ml (children 5 ml) 3 times a day.
Side effects:
Caution:
Not to be used for:
Not to be used with:
Contains: glycerol, honey, citric acid, terpeneless lemon oil, ipecacuanha.

Throaties Pastilles
(Ernest Jackson)

A pastille available in various flavours and used as an aromatic decongestant for coughs and colds.

Dose: suck 1 pastille when required. (Maximum ½ pack in 24 hours for children under 5 years, 1 pack in 24 hours for adults and older children.)
Side effects:
Caution:
Not to be used for:
Not to be used with:
Contains: benzoin tincture, menthol. (Throaties Extra also contain aniseed oil.)

Tixylix Chesty Cough
(Intercare)

A linctus used as an expectorant to loosen chesty coughs in children.

Dose: 2.5-10 ml according to age.
Side effects:
Caution:
Not to be used for: children under 1 year.
Not to be used with: cough suppressants.
Contains: guaiphenesin.

Tixylix Cough & Cold
(Intercare)

A linctus used as a sympathomimetic decongestant, opiate cough suppressant, and antihistamine treatment for dry coughs and nasal congestion in children.

Dose: 2.5-10 ml up to 3 times a day, according to age.
Side effects: drowsiness, constipation, dependence, rapid or abnormal heart rate, dry mouth, excitement, anxiety, shaking hands.
Caution: asthmatics and children taking other medicines should be seen by a doctor or pharmacist before using this product.
Not to be used for: children under 1 year, or for patients with high blood pressure, overactive thyroid, heart disease, diabetes.
Not to be used with: MAOIs, tricyclic antidepressants, beta-blockers, antihypertensives, other sedating medicines.
Contains: pseudoephedrine hydrochloride, chlorpheniramine maleate, pholcodine.

Tixylix Daytime
(Intercare)

A linctus used as an opiate cough suppressant to treat dry coughs in children.

Dose: 2.5-10 ml every 6 hours, according to age.
Side effects: constipation, dependence.
Caution: asthmatics and children taking other medicines should be seen by a doctor or pharmacist before using this product.
Not to be used for: children under 1 year.
Not to be used with: MAOIs.
Contains: pholcodine.

Tixylix Night-time
(Intercare)

A linctus used as an opiate cough suppressant and antihistamine treatment for dry coughs in children, particularly at night.

Dose: 2.5-10 ml 2-3 times a day, according to age.
Side effects: drowsiness, constipation, dependence.

Caution: asthmatics and children taking other medicines should be seen by a doctor or pharmacist before using this product.
Not to be used for: children under 1 year, or for more than 7 days (except on medical advice).
Not to be used with: MAOIs, other sedating medicines.
Contains: pholcodine, promethazine hydrochloride.

Triogesic see **Sinutab**
(Intercare)

Triominic
(Intercare)

A tablet used as an antihistamine and sympathomimetic decongestant treatment for nasal congestion and allergic rhinitis (including hayfever).

Dose: adults 1 tablet (children aged 6-12 years ½ tablet) up to 4 times a day.
Side effects: drowsiness, rapid or abnormal heart rate, dry mouth, excitement, anxiety, shaking hands.
Caution: asthmatics should consult a doctor or pharmacist before using this product, because prescribed medication may be affected.
Not to be used for: children under 6 years, or for patients with high blood pressure, overactive thyroid, heart disease, diabetes.
Not to be used with: MAOIs, tricyclic antidepressants, beta-blockers, antihypertensives, other sedating medicines, alcohol.
Contains: phenylpropanolamine hydrochloride, pheniramine maleate.

Tunes
(Mars)

A medicated sweet available in various flavours, used as an aromatic decongestant to assist breathing when congested.

Dose: 1 sucked when required. Adults: maximum of 6 packs (older children 4 packs, younger children 2 packs) in 24 hours.
Side effects:
Caution:
Not to be used for:
Not to be used with:
Contains: menthol.

Unichem Catarrh Pastilles see **Ernest Jackson's Catarrh Pastilles**
(Unichem)

Unichem Cold Relief Capsules see **Lemsip Capsules**
(Reckitt & Colman)

Unichem Cold Relief Powders see **Lemplus Powders**
(Unichem)

Unichem Day Cold Relief
(Unichem)

A liquid used as an analgesic, sympathomimetic decongestant and cough suppressant to treat headache, runny nose, sore throat, tickly cough, fever, and pain associated with colds and influenza.

Dose: adults 30 ml liquid every 4 hours (up to 4 times a day); children aged 6-12 years, half the adult dose.
Side effects: rapid or abnormal heart rate, dry mouth, excitement, anxiety, shaking hands, constipation, dependence.
Caution: asthmatics or patients already receiving medical advice or treatment (or who have chronic bronchitis) should consult a doctor before using this product.
Not to be used for: children under 6 years or patients with high blood pressure, overactive thyroid, heart disease, diabetes.

Not for prolonged use.

Not to be used with: MAOIs, tricyclic antidepressants, beta-blockers, antihypertensives, other medicines containing paracetamol.

Contains: pholcodine, pseudoephedrine hydrochloride, paracetamol.

Unichem Night Cold Relief
(Unichem)

A liquid used as an analgesic, sympathomimetic decongestant, antihistamine, and cough suppressant to treat headache, runny nose, sore throat, tickly cough, pain, and fever associated with colds and influenza at night-time.

Dose: 30 ml liquid at night.

Side effects: rapid or abnormal heart rate, dry mouth, excitement, anxiety, shaking hands, constipation, dependence, drowsiness.

Caution: asthmatics or patients already receiving medical advice or treatment (or who have chronic bronchitis) should consult a doctor before using this product.

Not to be used for: children under 12 years or patients with high blood pressure, overactive thyroid, glaucoma, enlarged prostate, heart disease, diabetes. Not for prolonged use.

Not to be used with: MAOIs, tricyclic antidepressants, beta-blockers, antihypertensives, other medicines containing paracetamol, other sedating medicines, alcohol.

Contains: pholcodine, pseudoephedrine hydrochloride, paracetamol, diphenhydramine hydrochloride.

Uniflu & Gregovite C
(Unigreg)

A lilac Uniflu tablet and a yellow Gregovite C tablet used as an analgesic, opiate, sympathomimetic decongestant stimulant and antihistamine treatment for cold and flu symptoms.

Dose: 1 each of the tablets every 6 hours (maximum of 4 Uniflu tablets in 24 hours for adults, or 3 in 24 hours for children over 12 years).

Side effects: constipation, drowsiness, anxiety, shaking hands, irregular or rapid heart rate, dry mouth, excitement, dependence.

Caution: asthmatics should consult a doctor before using this product.

Not to be used for: children under 12 years, or for patients suffering from heart disease, overactive thyroid, high blood pressure, or diabetes.

Not to be used with: MAOIs, alcohol, tricyclic antidepressants, beta-blockers, antihypertensives, other sedating medicines, other medicines containing paracetamol.

Contains: Uniflu tablets: paracetamol, codeine phosphate, caffeine, diphenhydramine hydrochloride, phenylephrine hydrochloride; Gregovite C tablets: vitamin C.

Valda Pastilles see entry in 'Diseases of the mouth and throat' section
(Seton Healthcare)

Vegetable Cough Remover
(Potters)

A mixture used as a herbal expectorant and antispasmodic remedy to relieve the symptoms of coughs.

Dose: adults 10 ml 3-4 times a day; children over 8 years 5 ml 3 times a day; children aged 5-7 years 5 ml twice a day.

Side effects:

Caution: pregnant women and nursing mothers should consult a doctor before using this product.

Not to be used for: children under 5 years.

Not to be used with:
Contains: black cohosh, ipecacuanha, lobelia, pleurisy root, scullcap, elecampane, horehound, hyssop.

Venos Dry Cough
(SmithKline Beecham Healthcare)

A mixture used as a soothing treatment for dry hacking coughs.

Dose: adults 10 ml every 2-3 hours. (Children aged 3-12 years half the adult dose.)
Side effects:
Caution: children under 3 years should be seen by a doctor before using this product.
Not to be used for:
Not to be used with:
Contains: liquid glucose, treacle.

Venos Expectorant
(SmithKline Beecham Healthcare)

A mixture used as an expectorant to treat chesty coughs.

Dose: adults 10 ml every 2-3 hours; children aged 3-12 years, half the adult dose.
Side effects:
Caution:
Not to be used for: children under 3 years.
Not to be used with:
Contains: guaiphenesin, liquid glucose, treacle.

Venos Honey and Lemon
(SmithKline Beecham Healthcare)

A mixture used as a soothing treatment for dry tickly coughs.

Dose: 5-15 ml every 2-3 hours (according to age). Maximum dose 120 ml in 24 hours for adults, 20-60 ml in 24 hours for children (according to age).
Side effects:
Caution:
Not to be used for: children under 1 year.
Not to be used with:
Contains: lemon juice, purified honey, liquid glucose.

Vicks Action
(Procter & Gamble)

A tablet used as a non-steroidal anti-inflammatory and sympathomimetic decongestant treatment for pain, headache, fever, sore throat, blocked nose and sinuses.

Dose: 2 tablets initially, then 1 or 2 tablets every 4 hours if required. (Maximum of 6 tablets per day.) Maximum suggested treatment period 3 days.
Side effects: stomach discomfort, nausea, diarrhoea, stomach ulcers, rapid or abnormal heart rate, dry mouth, anxiety, excitement, shaking hands, rash, rarely blood disorders.
Caution: elderly patients may require reduced doses. Asthmatics, pregnant women, nursing mothers, and patients taking other medication should consult a doctor before taking this product.
Not to be used for: children under 12 years, patients with stomach ulcers or other stomach disorder, heart disease, glaucoma, enlarged prostate, asthma, allergy to aspirin or anti-inflammatory drugs, high blood pressure, overactive thyroid, or diabetes.
Not to be used with: antihypertensives, MAOIs, tricyclic antidepressants, beta-blockers, some antibiotics.
Contains: ibuprofen, pseudoephedrine hydrochloride.

Vicks Coldcare see **Day Nurse Capsules**
(Procter & Gamble)

Vicks Medinite
(Proctor & Gamble)

A liquid used as a sympathomimetic decongestant, opiate cough suppressant, analgesic, and antihistamine treatment for pain, dry cough and, nasal congestion.

Dose: adults 30 ml (children aged 10-12 years 15 ml) at bedtime.
Side effects: rapid or abnormal heart rate, dry mouth, excitement, anxiety, shaking hands, constipation, dependence.
Caution: pregnant women, asthmatics, and patients receiving medical treatment or prescribed medicines should consult a doctor before using this product.
Not to be used for: children under 10 years, or for patients with high blood pressure, overactive thyroid, heart disease, diabetes.
Not to be used with: MAOIs, tricyclic antidepressants, beta-blockers, antihypertensive, other sedating medicines, alcohol, other medicines containing paracetamol.
Contains: dextromethorphan hydrobromide, pseudoephedrine hydrochloride, doxylamine succinate, paracetamol.

Vicks Original Formula (Chesty Cough)
(Proctor & Gamble)

A liquid used as an expectorant and antiseptic to treat chesty coughs.

Dose: adults 10 ml (children aged 6-12 years 5 ml) every 3 hours if needed.
Side effects:
Caution:

442

Not to be used for: children under 6 years.
Not to be used with:
Contains: guaiphenesin, cetylpyridinium chloride.

Vicks Original Formula (Dry/Tickly Cough)
(Proctor & Gamble)

A liquid used as a soothing and aromatic decongestant treatment for dry coughs associated with colds.

Dose: adults 10 ml (children aged 6-12 years 5 ml) every 3-4 hours, up to 6 times a day.
Side effects:
Caution:
Not to be used for: children under 6 years.
Not to be used with:
Contains: levomenthol, honey.

Vicks Vaposyrup Chesty Cough
(Proctor & Gamble)

A liquid used as an expectorant to treat chesty coughs and congestion in the upper chest.

Dose: adults 15 ml (children aged 6-11 years 10 ml, children aged 2-5 years 5 ml) up to 6 times a day.
Side effects:
Caution: children under 2 years should be seen by a doctor before using this medicine.
Not to be used for:
Not to be used with:
Contains: guaiphenesin.

Vicks Vaposyrup Chesty Cough and Blocked Nose
(Proctor & Gamble)

A liquid used as a sympathomimetic decongestant and expectorant to treat chesty coughs and blocked nose.

Dose: adults 15 ml (children aged 6-11 years 5 ml) up to 4 times a day, for a maximum of 7 days.
Side effects: rapid or abnormal heart rate, dry mouth, excitement, anxiety, shaking hands.
Caution: pregnant women, asthmatics, and patients receiving medical treatment or taking prescribed medication should consult a doctor before using this product.
Not to be used for: children under 6 years, patients with high blood pressure, overactive thyroid, heart disease, diabetes.
Not to be used with: MAOIs, tricyclic antidepressants, beta-blockers, antihypertensives.
Contains: guaiphenesin, phenylpropanolamine hydrochloride.

Vicks Vaposyrup Children's Dry Cough
(Proctor & Gamble)

A liquid used as an opiate cough suppressant to treat dry tickly coughs.

Dose: children aged 3-5 years 7.5 ml (aged 6-11 years 15 ml) up to 4 times a day.
Side effects: constipation, dependence.
Caution: children under 3 years, asthmatics, and patients taking other medications should consult a doctor before using this product.
Not to be used for:
Not to be used with: MAOIs.
Contains: dextromethorphan.

Vicks Vaposyrup Dry Cough
(Proctor & Gamble)

A liquid containing an opiate cough suppressant, used to treat dry coughs and to coat the throat.

Dose: adults 15 ml (children aged 6-11 years 5 ml) up to 4 times a day.
Side effects: constipation, dependence.
Caution: children under 6 years and asthmatics should consult a doctor before using this product.
Not to be used for:
Not to be used with: MAOIs.
Contains: dextromethorphan hydrobromide.

Vicks Vaposyrup Dry Cough and Blocked Nose
(Proctor & Gamble)

A liquid containing an opiate cough suppressant and sympathomimetic decongestant, used to treat dry coughs and blocked nose.

Dose: adults 15 ml (children aged 6-11 years 5 ml) up to 4 times a day.
Side effects: rapid or abnormal heart rate, dry mouth, excitement, anxiety, shaking hands, constipation, dependence.
Caution: pregnant women, asthmatics, and patients receiving medical treatment or taking prescribed medicines should consult a doctor before using this product.
Not to be used for: patients with high blood pressure, overactive thyroid, heart disease, diabetes.
Not to be used with: MAOIs, tricyclic antidepressants, beta-blockers, antihypertensives.
Contains: dextromethorphan hydrobromide, phenyl-propanolamine hydrochloride.

Victory V
(Ernest Jackson)

A lozenge used as a soothing, expectorant, and aromatic decongestant preparation to treat coughs and sore throats.

Dose: 1 lozenge sucked when required. (Maximum 4 packets in 24 hours.)
Side effects:
Caution:
Not to be used for:
Not to be used with:
Contains: menthol, liquorice powder.

Weleda Cough Drops
(Weleda)

A liquid used as a herbal remedy to relieve the symptoms of irritating coughs.

Dose: 10-20 drops every 2 hours, taken in warm water.
Side effects:
Caution:
Not to be used for: children, pregnant women, or nursing mothers.
Not to be used with: some homeopathic remedies.
Contains: angelica root, cinnamon, clove, coriander, lemon oil, lemon balm, nutmeg, aqua cherry laurel, alcohol.

Weleda Cough Elixir
(Weleda)

A liquid used as a natural herbal expectorant to treat coughs.

Dose: adults 10 ml (children aged 6-12 years 5 ml) every 3-4 hours (up to 4 times a day).

Side effects:
Caution:
Not to be used for: children under 6 years, or for diabetics.
Not to be used with:
Contains: aniseed, thyme, horehound, marshmallow, ipecacuanha, drosera, pulsatilla.

Zubes
(Ernest Jackson)

A lozenge available in various flavours, and used as an aromatic decongestant to treat coughs and congestion.

Dose: suck one lozenge every 30 minutes (adults), every hour (children over 6 years), or every 2 hours (children under 6 years).
Side effects:
Caution:
Not to be used for:
Not to be used with:
Contains: menthol. (Some flavours also contain aniseed oil, citric acid, or lemon oil.)

Respiratory conditions

2 Inhaled remedies

Runny nose is usually due to allergy, such as hayfever (see 'Allergic disorders' section), or the common cold (see 'Respiratory conditions – cough and cold remedies' section). Sinusitis may present as persistent runny nose, or as tender, congested areas of the face (resulting in headache) if the sinus entrances are blocked. Steam inhalations help to widen the narrow sinus passages, allowing the trapped catarrh to clear, and the heat helps to relieve discomfort. (Aromatic products such as menthol are also of help in clearing nasal congestion, and may be used in hot water to add to the steam inhaled.) Sinusitis that persists for more than a few days may be the result of infected catarrh, in which case a doctor should be consulted.

Persistent nasal drip and sinus congestion may respond to sympathomimetic drugs which narrow the blood vessels and restrict leaking of fluid into the nose. These drugs, when applied inside the nose, should not be used repeatedly or for longer than 1 week.

Afrazine
(Schering-Plough)

A spray used as a sympathomimetic decongestant for blocked nose.

Dose: adults and children over 5 years 2-3 sprays in each nostril twice a day. Use for a maximum of 7 days.
Side effects: itching nose, headache, rapid heart rate.
Caution: pregnant women and patients suffering from heart disease should consult a doctor before using this product.
Not to be used for: children under 5 years.
Not to be used with: MAOIs.
Contains: oxymetazoline hydrochloride.

---

benzoin tincture compound see **friars' balsam BP**

Boots Decongestant Nasal Spray see **Sudafed Nasal Spray**
(Boots)

Boots Vapour Rub see **Vicks Vaporub**
(Boots)

Boots Vapour Stick see **Vicks Vaporub**
(Boots)

Catarrh Cream
(Weleda)

A cream used as an aromatic herbal decongestant to relieve the symptoms of catarrhal congestion and inflamed nasal passages.

Dose: insert a small quantity into each nostril as required.

Side effects:
Caution:
Not to be used for: children under 3 years or pregnant women.
Not to be used with: homeopathic remedies.
Contains: aesculin, barberry, blackthorn, bryonia 3x, camphor, echinacea, mercurius sulphuratus 5x, eucalyptus oil, thyme oil.

Cupal Baby Chest Rub
(Cupal)

An ointment used as an aromatic decongestant to treat congestion and catarrh in babies and children.

Dose: apply to chest, throat, and back twice a day.
Side effects: irritation.
Caution: keep away from the eyes.
Not to be used for: babies under 3 months, or for application to the nostrils.
Not to be used with:
Contains: turpentine oil, menthol, eucalyptus oil.

Dristan Spray
(Whitehall Laboratories)

A spray used as a sympathomimetic decongestant treatment for nasal catarrh due to colds, hayfever, or allergy.

Dose: 1 or 2 sprays (according to age) into each nostril every 8-12 hours. Use for a maximum of 7 days.
Side effects: stinging or irritation, rapid or abnormal heart rate.
Caution: pregnant women and patients suffering from heart disease should consult a doctor before using this product.
Not to be used for: children under 6 years.
Not to be used with: MAOIs.
Contains: oxymetazoline hydrochloride.

Easy Breathers*
(Robinson Healthcare)

A tissue impregnated with aromatic decongestants.

Dose: hold the tissue under the nose and breathe in the vapours.
Side effects:
Caution: avoid contact with the eyes.
Not to be used for: children under 6 months.
Not to be used with:
Contains: camphor, menthol, methylsalicylate equivalent, nutmeg oil, pine oil.

---

ephedrine nasal drops BP

A nose drop available in two strengths (0.5 % and 1 %) and used as a sympathomimetic decongestant to treat congestion in the nose.

Dose: 1-2 drops in each nostril up to 3-4 times a day when required. (Children should use the weaker strength product.)
Side effects: irritation, congestion, and less effect after excessive use.
Caution: asthmatics and children under 3 years should be seen by a doctor before using this product. Avoid swallowing the solution.
Not to be used for: more than 5 days (except on medical advice).
Not to be used with: MAOIs.
Contains: ephedrine hydrochloride.

---

eucalyptus oil BP

An oil used as an aromatic decongestant to clear blocked nose.

Dose: place a few drops on to a handkerchief and inhale the

vapour, or add a few drops to hot (not boiling) water and inhale the steam.
Side effects: contact with skin may cause irritation.
Caution: avoid the eyes.
Not to be used for:
Not to be used with:
Contains: eucalyptus oil.

Fenox
(Seton Healthcare)

A nasal spray or drops used as a sympathomimetic decongestant to treat nasal congestion.

Dose: adults 4-5 drops or two sprays in each nostril twice a day (or every 4 hours if needed). Children aged 5-12 years use half adult dose.
Side effects:
Caution: patients suffering from high blood pressure or heart disease, or taking other medication should consult a doctor before using this product.
Not to be used for: children under 5 years, or for more than 7 days.
Not to be used with: MAOIs.
Contains: phenylephrine hydrochloride.

---

friars' balsam BP

A liquid containing an aromatic decongestant to relieve nasal congestion.

Dose: add 5 ml to 1 pint of hot (not boiling) water and inhale the vapour.
Side effects:
Caution:
Not to be used for: infants under 3 months.

Not to be used with:
Contains: compound benzoin tincture BP.

Hills Inhalant Capsules
(Windsor Healthcare)

A capsule containing aromatic decongestants in oil, used to relieve nasal congestion.

Dose: sprinkle the contents of 1 capsule on to a handkerchief and hang out of reach of young children. (Older children and adults may have contents applied to clothing or added to hot water and used as a steam inhalation.)
Side effects:
Caution: not to be swallowed. Avoid contact with eyes, nostrils, and skin.
Not to be used for: children under 3 months.
Not to be used with:
Contains: natural menthol, pine oil, eucalyptus oil, lemon oil.

Karvol
(Crookes Healthcare)

A capsule containing aromatic decongestants in oil, used to relieve nasal congestion.

Dose: sprinkle the contents of one capsule on to a handkerchief and hang out of reach of young children. (Older children and adults may have contents applied to bedding or added to hot water and used as a steam inhalation.)
Side effects:
Caution: not to be swallowed. Avoid contact with eyes, nostrils, and skin.
Not to be used for: children under 3 months.
Not to be used with:
Contains: chlorbutol, levomenthol, pine oil sylvestris, terpineol,

thymol, pumilio pine oil.

Labmist*
(LAB)

A nasal spray used to treat dryness of the nasal passages (including that caused by central heating and low humidity) in adults, and to clear children's noses.

Dose:
Side effects:
Caution:
Not to be used for:
Not to be used with:
Contains: sodium chloride.

Mackenzies Smelling Salts
(Cox Pharmaceuticals)

A solution used as an aromatic decongestant to treat catarrh and head colds.

Dose: inhale as required.
Side effects:
Caution:
Not to be used for: children under 3 months.
Not to be used with:
Contains: strong ammonia solution, eucalyptus oil.

menthol crystals

A crystal used as an aromatic decongestant to treat congestion in the nose.

Dose: place a few crystals in hot water and inhale the vapour.
Side effects:

Caution: avoid contact with the eyes or skin.
Not to be used for:
Not to be used with:
Contains: menthol.

---

menthol and benzoin inhalation BP

A liquid containing an aromatic decongestant to relieve nasal congestion.

Dose: add 5 ml to 1 pint of hot (not boiling) water and inhale the vapour.
Side effects:
Caution:
Not to be used for: infants under 3 months.
Not to be used with:
Contains: menthol, benzoin.

---

menthol and eucalyptus inhalation BP 1980

A liquid containing an aromatic decongestant to relieve nasal congestion.

Dose: add 5 ml to 1 pint of hot (not boiling) water and inhale the vapour.
Side effects:
Caution:
Not to be used for: infants under 3 months.
Not to be used with:
Contains: menthol, eucalyptus oil.

Mentholair*
(Mentholatum)

A liquid containing aromatic decongestants, used in the bath to release aromatic vapours into the atmosphere, and help relieve symptoms of nasal congestion.

Dose: one measure added to hot bath water.
Side effects:
Caution:
Not to be used for:
Not to be used with:
Contains: menthol, eucalyptus, peppermint, rosemary, lavender.

Mentholatum
(Mentholatum)

An ointment used as an aromatic decongestant to treat congestion associated with colds. (For use in treating muscular disorders see 'Joint and muscle disorders' section. For use in treating skin problems see 'Skin disorders' section.)

Dose: apply to the chest, throat, and back 2-3 times a day, or add to hot water and inhale the vapour.
Side effects:
Caution: avoid the eyes, nose, and delicate skin.
Not to be used for: children under 1 year.
Not to be used with:
Contains: menthol, camphor, methyl salicylate.

Nostroline
(Bioglan)

An ointment used as an aromatic decongestant to relieve blocked and sore nose.

Dose: apply inside the nostrils every 4 hours. (May also be rubbed on to chest.)
Side effects: irritation.
Caution:

Not to be used for: children under 10 years.
Not to be used with:
Contains: eucalyptol, menthol, geranium oil.

Olbas Oil
(Lane)

A non-greasy oil used as an aromatic decongestant to relieve bronchial and nasal congestion. (For use as an application for muscular pain see 'Joint and muscle disorders' section.)

Dose: adults 3-4 drops (children aged over 2 years 1-2 drops) applied to a tissue and inhaled, or add to hot water for steam inhalation. (For children aged 3 months-2 years, apply 1 drop to a tissue and hang out of reach of child.)
Side effects: stinging, rash.
Caution: avoid contact with the eyes, and with plastic or delicate surfaces. Children should be strictly supervised with this product, particularly if used in hot water.
Not to be used for: babies under 3 months, or on broken skin.
Not to be used with:
Contains: cajuput oil, clove oil, eucalyptus oil, juniper berry oil, menthol, mint oil, wintergreen oil.

Oleum Rhinale
(Weleda)

An oil used as a herbal remedy to relieve the symptoms of catarrh, sinus congestion, and dry rhinitis.

Dose: 2-4 drops distilled into and around the opening of each nostril twice a day.
Side effects:
Caution:
Not to be used for:
Not to be used with: homeopathic remedies.

Contains: marigold, mercurius sulphuratus ruber 3x, peppermint oil, eucalyptus oil.

Otrivine
(Zyma Healthcare)

An adult-strength nose drop and spray (0.1 %) and a children's formula nose drop (0.05 %) used as a sympathomimetic decongestant to relieve nasal congestion, rhinitis, and sinusitis.

Dose: adults 2-3 drops or 1 spray in each nostril 2-3 times a day, children 1-2 drops of children's formula in each nostril once or twice a day. Use for a maximum of 7 days.
Side effects: stinging, sneezing, dry nose, headache, heart rhythm disturbance.
Caution: pregnant women and patients with heart disease should consult a doctor before using this product. Children under 2 years should be treated only on the advice of a doctor.
Not to be used for: babies under 3 months, or for patients who have undergone surgery on parts of the skull and brain.
Not to be used with: MAOIs.
Contains: xylometazoline hydrochloride.

Penetrol Inhalant
(Seton Healthcare)

A liquid used as an aromatic decongestant to relieve nasal congestion.

Dose: add a few drops to a handkerchief and inhale the vapour.
Side effects:
Caution: avoid contact with eyes.
Not to be used for: children under 3 months.
Not to be used with:
Contains: menthol, peppermint oil.

---

peppermint oil*

A liquid used as an aromatic decongestant to relieve the symptoms of nasal congestion when inhaled. (For use as a stomach-calming product see 'Stomach preparations' section.)

Dose: sprinkle a few drops on a handkerchief, or add a few drops to hot (not boiling) water and inhale the vapour.
Side effects:
Caution:
Not to be used for:
Not to be used with:
Contains: peppermint.

Snufflebabe
(Pickles)

A mild vapour rub containing aromatic decongestants, used to treat congestion in small children.

Dose: rub on to chest and throat, or apply to a handkerchief placed in the child's clothing. (For very young children, tie the handkerchief out of reach.)
Side effects:
Caution: children under 3 months should be seen by a doctor before using this product. Keep away from eyes.
Not to be used for: application to nostrils.
Not to be used with:
Contains: eucalyptus oil, menthol, thyme oil.

---

sodium chloride nasal drops

Drops used to liquefy mucous secretions and clear nasal congestion.

Dose: 1-2 drops in each nostril when required. (Babies should

be treated before feeds.)
Side effects:
Caution: babies should be seen by a doctor before starting treatment.
Not to be used for:
Not to be used with:
Contains: sodium chloride.

Sudafed Nasal Spray
(Wellcome)

A spray used as a sympathomimetic decongestant treatment for colds, hayfever, allergy, or sinusitis.

Dose: 1 or 2 sprays into each nostril 2 or 3 times a day, as required.
Side effects: stinging or irritation.
Caution: pregnant women, nursing mothers, and patients using other medications should consult a doctor before using this product.
Not to be used for: children under 6 years.
Not to be used with: MAOIs.
Contains: oxymetazoline hydrochloride.

Tixylix Decongestant Inhalant
(Intercare)

A capsule containing aromatic decongestants, used to treat nasal congestion.

Dose: sprinkle the contents of one capsule on to a handkerchief and hang out of reach of young children. (Older children and adults may have contents applied to bedding or added to hot water and used as a steam inhalation.)
Side effects:
Caution: not to be swallowed. Avoid contact with eyes, nostrils,

and skin.
Not to be used for: children under 3 months.
Not to be used with:
Contains: camphor, menthol, turpentine oil, eucalyptus oil.

Vicks Inhaler
(Procter & Gamble)

An aromatic decongestant in a stick used to clear stuffy nose.

Dose: insert stick into nostril and inhale the vapour when required.
Side effects:
Caution:
Not to be used for:
Not to be used with:
Contains: menthol, camphor, oil of pine needles.

Vicks Sinex
(Procter & Gamble)

A nasal spray used as a sympathomimetic decongestant and aromatic decongestant to treat nasal congestion.

Dose: 1-2 sprays every 6-8 hours for up to 7 days.
Side effects:
Caution:
Not to be used for: children under 6 years.
Not to be used with: MAOIs.
Contains: oxymetazoline hydrochloride, menthol, eucalyptol.

Vicks Vaporub
(Procter & Gamble)

An aromatic decongestant rub used to treat nasal congestion due to colds.

Dose: rub on to chest and back. (Adults and older children may also rub on to throat, or may add it to hot water to use as a steam inhalation.)
Side effects:
Caution: do not use inside nostrils.
Not to be used for: children under 6 months.
Not to be used with:
Contains: menthol, camphor, eucalyptus oil, turpentine oil.

Wright's Vaporizer
(LRC)

An electrical vaporizing kit, used as a source of aromatic vapour to treat coughs, colds, and other upper respiratory tract infections at night.

Dose: 10 ml heated in the vaporizer at night. (Maximum of 10 ml in 8 hours.)
Side effects:
Caution: children under 2 years should not be treated except on the advice of a doctor or pharmacist.
Not to be used for:
Not to be used with:
Contains: chlorocresol.

462

Respiratory conditions

3   Bronchodilators

Bronchodilators, such as theophylline, open up the respiratory muscles controlling the size of the airways. Doctors prescribe them for use in asthma and related conditions, but they may be purchased over the counter in products used to treat bronchial coughs associated with wheezing. Any patient with wheezing or breathing difficulty, however, should consult a doctor rather than self-medicate. In particular, asthmatics should not use these products before taking medical advice because they may interfere with their usual asthma treatment.

Anestan
(Seton Healthcare)

A tablet used as a bronchodilator and sympathomimetic decongestant to treat wheezing and reversible bronchospasm associated with asthma.

Dose: 1-2 tablets when required. (Maximum of 4 tablets in 24 hours.)

Side effects: rapid or abnormal heart rate, dry mouth, excitement, anxiety, shaking hands, nausea, upset stomach, convulsions, sleeplessness, headache.

Caution: all users (but especially asthmatics, pregnant women, nursing mothers, the elderly, and patients taking other medications or suffering from epilepsy or fever) are advised to consult a doctor before using this product.

Not to be used for: children under 12 years and patients with high blood pressure, overactive thyroid, heart disease, diabetes, or porphyria (a blood disorder).

Not to be used with: MAOIs, tricyclic antidepressants, beta-blockers, antihypertensives, cimetidine, some anti-angina medications, some antibiotics, some anti-epileptics, some anti-asthma treatments, some antifungals, lithium, some oral contraceptives, cimetidine.

Contains: ephedrine hydrochloride, theophylline.

Do-do
(Zyma Healthcare)

A tablet used as a bronchodilator, stimulant, and sympathomimetic decongestant treatment for bronchial coughs, wheezing, and breathlessness.

Dose: 1 tablet up to 4 times a day. (Children over 12 years 1 tablet up to 3 times a day.)

Side effects: rapid or abnormal heart rate, dry mouth, excitement, anxiety, shaking hands, nausea, upset stomach, convulsions, sleeplessness, headache.

Caution: all users (but especially asthmatics, pregnant women, nursing mothers, the elderly, and patients taking other medications or suffering from epilepsy or fever) are advised to consult a doctor before using this product. Children under 12 years may only be treated after a doctor's recommendation.

Not to be used for: patients with high blood pressure, overactive thyroid, heart disease, diabetes, or porphyria (a blood disorder).

Not to be used with: MAOIs, tricyclic antidepressants, beta-blockers, antihypertensives, cimetidine, some anti-angina medications, some antibiotics, some anti-epileptics, some anti-asthma treatments, some anti-fungals, lithium, some oral contraceptives, excess tea or coffee.

Contains: ephedrine, caffeine, theophylline.

Franolyn For Chesty Coughs
(Centra Healthcare)

A liquid used as a sympathomimetic decongestant, bronchodilator, and expectorant to treat cough associated with bronchospasm (as in asthma, bronchitis, or hayfever).

Dose: adults 10 ml (children aged 7-12 years 5 ml) up to 4 times a day.

Side effects: rapid or abnormal heart rate, dry mouth, excitement, anxiety, shaking hands, nausea, upset stomach, convulsions, sleeplessness, headache.

Caution: all users (but especially asthmatics, pregnant women, nursing mothers, the elderly, and patients taking other medications or suffering from epilepsy or fever) are advised to consult a doctor before using this product. Children under 7 years may only be treated after a doctor's recommendation.

Not to be used for: patients with high blood pressure, overactive thyroid, heart disease, diabetes, or porphyria (a blood disorder).

Not to be used with: MAOIs, tricyclic antidepressants, beta-blockers, antihypertensives, cimetidine, some anti-angina medications, some antibiotics, some anti-epileptics, some anti-asthma treatments, some antifungals, lithium, some oral contraceptives.

Contains: guaiphenesin, theophylline, ephedrine.

Allergic disorders

Allergies can manifest themselves in many different forms, the commonest being skin rashes (as in urticaria or insect bites) and eye/nose irritation (as in hayfever). Anti-allergy treatments can either work at reducing the symptoms (i.e. cooling the skin with calamine, or unblocking the nose with decongestants), or can aim to reduce the allergy itself (with the products listed in this section). Some products combine anti-allergy ingredients with symptom-relieving ingredients. (In particular, decongestants are often found in antihistamine hayfever remedies.)

Antihistamines are available as creams (such as Anthisan) or tablets (such as Piriton) and work by reducing the histamine response produced by the body because of the allergy. Tablet forms are useful if the allergy is widespread or if swelling of the tissues has occurred, and creams are suitable for more localized skin allergies. (Severe swelling or any swelling of the mouth or throat should always be referred urgently to a doctor, however.) Many antihistamines have a sedative effect, but the newer ones are less likely to cause this problem. Note that antihistimines and anti-depressants should be used with care when driving or operating machinery, or if the patient is involved in important decision-making. Note, too, that the sedative effects of other drugs my be potentiated. (See individual product entries for details.)

Sodium cromoglycate is another useful anti-allergy ingredient, and can be found in the form of eye drops and nose drops or sprays, for eye and nose allergies (especially hayfever). This type of product needs to be used regularly throughout exposure to be effective. Topical steroid nose preparations (such as Beconase Hayfever) also need to be used regularly to produce an effect.

Sedating antihistamines are used as over-the-counter products to treat insomnia (see 'Sleeping problems' section). Some antihistamines are also used to treat and prevent travel sickness (see 'Stomach preparations' section).

Actifed see entry in 'Respiratory conditions – cough and cold remedies' section
(Warner Wellcome Consumer Healthcare)

Allereze
(Intercare)

A tablet used as an antihistamine to treat hayfever and other allergies, insect bites and stings.

Dose: ½-1 tablet twice a day, according to age.
Side effects: drowsiness.
Caution:
Not to be used for: children under 3 years, pregnant women, nursing mothers.
Not to be used with: other sedating drugs, alcohol.
Contains: clemastine.

Allereze Clear see **Triludan**
(Intercare)

Allereze Plus
(Intercare)

Tablets used as an antihistamine and decongestant treatment for hayfever and allergies with sinus or nasal congestion.

Dose: 1 tablet every 6 hours.
Side effects: rapid or abnormal heart rate, dry mouth, excitement, anxiety, shaking hands, drowsiness.
Caution: asthmatics should consult a doctor or pharmacist before using this product, because prescribed medication may be affected.
Not to be used for: children under 12 years, pregnant women, nursing mothers, and patients with high blood pressure, overactive thyroid, heart disease, diabetes.
Not to be used with: MAOIs, tricyclic antidepressants, beta-

blockers, antihypertensives, alcohol, other sedating medicines.
Contains: clemastine, phenylpropanolamine hydrochloride.

Anthisan
(Rhone-Poulenc Rorer Family Health)

An antihistamine cream used to relieve allergic skin reactions, including insect bites, stings, and nettle rash.

Dose: apply to the affected area 2-3 times a day for up to 3 days.
Side effects: rarely allergy.
Caution:
Not to be used for: areas of broken skin or eczema.
Not to be used with:
Contains: mepyramine maleate.

Beconase Hayfever
(Allen and Hanburys)

A spray used as a steroid treatment for sneezing and a runny, itchy, or blocked nose associated with hayfever. Doctors may prescribe this medication for different disorders. Self-medication should be limited to the conditions and doses stated.

Dose: 2 sprays into each nostril night and morning.
Side effects: irritation in throat or nose, nosebleeds.
Caution: pregnant women, nursing mothers, and patients with nasal infection or glaucoma should consult a doctor before using this product.
Not to be used for: children under 12 years.
Not to be used with:
Contains: beclomethasone dipropionate.

Boots Antihistamine Tablets see Triludan
(Boots)

Boots Hayfever Allergy Eye Drops see **Opticrom Allergy**
(Boots)

Boots One-a-day Antihistamine Tablets see **Triludan Forte**
(Boots)

Boots Pharmacy Skincare no. 5
(Boots)

A cream used as an antihistamine treatment to relieve pain
and irritation from insect bites and stings.

Dose: apply 2-3 times a day for up to 3 days.
Side effects: allergy.
Caution:
Not to be used for: application to broken skin or eczema.
Not to be used with:
Contains: mepyramine maleate.

Brol-eze see **Opticrom Allergy**
(Rhone-Poulenc Rorer Family Health)

Buttercup Pol 'N' Count
(Charwell Health Care)

A herbal remedy used to treat runny nose and eyes due to
hayfever.

Dose: 2 tablets 3 times a day.
Side effects:
Caution:
Not to be used for: children.
Not to be used with:
Contains: garlic, echinacea.

Caladryl
(Warner Wellcome Consumer Healthcare)

A cream or lotion used as an antihistamine and soothing preparation to relieve skin irritation and itching, shingles, prickly heat, and insect bite reactions.

Dose: apply 3-4 times a day.
Side effects: rash, burning.
Caution: avoid using near the eyes. Pregnant women and nursing mothers should consult a doctor before using this product.
Not to be used for: raw or broken skin, or for application to chicken pox, measles, or large areas of skin.
Not to be used with:
Contains: diphenhydramine hydrochloride, camphor, zinc oxide. (The lotion also contains calamine.)

Calimal see Piriton Tablets
(Sussex)

Clariteyes see Opticrom Allergy
(Schering-Plough Consumer Health)

Clarityn
(Schering-Plough Consumer Health)

A tablet used as an antihistamine treatment for allergic rhinitis, hayfever, and other allergies.

Dose: 1 tablet a day.
Side effects: rarely tiredness, headache, nausea.
Caution:
Not to be used for: children under 12 years, pregnant women, nursing mothers.
Not to be used with:

Contains: loratadine.

Dimotapp see entry in 'Respiratory conditions – cough and cold remedies' section
(Whitehall Laboratories)

Dristan see entry in 'Respiratory conditions – cough and cold remedies' section
(Whitehall Laboratories)

Eskornade see entry in 'Respiratory conditions – cough and cold remedies' section
(Goldshield Healthcare)

Gencydo
(Weleda)

A paint and ointment used to relieve the symptoms of hayfever.

Dose: apply the paint inside the nostrils several times a day. (May also be diluted 1:5 with water and used as a nasal spray.) Apply the ointment into each nostril twice a day, especially before retiring, or more often if required.
Side effects:
Caution:
Not to be used for:
Not to be used with:
Contains: concentrated lemon juice, quince seeds, glycerin, boric acid.

Haycrom Hayfever see **Opticrom Allergy**
(Norton Consumer)

Haymine
(Pharmax)

A tablet used as an antihistamine and sympathomimetic decongestant treatment for allergies, including hayfever and allergic skin conditions.

Dose: 1 tablet in the morning and 1 tablet at night if needed.
Side effects: drowsiness, rapid or abnormal heart rate, dry mouth, excitement, anxiety, shaking hands.
Caution: asthmatics and patients taking other medications should consult a doctor before using this product.
Not to be used for: children under 12 years, or for patients suffering from overactive thyroid, high blood pressure, heart disease, diabetes.
Not to be used with: alcohol, MAOIs, tricyclic antidepressants, beta-blockers, antihypertensives, other sedating medicines.
Contains: chlorpheniramine maleate, ephedrine hydrochloride.

Hismanal
(Janssen)

A tablet used as an antihistamine treatment for hay fever, allergic rhinitis, and skin allergies.

Dose: 1 daily.
Side effects: rarely drowsiness, weight gain, abnormal heart rhythm, convulsions, hepatitis.
Caution: women of child-bearing age should take steps to avoid pregnancy during, and for some weeks after, treatment.
Not to be used for: children under 12 years, pregnant women, nursing mothers, and patients with low blood potassium level.
Not to be used with: some antibiotics, tricyclic antidepressants, and some antifungal treatments.
Contains: astemizole.

Opticrom Allergy
(Fisons)

Eye drops used as an anti-allergy treatment for itchy eyes due to seasonal allergy (including hayfever). Doctors may prescribe this medication for different disorders. Self-medication should be limited to the conditions and doses stated.

Dose: 1-2 drops in each eye 4 times a day.
Side effects: stinging, irritation.
Caution: pregnant women, nursing mothers, and patients needing to use the drops for more than 3 consecutive months should consult their doctor.
Not to be used for: patients who wear soft contact lenses.
Not to be used with:
Contains: sodium cromoglycate.

Optrex Hayfever Allergy
(Crookes Healthcare)

Eye drops used as an anti-allergy treatment for eyes in patients suffering from seasonal allergy (hayfever). Doctors may prescribe this medication for different disorders. Self-medication should be limited to the conditions and doses stated.

Dose: 1 or 2 drops in each eye 4 times a day.
Side effects: temporary stinging.
Caution: pregnant women, nursing mothers, and patients needing to use the drops for more than 3 consecutive months should consult their doctor.
Not to be used for: children under 5 years, or for patients who wear soft contact lenses.
Not to be used with:
Contains: sodium cromoglycate.

Otrivine-Antistin
(CIBA Vision Ophthalmics)

Drops used as a sympathomimetic, antihistamine treatment for allergic conjunctivitis (hayfever).

Dose: adults 1-2 drops into the eye 2-3 times a day; children over 5 years 1 drop 2-3 times a day.
Side effects: temporary smarting, headache, drowsiness, blurred vision, allergy.
Caution: patients suffering from high blood pressure, overactive thyroid, dry eyes, coronary disease, or diabetes should consult a doctor before using this product. Patients with existing or previous eye disease, glaucoma, eye pain, or visual disturbance should also seek medical advice.
Not to be used for: children under 5 years or for patients suffering from glaucoma or who wear soft contact lenses.
Not to be used with: MAOIs, some antihypertensives.
Contains: xylometazoline hydrochloride, antazoline sulphate.

Phenergan
(M & B)

An elixir and tablet (available in 2 strengths) and used as an antihistamine to treat allergies and travel sickness. (Doctors may prescribe this product for other conditions. Self-medication should be restricted to the conditions and doses stated, however.)

Dose: adults 10-75 mg at bedtime, or in divided doses through the day. (Children 5-25 ml elixir at bedtime, or in divided doses, according to age.)
Side effects: drowsiness, reduced reactions, dizziness, disorientation, sensitivity to light, shaking, rigidity, dry mouth, difficulty passing water, headache, confusion, restlessness.
Caution: avoid exposure to strong sunlight while taking this medicine. Pregnant women, nursing mothers, asthmatics, and patients with glaucoma, bronchitis, epilepsy, heart disease, or who take other medicines, should consult a doctor before using this product. Do not use for more than 7 days, except on the advice of a doctor.

Not to be used for: children under 2 years. (The liquid is not suitable for diabetics.)
Not to be used with: other sedating drugs, alcohol, MAOIs, pregnancy tests, allergy tests.
Contains: promethazine hydrochloride.

Piriton
(A & H)

A tablet and liquid used as an antihistamine treatment for allergies, including skin allergies and hayfever.
Dose: adults 1 tablet or 10 ml liquid every 4-6 hours; children 6-12 years half adult dose, 1-5 years 2.5 ml liquid 2-6 times a day according to age.
Side effects: drowsiness, rarely reduced reactions, dizziness, excitation, upset stomach, dry mouth, difficulty passing urine, jaundice, palpitations, noises in the ears, allergy, blood disorder.
Caution: pregnant women, nursing mothers, and patients suffering from epilepsy, glaucoma, enlarged prostate, overactive thyroid, or chest disease should consult a doctor before using this product.
Not to be used for: children under 1 year.
Not to be used with: MAOIs, alcohol, other sedating medicines.
Contains: chlorpheniramine maleate.

Pollon-eze see Hismanal
(Janssen)

Q-Mazine
(Seton Healthcare)

A sugar-free elixir used as an antihistamine to treat allergies and travel sickness.

Dose: children 5-25 ml (according to age) once daily at bedtime, or in divided doses (as directed on the pack).

Side effects: drowsiness, reduced reactions, dizziness, disorientation, sensitivity to light, shaking, rigidity, dry mouth, difficulty passing water, headache, confusion, restlessness.

Caution: avoid exposure to strong sunlight while taking this medicine. Pregnant women, nursing mothers, asthmatics, and patients with glaucoma, bronchitis, epilepsy, heart disease, or who take other medicines, should consult a doctor before using this product. Do not use for more than 7 days, except on the advice of a doctor.

Not to be used for: children under 1 year.

Not to be used with: other sedating drugs, alcohol, MAOIs, pregnancy tests, allergy tests.

Contains: promethazine hydrochloride.

Resiston-One
(Fisons)

A nasal spray used as an anti-allergy product to treat and prevent the symptoms of hayfever.

Dose: 1 spray in each nostril 4 times a day. (Use continuously throughout hayfever season.)

Side effects: temporary irritation of the nose.

Caution: pregnant women and patients taking other medicines should consult a doctor before using this product.

Not to be used for: children under 5 years.

Not to be used with:

Contains: sodium cromoglycate, xylometazoline hydrochloride.

Rynacrom
(Fisons)

A nasal spray and nose drops used as an anti-allergy product to prevent hayfever and other forms of rhinitis.

Dose: 1 spray or 2 drops into each nostril 2-4 times a day. Use regularly.

Side effects: temporary itching nose, rarely breathlessness, wheezing.

Caution: pregnant women should consult a doctor before using this product.

Not to be used for:

Not to be used with:

Contains: sodium cromoglycate.

Rynacrom Compound see **Resiston-One**
(Fisons)

Seldane see **Triludan Forte**
(Marion Merrell Dow)

Sudafed Plus see entry in 'Respiratory conditions – cough and cold remedies' section.
(Warner Wellcome Consumer Healthcare)

Swarm
(Pickles)

A cream used as a soothing, antihistamine, and astringent treatment for insect bites and stings.

Dose: use as required.

Side effects:

Caution:

Not to be used for:

Not to be used with:

Contains: witch hazel, calamine, dibromopropamidine isethionate.

Syntaris Hayfever
(Roche Consumer Health)

A steroid nasal spray used to treat and prevent hayfever symptoms in the nose. Doctors may prescribe this medication for different disorders. Self-medication should be limited to the conditions and doses stated.

Dose: adults 2 sprays into each nostril night and morning; children aged 12-16 years 1 spray in each nostril up to 3 times a day. (Use the smallest dose necessary to control the symptoms.)

Side effects: irritation in throat or nose, nose bleeds, hoarseness, aftertaste, altered taste and smell.

Caution: patients with nose bleeds or who have had recent nasal surgery or nasal ulcers should consult a doctor before using this product.

Not to be used for: children under 12 years, pregnant women, nursing mothers, and patients with nasal infection.

Not to be used with: corticosteroid tablet treatments.

Contains: flunisolide.

Terfenor see Triludan
(Baker Norton Pharmaceuticals)

Triludan
(Marion Merrell Dow)

A tablet supplied at a strength of 60 mg (Triludan) and 120 mg (Triludan Forte) and used as an antihistamine treatment for allergies including hay fever and skin allergies.

Dose: for skin allergy, 120 mg once a day or 60 mg twice a day (not suitable for children). For hayfever, adults should initially take 60 mg once a day or 30 mg twice a day (children aged 6-12 years half adult dose), and the dose may be doubled if needed.

Side effects: heart rhythm disturbance, allergy, sweating, headache, trembling, dizziness, disturbed sleep, fainting, wheezing, fits, hair loss, sensitivity to sunlight, mental changes, jaundice, pain, tingling, visual disturbances, menstrual disorder.
Caution: pregnant women and nursing mothers should consult a doctor before using this product.
Not to be used for: children under 6 years (for hayfever) or children under 12 years (for skin allergy).
Not to be used with: some antibiotics, antifungal drugs, heart drugs, other antihistamines, diuretics, some drugs for psychiatric disorders,
Contains: terfenadine.

Triominic see entry in 'Respiratory Conditions – cough and cold remedies' section
(Intercare)

Unichem Antihistamine Tablets see **Triludan Tablets**
(Unichem)

Wasp-eze Ointment
(Seton Healthcare)

An ointment used as an antihistamine treatment for insect bites and stings.

Dose: apply every hour if needed, for up to 24 hours.
Side effects: allergy.
Caution:
Not to be used for: children under 1 year, or for areas of eczema.
Not to be used with:
Contains: antazoline hydrochloride.

Wasp-eze Spray
(Seton Healthcare)

An antihistamine and local anaesthetic spray used as a first-aid treatment for stings.

Dose: spray after removing sting, then repeat after 15 minutes if necessary.
Side effects:
Caution: patients with any known allergy should consult a doctor.
Not to be used for: areas of broken skin, or near the eyes.
Not to be used with:
Contains: mepyramine maleate, benzocaine.

Zirtek
(UCB Pharma)

A tablet used as an antihistamine treatment to relieve the symptoms of hayfever and skin allergies.

Dose: 1 tablet each day.
Side effects: headache, upset stomach, agitation, dry mouth, dizziness.
Caution: pregnant women, nursing mothers, and patients receiving medical advice or treatment should consult a doctor before using this product.
Not to be used for: children under 12 years.
Not to be used with: excessive alcohol.
Contains: cetirizine dihydrochloride.

Anti-smoking treatments

Many anti-smoking products are now available to assist smokers when they decide to give up cigarettes. Most contain nicotine to replace the nicotine that would have been obtained from smoking, but some are designed to calm the ex-smoker and to relieve stress.

Nicotine replacement products may be in the form of lozenges to suck, patches to put on the skin, or chewing gum. All of these products should be viewed only as a short-term aid to stopping smoking because ingestion of nicotine in these ways can in itself be harmful over a period of time, and the aim must therefore be to reduce the dependence on these aids and to stop using them within a few weeks.

Most of the patch products are designed for a maximum of 3 months' use, and the dose needed will depend on the number of cigarettes smoked. (Patch therapy is not generally suitable for smokers using less than 10 cigarettes a day.) The patch is worn either for 16 hours (and removed at night) or left in place for 24 hours. (The latter is useful if early morning craving for a cigarette is common.) It is essential not to smoke while wearing the patch, or to cut the patch to reduce the dose. (Smaller patches are available for reduced doses.) It is not suitable for occasional smokers.

Nicotine chewing gum therapy can be tailored to match the exact smoking pattern of the individual, and is therefore more flexible, but the gum can be a problem to people wearing dentures. The recommended technique is to chew the gum, and then 'park' it inside the mouth, then repeat the chewing and parking pattern several times. The treatment should continue for about 3 months, and then be reduced and stopped.

Nicotine can have a profound effect on the absorption and distribution of various drugs in the body, so anyone receiving regular prescription medication should consult their doctor or pharmacist, in case their reduced nicotine intake (as they give up) will affect their treatment. Any patient suffering from heart or circulation disorders, thyroid disease, diabetes, high blood pressure, stomach ulcer, or skin disease should consult a doctor before using nicotine products, because their conditions may be affected by the treatment.

Antismoking Tablets
(Potters)

A tablet used as a herbal remedy which gives similar effects to nicotine, to help reduce addiction to tobacco smoking.

Dose: 1 tablet taken every hour all day. (Suck the tablet for 30 seconds, then swallow whole.) Do not exceed 10 tablets per day.
Side effects: high doses cause nausea and vomiting.
Caution:
Not to be used for: children, pregnant women, or nursing mothers.
Not to be used with: tobacco products.
Contains: lobelia.

Nicobrevin*
(Intercare)

A capsule used as a supporting treatment for those giving up smoking.

Dose: 3 daily, reducing to 1 daily, as directed.
Side effects:
Caution:
Not to be used for: pregnant women, children.
Not to be used with: sedating medicines.
Contains: methyl valerate, quinine, camphor, eucalyptus oil.

Niconil
(Elan Pharma)

A patch available in two sizes, used to provide nicotine replacement through the skin (24 hours a day), to relieve withdrawal symptoms in people dependent on nicotine.

Dose: 1 22 mg patch daily for 4 weeks, then 1 11 mg patch for at least a further 2 weeks. (Total maximum treatment period 12 weeks.) Those smoking fewer than 20 cigarettes a day should use lower doses – consult a pharmacist or doctor for advice.

Side effects: redness and itching of skin at patch site, nausea, headaches, nightmares, dizziness, sleep disturbance.

Caution: patients suffering from heart or circulation disorders, thyroid disease, diabetes, high blood pressure, stomach ulcer, or skin disease should consult a doctor before using this product.

Not to be used for: non-smokers, children under 18 years, pregnant women, nursing mothers.

Not to be used with: cigarettes, other nicotine-replacement products. The doses of certain other medications may need to be adjusted. (Consult a doctor if receiving medical treatment.)

Contains: nicotine.

Nicorette Gum
(Pharmacia)

A chewing gum available in two strengths, 2 mg and 4 mg (Nicorette Plus), used to provide nicotine replacement to help smokers who wish to stop smoking.

Dose: chew 1 piece of gum when there is the urge to smoke. (Maximum of 15 pieces of either strength per day.) Use for 3 months, then gradually reduce usage. The 4 mg gum is recommended for smokers using more than 20 cigarettes per day.

Side effects: nausea, headaches, bitter taste, hiccups, sore throat, heartburn, nightmares, dizziness, sleep disturbance, palpitations, chest pain, leg pain.

Caution: patients suffering from heart or circulation disorders, thyroid disease, diabetes, high blood pressure, stomach ulcer, or skin disease should consult a doctor before using this product.

Not to be used for: non-smokers, children under 18 years,

pregnant women, nursing mothers.

Not to be used with: cigarettes, other nicotine-replacement products. The doses of certain other medications may need to be adjusted. (Consult a doctor if receiving medical treatment.)

Contains: nicotine.

Nicorette Patch
(Pharmacia)

A patch available in three sizes, used to provide nicotine replacement through the skin (16 hours a day), to help smokers who wish to stop smoking.

Dose: one 15 mg patch daily for 8 weeks (removing the patch at night), then one 10 mg patch daily for 2 weeks, then one 5 mg patch daily for 2 weeks. Those smoking fewer than 20 cigarettes a day should use lower doses – consult a doctor or pharmacist for advice.

Side effects: redness and itching of skin at patch site, nausea, headaches, nightmares, dizziness, sleep disturbance, palpitations, chest pain, leg pain.

Caution: patients suffering from heart or circulation disorders, thyroid disease, diabetes, high blood pressure, stomach ulcer, or skin disease should consult a doctor before using this product.

Not to be used for: non-smokers, children under 18 years, pregnant women, nursing mothers.

Not to be used with: cigarettes, other nicotine-replacement products. The doses of certain other medications may need to be adjusted. (Consult a doctor if receiving medical treatment.)

Contains: nicotine.

Nicotinell Gum
(Zyma Healthcare)

A chewing gum used to provide nicotine replacement to help

smokers who wish to stop smoking.

Dose: chew 1 piece of gum when there is the urge to smoke. (Maximum of 15 pieces of either strength per day.) Use for 3 months, then gradually reduce usage. The 4 mg gum is recommended for smokers using more than 20 cigarettes per day.

Side effects: nausea, headaches, bitter taste, hiccups, sore throat, heartburn, nightmares, dizziness, sleep disturbance, palpitations, chest pain, leg pain.

Caution: patients suffering from heart or circulation disorders, thyroid disease, diabetes, high blood pressure, stomach ulcer, or skin disease should consult a doctor before using this product.

Not to be used for: non-smokers, children under 18 years, pregnant women, nursing mothers.

Not to be used with: cigarettes, other nicotine-replacement products. The doses of certain other medications may need to be adjusted. (Consult a doctor if receiving medical treatment.)

Contains: nicotine.

Nicotinell Patches
(Zyma Healthcare)

A patch available in three sizes, used to treat nicotine dependence, by replacing nicotine through the skin (24 hours a day).

Dose: smokers using more than 20 cigarettes per day, start with the largest patch (30 cm or 21 mg). [If smoking less, start with the medium patch (20 cm or 14 mg).] Replace daily for 1 month, then reduce to next smallest patch, until the smallest size (10 cm or 7 mg) has been used for 1 month. Maximum total treatment period: 3 months (unless doctor advises otherwise).

Side effects: redness and itching of skin at patch site, nausea, headaches, dizziness, sleep disturbance.

Caution: patients suffering from heart or circulation disorders, thyroid disease, diabetes, high blood pressure, stomach ulcer, or skin disease should consult a doctor before using this product.

Not to be used for: non-smokers, children under 18 years, pregnant women, nursing mothers.

Not to be used with: cigarettes, other nicotine-replacement products. The doses of certain other medications may need to be adjusted. (Consult a doctor if receiving medical treatment.)

Contains: nicotine.

Resolution*
(Phoenix Health)

A lozenge used as a tobacco substitute.

Dose: 1 lozenge dissolved in the mouth instead of smoking a cigarette.

Side effects:

Caution: do not chew, suck, or swallow.

Not to be used for:

Not to be used with:

Contains: nicotine, vitamin A, vitamin C, vitamin E.

Stoppers*
(Charwell)

A lozenge used as a tobacco substitute.

Dose: 1 lozenge dissolved in the mouth instead of smoking a cigarette.

Side effects:

Caution: do not chew, suck, or swallow.

Not to be used for:

Not to be used with:

Contains: nicotine.

Joint and muscle disorders

Sprains, strains, sports injuries, and other rheumatic conditions, such as frozen shoulder, fibrositis, and lumbago, respond to simple pain killers or analgesics (see 'Simple pain killers' section) or the application of an externally applied preparation, such as Algipan, Transvasin, or Radian B. (Unlicensed bath additives containing similar ingredients are also available. These are not included here, but can be useful where soaking in a warm bath is beneficial.) The effect of these products is to relax the muscle spasm and to have a local anaesthetic effect. Ibuprofen (see 'Simple pain killers' section) is useful as a good general anti-inflammatory product, and is available in various cream products for external application.

Night cramps may respond to Crampex, but persistent cramp, or cramp in children, should be referred to a doctor.

Hot, swollen joints may indicate arthritis, which should be investigated fully by a medical practitioner.

Algesal
(Duphar)

A cream used as an analgesic rub to treat rheumatic and musculoskeletal conditions, such as lumbago, sciatica, and sprains.

Dose: massage into the affected area 3 times a day.
Side effects:
Caution: patients allergic to aspirin may react to this product.
Not to be used for: children under 6 years, or on broken skin.
Not to be used with:
Contains: diethylamine salicylate.

Algipan see Ralgex
(Whitehall)

Allcock's Porous Capsicum Plaster
(Richards & Appleby)

An adhesive plaster, impregnated with rubefacients and counter-irritants, and used to relieve muscular pain.

Dose: trim to size, warm, and place on to affected area. Leave in place for up to a week.
Side effects: skin irritation.
Caution:
Not to be used for: children under 10 years.
Not to be used with:
Contains: burgundy pitch, frankincense, orris root, capsicum, white beeswax, camphor, gum elemi, gum myrrh.

Arnica Cream
(Nelsons)

A cream used as a herbal remedy to treat bruises.

Dose: apply as needed.
Side effects:
Caution:
Not to be used for:
Not to be used with:
Contains: arnica.

Arnica Lotion/Ointment
(Weleda)

A lotion and ointment used as a herbal remedy to relieve the symptoms of muscular pain, stiffness, sprains, and bruises.

Dose: dilute 1 dessertspoonful of lotion in ½ pint water and bathe or apply as a compress. Repeat as needed once or twice a day. (A tablespoonful in a warm bath will help relieve muscles after exercise.) The ointment should be applied with massage 3-4 times a day. Apply immediately after injury to prevent bruising.
Side effects: allergy.
Caution:
Not to be used for: pregnant women, or for application to broken skin.
Not to be used with:
Contains: arnica.

Arnica Ointment see Arnica Lotion
(Weleda)

Backache Tablets
(Potters)

A tablet used as a herbal urinary antiseptic and diuretic remedy to treat the symptoms of backache. (This formula arises from the herbalist's view that the urinary system must also be toned to deal with backache.)

Dose: 2 tablets 3 times a day.
Side effects:
Caution:
Not to be used for: children, or pregnant women.
Not to be used with:
Contains: gravel root, hydrangea root, buchu, uva ursi.

Balmosa
(Pharmax Healthcare)

A cream used as an analgesic rub to treat muscular rheumatism, fibrositis, lumbago, sciatica, unbroken chilblains.

Dose: massage into the affected area as needed.
Side effects: irritation.
Caution: patients allergic to aspirin may react to this product.
Not to be used for: areas near the eyes, on broken or inflamed skin, or on membranes (such as the mouth).
Not to be used with:
Contains: levomenthol, camphor, methyl salicylate, capsicum oleoresin.

Belladonna Plaster
(Cuxson Gerrard)

An adhesive cloth plaster, available in two sizes, impregnated with a counter-irritant, and used to relieve muscular and rheumatic pain, strains, stiffness, and lumbago.

Dose: apply to affected area, and leave in place for 2-3 days.
Side effects:
Caution:
Not to be used for: children under 10 years.
Not to be used with:
Contains: belladonna alkaloids (hyoscyamine).

Bio-Strath Willow Formula
(Cedar Health)

A liquid used as a herbal remedy to relieve the symptoms of backache, lumbago, sciatica, fibrositis, and muscular pain.

Dose: 50 drops (1.5 ml) in a little water 3 times a day before meals, or as directed by a doctor.
Side effects:
Caution:
Not to be used for: children, pregnant women, or nursing mothers.
Not to be used with:
Contains: yeast, willow bark, primula root.

BN Liniment
(3M Health Care)

A liniment used as a rubefacient to treat muscular and rheumatic pain, neuralgia, sciatica, sprains, and stiffness.

Dose: apply and massage into affected area 2-3 times a day. (For children, dilute with an equal amount of olive oil before use.)
Side effects:
Caution: keep away from the eyes.
Not to be used for: children under 6 years, or on broken or sensitive skin areas.
Not to be used with:
Contains: turpentine oil, strong ammonia solution, ammonium chloride.

Boots Herbal Rheumatic Pain Tablets
(Boots)

A tablet used as a herbal remedy to relieve symptoms of

muscular and rheumatic pain, lumbago, and fibrositis.

Dose: 3 tablets 3 times a day before food.
Side effects:
Caution:
Not to be used for: children under 12 years, pregnant women, and nursing mothers.
Not to be used with:
Contains: celery leaf, buckbean, black cohosh.

Boots Icy Gel Muscle Rub*
(Boots)

A gel used to freeze the skin and relieve tension and discomfort.

Dose: apply as needed.
Side effects: irritation.
Caution: avoid contact with the eyes and sensitive skin parts.
Not to be used for: children under 5 years, or on broken skin.
Not to be used with:
Contains:

Boots Pain Relief Balm
(Boots)

A non-greasy balm used to relieve muscular and rheumatic pain.

Dose: apply to affected area and repeat when necessary.
Side effects:
Caution: avoid eyes and sensitive parts of body. Patients who are allergic to aspirin may react to this product.
Not to be used for: children under 12 years, or on broken skin.
Not to be used with:
Contains: glycol monosalicylate, ethyl nicotinate, nonyic acid,

vanillylamide.

Boots Pain Relief Embrocation
(Boots)

A liquid used to relieve muscular and rheumatic pain (including pain associated with sports injuries).

Dose: apply twice a day.
Side effects:
Caution: avoid eyes and other sensitive parts.
Not to be used for: areas of broken skin.
Not to be used with:
Contains: camphor, turpentine oil.

Boots Pain Relief Warming Spray see PR Heat Spray
(Boots)

celery tablets
(licensed product available from Gerard House and 'Heath and Heather')

A tablet used as a herbal remedy to treat the symptoms of rheumatic pain.

Dose: (as specified for each individual product).
Side effects:
Caution: pregnant women and nursing mothers should consult a doctor before using this product.
Not to be used for: children.
Not to be used with:
Contains: celery.

Chymol see entry in 'Skin disorders' section
(Waterhouse)

Comfrey Ointment
(Potters)

An ointment used as a herbal remedy to relieve the symptoms
of bruises and sprains.

Dose: apply twice a day after bathing, for a maximum of 10
days.
Side effects:
Caution:
Not to be used for: pregnant women or nursing mothers.
Not to be used with:
Contains: comfrey.

---

copper bracelet*

A bracelet made of copper, and worn to help relieve the
symptoms of arthritis and rheumatism.

Copper Ointment
(Weleda)

An ointment used to relieve muscular rheumatic pain.

Dose: apply thinly with massage once or twice a day.
Side effects:
Caution:
Not to be used for:
Not to be used with:
Contains: cuprum metallicum praep.

Copperplast*

A copper patch made applied to the skin every 7 days to help relieve the symptoms of arthritis and rheumatism.

Crampex
(Napp Consumer Products)

Tablets used to prevent muscle cramp at night.

Dose: 1-2 tablets before bedtime.
Side effects: flushing of face and upper body.
Caution: patients suffering from heart or circulation disorders should consult a doctor before using this product.
Not to be used for: children.
Not to be used with: other products containing vitamin D.
Contains: nicotinic acid, calcium gluconate, vitamin D_3.

Cremalgin
(Rhone-Poulenc Rorer Family Health)

A balm used as an analgesic and rubefacient rub to treat rheumatism, fibrositis, lumbago, sciatica, and muscle stiffness.

Dose: massage into the affected area 2-3 times a day.
Side effects: may be irritant.
Caution:
Not to be used for: areas near the eyes, broken or inflamed skin, or on membranes (such as the mouth). Patients allergic to aspirin may react to this product.
Not to be used with:
Contains: methyl nicotinate, glycol monosalicylate, capsicin.

Deep Freeze Cold Gel*
(Mentholatum)

A gel used as a cold muscle rub after exercise for tired muscles.

Dose: use when required.
Side effects:
Caution: avoid the eyes.
Not to be used for: broken skin.
Not to be used with:
Contains: menthol.

Deep Freeze Spray
(Mentholatum)

A spray used as a cold treatment to relieve the symptoms of muscular stiffness, sprains, cramp, and rheumatic pain.

Dose: spray for 3-5 seconds up to 3 times a day.
Side effects:
Caution: avoid inhaling the spray, and avoid the eyes, nose, and sensitive skin areas. Use in a well-ventilated space.
Not to be used for: children under 6 years, or for broken skin, the head, neck, fingers or toes.
Not to be used with:
Contains: dichlorodifluromethane, trichlorofluoromethane.

Deep Heat
(Mentholatum)

A spray, liniment, rub, and maximum-strength rub, used as an analgesic to treat rheumatic pain, and muscular aches and strains. (The rubs are also used to treat bruises.)

Dose: apply 2-3 times a day (or up to 4 times a day for liniment).
Side effects: irritation.

Caution: avoid using on broken or sensitive skin, or near the eyes. The spray should not be used on the face, neck, or shoulders. Patients who are allergic to aspirin may react to this product.
Not to be used for: children under 5 years.
Not to be used with:
Contains: methyl salicylate. (The liniment and maximum-strength rub also contain menthol. The spray also contains methyl nicotinate, 2-hydroxyethyl salicylate, and ethyl salicylate. The rub also contains menthol, eucalyptus oil, and turpentine oil.)

Deep Relief
(Mentholatum)

A gel used as a non-steroidal anti-inflammatory treatment for pain and inflammation associated with backache, muscular pain, sprains, strains, lumbago, fibrositis.

Dose: massage into affected area up to 3 times a day.
Side effects: redness and tingling.
Caution: avoid contact with broken skin, lips, and eyes. Patients with a history of kidney problems, asthma, or allergy to aspirin should contact a doctor before using this product.
Not to be used for: children under 14 years, pregnant women, nursing mothers.
Not to be used with: other non-steroidal anti-inflammatory treatments (including those taken by mouth).
Contains: ibuprofen, menthol.

Difflam
(3M Healthcare)

A cream used as a non-steroidal anti-inflammatory rub to relieve pain and inflammation of sprains, strains, arthritis, and bruises.

Dose: massage gently into the affected area 3 times a day for up to 10 days.

Side effects: itching, reddening of the skin, sensitivity to sunlight.

Caution: avoid contact with eyes and mouth. Pregnant women, nursing mothers, and patients using other medication should consult a doctor before using this product.

Not to be used for: areas or broken skin.

Not to be used with:

Contains: benzydamine hydrochloride.

Dragon Balm Ointment
(Gerard House)

An ointment used as a herbal remedy to relieve the symptoms of rheumatism and allied conditions.

Dose: apply as required.

Side effects:

Caution:

Not to be used for: children under 6 years.

Not to be used with:

Contains: camphor, menthol, turpentine oil, nutmeg oil, eucalyptus oil, cassia oil, pine oil, thymol, guaiacol, balsam of Peru.

Dubam
(Norma Chemicals)

An aerosol used as a topical analgesic and rubefacient to relieve muscular pain.

Dose: spray on to the affected area for 2 seconds up to 4 times a day.

Side effects: may be irritant.

Caution: avoid inhaling the spray.

Not to be used for: areas near the eyes, the face, or on broken or inflamed skin, or on membranes (such as the mouth).
Not to be used with:
Contains: glycol monostearate, methyl salicylate, ethyl salicylate, methyl nicotinate.

Ellimans Embrocation
(Seton Healthcare)

An embrocation used as a rubefacient and counter-irritant to relieve the symptoms of muscular and rheumatic pain, stiffness, and sciatica.

Dose: apply every 3 hours for one day, then use twice a day.
Side effects:
Caution: keep away from the eyes and other sensitive skin areas.
Not to be used for: children under 12 years, or for broken skin.
Not to be used with:
Contains: turpentine oil, acetic acid.

---

evening primrose oil* see entry in 'Skin disorders' section

Feldene P
(Charwell Health Care)

A non-steroidal anti-inflammatory gel used to relieve muscular and joint pain, including rheumatic and back pain.

Dose: apply up to 4 times a day.
Side effects:
Caution: avoid contact with eyes, lips, and inflamed or broken skin.
Not to be used for: children, or for patients with allergy to anti-inflammatory drugs.

Not to be used with: other non-steroidal anti-inflammatory treatments (including those taken by mouth).
Contains: piroxicam.

Fiery Jack
(Pickles)

A cream and ointment used as a rubefacient to treat muscular and rheumatic pain.

Dose: apply twice a day.
Side effects:
Caution: the cream may cause a reaction in patients allergic to aspirin or salicylates.
Not to be used for: areas of broken skin.
Not to be used with:
Contains: capsicum oleoresin. (The cream also contains methyl nicotinate, glycol salicylate, and diethylamine salicylate.)

Germolene Antiseptic Ointment
(SmithKline Beecham Consumer)

An antiseptic, soothing, protective, and analgesic ointment used to treat aching muscles. (For use in treating minor wounds, burns and scalds, blisters, and sore skin, see entry in 'Antiseptics' section.)

Dose: apply to affected area and massage when required.
Side effects:
Caution: patients who are allergic to aspirin may react to this product.
Not to be used for:
Not to be used with:
Contains: lanolin, white soft paraffin, yellow soft paraffin, light liquid paraffin, starch, zinc oxide, methyl salicylate, octaphonium chloride, phenol.

Goddards White Oil Embrocation
(LRC Products)

An embrocation used as a rubefacient and counter-irritant to relieve the symptoms of muscular and rheumatic pain, and pain from bruises, strains, stiff muscles, or unbroken chilblains.

Dose: apply once or twice a day.
Side effects:
Caution:
Not to be used for: children, or for broken skin.
Not to be used with:
Contains: turpentine oil, acetic acid, dilute ammonia solution.

Heath & Heather Rheumatic Pain Tablets
(Ferrosan Healthcare)

A herbal remedy used to relieve the symptoms of backache, lumbago, fibrositis, and rheumatic pain.

Dose: 1 tablet 3 times a day.
Side effects: stomach upset.
Caution: pregnant women should consult a doctor before using this product.
Not to be used for: children.
Not to be used with:
Contains: guaiacum resin, bogbean, celery seed.

Ibugel see Ibuleve
(Dermal)

Ibuleve
(Dendron)

A clear gel and spray used as a non-steroidal anti-inflammatory treatment for pain and inflammation associated with backache, rheumatic and muscular pain, sprains, and strains. (The gel is also used to treat neuralgia.)

Dose: massage gel into affected area or use 5-10 sprays up to 3 times a day.
Side effects:
Caution: avoid contact with broken skin, lips, and eyes. Patients with a history of kidney problems, asthma, or allergy to aspirin, or stomach ulcers should contact a doctor before using this product.
Not to be used for: children under 14 years, pregnant women, nursing mothers.
Not to be used with: other non-steroidal anti-inflammatory treatments (including those taken by mouth).
Contains: ibuprofen.

Ibuspray
(Dermal)

A spray used as a non-steroidal anti-inflammatory treatment for pain and inflammation in soft tissues, such as backache, muscular pain, and sprains.

Dose: apply 5-10 sprays and massage the area 3-4 times a day.
Side effects:
Caution: avoid contact with eyes, nose, lips, and inflamed or broken skin. Patients with stomach ulcers, a history of kidney disorders, or allergy to aspirin should see a doctor before using this product.
Not to be used for: children under 14 years, pregnant women, nursing mothers, or patients with allergy to anti-inflammatory drugs.
Not to be used with: other non-steroidal anti-inflammatory treatments (including those taken by mouth).
Contains: ibuprofen.

Intralgin
(3M Healthcare)

A gel used as an analgesic rub to treat muscle pain.

Dose: massage gently into the affected area as needed.
Side effects: may be irritant.
Caution:
Not to be used for: areas near the eyes, broken or inflamed skin, or on membranes (such as the mouth).
Not to be used with:
Contains: salicylamide, benzocaine.

---

kelp products see entry in 'Miscellaneous' section

Lasonil
(Bayer)

An ointment used as an anti-inflammatory preparation to treat bruises, sprains, and soft tissue injuries.

Dose: apply 2-3 times a day.
Side effects:
Caution: women in the first 3 months of pregnancy should consult a doctor before using this product.
Not to be used for: broken or infected skin.
Not to be used with:
Contains: heparinoid, hyaluronidase.

Ligvites
(Gerard House)

A tablet used as a herbal analgesic and anti-inflammatory remedy to relieve symptoms of rheumatic pain and stiffness, backache, and lumbago.

Dose: 2 tablets twice a day after food.
Side effects:
Caution: nursing mothers are advised to consult a doctor before using this product.
Not to be used for: children under 12 years or pregnant women.
Not to be used with:
Contains: guaiacum resin, black cohosh, white willow bark, sarsaparilla, poplar bark.

Lloyds Cream
(Seton Healthcare)

An odourless cream used as an analgesic to treat muscular aches and pains.

Dose: apply up to three times a day.
Side effects:
Caution: children under 6 years should see a doctor before using this product. Patients allergic to aspirin may react to this product.
Not to be used for: broken or sensitive skin.
Not to be used with:
Contains: diethylamine salicylate.

Malted Kelp see entry in 'Miscellaneous' section
(Potters)

Massage Balm with Arnica
(Weleda)

A balm used as a herbal remedy to treat symptoms of rheumatic pain, muscular pain and stiffness, backache, fibrositis, bruises, cramps, and sprains.

Dose: massage into affected area 3-4 times a day.

Side effects: allergy.
Caution:
Not to be used for: pregnant women, or for application to broken skin.
Not to be used with:
Contains: silver birch, arnica, lavender oil, rosemary oil.

Mentholatum Balm
(Mentholatum)

An ointment used as an analgesic and rubefacient, applied to the skin to treat muscular pain, stiffness, and bruises. (For use in treating coughs and colds, see 'Respiratory conditions – inhaled remedies' section. For use in treating skin disorders, see 'Skin disorders' section.)

Dose: make a light application to the affected area 2-3 times a day.
Side effects:
Caution: avoid the eyes, nose, and delicate skin. Patients who are allergic to aspirin may react to this product.
Not to be used for: children under 1 year.
Not to be used with:
Contains: menthol, camphor, methyl salicylate.

Minalka see entry in 'Vitamins and minerals' section
(Cedar Health)

Movelat
(Panpharma)

A cream or gel used as a non-steroidal anti-inflammatory treatment for muscle and joint pain and inflammation, sprains, and strains.

Dose: apply up to 4 times a day.

Side effects:
Caution: avoid contact with eyes, lips, sensitive areas of skin, mucous membranes, and inflamed or broken skin. Some asthmatic patients may be adversely affected by this product.
Not to be used for: children, women in the first or last 3 months of pregnancy, or patients with allergy to aspirin or anti-inflammatory drugs.
Not to be used with:
Contains: mucopolysaccharide polysulphate, salicylic acid.

Nasciodine
(Castleowen)

A cream used as an analgesic and rubefacient to treat the symptoms of rheumatic and back pain, chilblains, sprains, strains, and bruises.

Dose: massage into the affected area 2-3 times a day.
Side effects:
Caution: avoid broken or inflamed skin. Patients who are allergic to aspirin may react to this product.
Not to be used for: children, pregnant women, or patients with an allergy to iodine. Not for prolonged use.
Not to be used with:
Contains: iodine, menthol, methyl salicylate, turpentine oil, camphor

---

Nella Red Oil
(Nella)

An oil supplied in a roll-on applicator, used as a rubefacient treatment for the symptoms of muscular and rheumatic pain, and lumbago.

Dose: apply every 3 hours or as required.
Side effects:

Caution: avoid broken or very sensitive skin. Children under 5 years should be seen by a doctor before using this product.
Not to be used for:
Not to be used with:
Contains: methyl nicotinate, clove oil, mustard oil, arachis oil.

New Zealand green lipped mussel*

A capsule of shellfish extract, used for its anti-inflammatory properties to maintain healthy joints.

Dose: (as specified for each individual product).
Side effects: allergy, stomach upset.
Caution: patients with high blood pressure are advised to consult a doctor before using this product.
Not to be used for: patients with allergy to shellfish.
Not to be used with:
Contains: minerals, B vitamins, amino acids.

Nine Rubbing Oils
(Potters)

An oil mixture used as a rubefacient treatment for the symptoms of muscular pain and stiffness, including backache, sciatica, lumbago, fibrositis, rheumatic pain, and strains.

Dose: rub into the affected part as required.
Side effects:
Caution:
Not to be used for: pregnant women, or for application to broken skin.
Not to be used with: homeopathic products.
Contains: amber oil, clove oil, eucalyptus oil, linseed oil, methyl salicylate, volatile mustard oil, rectified turpentine oil, thyme oil, peppermint oil, arachis oil.

Ointment for Strains
(Nelsons)

An ointment used as a herbal remedy to treat strains and sprains.

Dose: apply when required.
Side effects:
Caution:
Not to be used for:
Not to be used with:
Contains: ruta graveolens.

Olbas Oil
(Lane)

A non-greasy oil used as an analgesic and rubefacient applied to the skin to treat muscular pain and stiffness. (For use as a decongestant, see 'Respiratory conditions – inhaled remedies' section.)

Dose: massage into affected area 3 times a day.
Side effects: stinging, rash.
Caution: avoid contact with the eyes, and with plastic or delicate surfaces. Patients allergic to aspirin may react to this product.
Not to be used for: children, or on broken skin.
Not to be used with:
Contains: cajuput oil, clove oil, eucalyptus oil, juniper berry oil, menthol, mint oil, wintergreen oil.

---

omega 3 fish oils* see entry in 'Miscellaneous' section

Oruvail
(Rhone-Poulenc Rorer)

A gel used as a non-steroidal anti-inflammatory treatment for pain and swelling in sports injuries, sprains, strains, and rheumatic pain.

Dose: massage into affected area 3 times a day for up to 7 days.
Side effects: itching, rash.
Caution: avoid contact with eyes and lips. Pregnant women, nursing mothers, and patients with kidney disease or who are taking any other medication should consult a doctor before using this product.
Not to be used for: children under 12 years, patients with asthma, allergic disease, or allergy to aspirin or anti-inflammatory drugs. Do not apply if there is eczema or sore/broken skin at the site of the injury.
Not to be used with: other non-steroidal anti-inflammatory treatments (including those taken by mouth), and see caution above.
Contains: ketoprofen.

PR Freeze Spray*
(Crookes Healthcare)

A spray used as a cold treatment to relieve the symptoms of muscular discomfort, such as sprains and strains and bruises.

Dose: apply up to 3 times a day.
Side effects:
Caution: for short-term use only. Avoid inhaling the spray. Do not use in a confined space. Do not spray near eyes, nose, or sensitive skin areas. Do not use near painted or polished surfaces.
Not to be used for: children under 6 years, or on broken or irritated skin, the head, neck, fingers, or toes.
Not to be used with:
Contains: ethanol, dimethyl ether, methylal.

PR Heat Spray
(Crookes Healthcare)

A spray used as an analgesic and rubefacient to treat muscular and rheumatic pain, sprains, and bruises.

Dose: apply up to twice a day.
Side effects: irritation.
Caution: avoid the eyes, nose, and sensitive skin. Avoid inhaling the spray. Patients who are allergic to aspirin may react to this product.
Not to be used for: children under 5 years, or on broken skin.
Not to be used with:
Contains: methyl salicylate, ethyl nicotinate, camphor.

Proflex cream
(Zyma Healthcare)

A cream used as a non-steroidal anti-inflammatory treatment to relieve symptoms of muscular and rheumatic pain, backache, sprains, and strains.

Dose: massage into affected area up to 3 times a day.
Side effects: mild skin irritation.
Caution: pregnant women, nursing mothers, and patients receiving current medical treatment, or who suffer from asthma or allergy to aspirin should contact a doctor before using this product.
Not to be used for: children under 14 years, or on broken skin, the lips, or near the eyes.
Not to be used with: other non-steroidal anti-inflammatory treatments (including those taken by mouth).
Contains: ibuprofen.

Quool*
(Allmi-Care)

A patch applied to the skin as a cooling remedy to relieve muscular tension and discomfort.

Dose: apply the patch, and secure with a loose net bandage if necessary. Change the patch twice a day.
Side effects:
Caution:
Not to be used for: children under 12 years, or on cuts, infected skin, eczema, or sensitive skin.
Not to be used with:
Contains: menthol.

Radian-B
(Roche Consumer Health)

A muscle rub, spray, and lotion used as a rubefacient and analgesic to treat muscular and rheumatic aches and pains (including sports uses).

Dose: apply up to 3 times a day.
Side effects: irritation.
Caution: avoid eyes, irritated skin, and sensitive areas. The spray should not be used near painted or polished surfaces. Patients allergic to aspirin may react to these products.
Not to be used for: children under 6 years.
Not to be used with:
Contains: menthol, camphor. (The lotion and spray also contain ammonium salicylate and salicylic acid. The rub also contains methyl salicylate and capsicum.)

Ralgex
(SmithKline Beecham Consumer)

A stick, cream, and heat spray used as a rubefacient and analgesic to treat muscular and rheumatic pain and stiffness (including sprains, strains, sciatica, fibrositis, and lumbago).

Dose: apply up to 4 times a day.
Side effects:
Caution: avoid the eyes. Do not spray the head and neck. Avoid inhaling the spray. Patients allergic to aspirin may react to these products.
Not to be used for: children under 12 years, or on broken or sensitive skin.
Not to be used with:
Contains: glycol monosalicylate, methyl nicotinate. (The cream also contains capsicin. The stick also contains ethyl salicylate and menthol.)

Ralgex Freeze Spray
(SmithKline Beecham Consumer Healthcare)

A spray used as a cooling treatment, to relieve the symptoms of muscular and rheumatic pain and stiffness, sprains, strains, and bruises.

Dose: apply up to 4 times a day.
Side effects:
Caution: patients allergic to aspirin may react to this product.
Not to be used for:
Not to be used with:
Contains: isopentane, methoxymethane, glycol monosalicylate.

Reumalex
(Gerard House)

A tablet used as a herbal remedy to provide relief from symptoms of rheumatic aches and pains.

Dose: 2 tablets twice a day after food.
Side effects:
Caution: pregnant women and nursing mothers should consult a doctor before using this product.

Not to be used for: children.
Not to be used with:
Contains: white willow bark, guaiacum, black cohosh, sarsaparilla, poplar bark.

Rheumadoron 102A Drops
(Weleda)

A liquid used as a herbal remedy to relieve the symptoms of muscular rheumatic pain.

Dose: 5-10 drops 3-4 times a day.
Side effects:
Caution: do not exceed the stated dose.
Not to be used for: pregnant women or nursing mothers.
Not to be used with:
Contains: aconite 3x, arnica, birch, mandragora root 1x.

Rheumadoron Ointment
(Weleda)

An ointment used as a herbal remedy to relieve the symptoms of muscular rheumatic pain.

Dose: apply with massage twice a day.
Side effects: allergy.
Caution:
Not to be used for: application to broken skin.
Not to be used with:
Contains: wolfbane, arnica, birch, mandrake, rosemary oil.

Rheumasol
(English Grains Healthcare)

A tablet used as a herbal anti-inflammatory treatment for joint and muscle pain and stiffness.

Dose: 1 tablet 3 times a day with meals.
Side effects:
Caution:
Not to be used for: children.
Not to be used with:
Contains: guaiacum resin, prickly ash bark.

___

Rheumatic Pain Tablets
(Potters)

A tablet used as a herbal remedy to relieve the symptoms of rheumatic aches and pains.

Dose: 2 tablets 3 times a day,
Side effects:
Caution: patients who are prone to diarrhoea should use with caution.
Not to be used for: children, pregnant women, or nursing mothers.
Not to be used with:
Contains: bogbean, yarrow, burdock root, guaiacum resin, nutmeg.

___

Rhus Tox. Cream
(Nelsons)

A cream used as a herbal remedy to treat rheumatic disorders and strains.

Dose: apply when required, and massage into skin.
Side effects:
Caution:
Not to be used for:
Not to be used with:
Contains: rhus toxicondendron.

___

Rhus Tox. Ointment
(Weleda)

An ointment used as a herbal remedy to relieve the symptoms of rheumatic pain.

Dose: apply directly to the skin or on a dry dressing.
Side effects: allergy.
Caution:
Not to be used for:
Not to be used with:
Contains: rhus toxicodendron.

Ruta Ointment
(Weleda)

An ointment used as a herbal remedy to relieve the symptoms and aid the healing of strains and sprains.

Dose: apply directly to the skin or on a dry dressing.
Side effects: allergy.
Caution:
Not to be used for:
Not to be used with:
Contains: rue tincture.

---

royal jelly* see entry in 'Vitamins and minerals' section

Salonair
(Salonpas)

An aerosol used as an analgesic and rubefacient rub to relieve muscular and rheumatic pain.

Dose: spray on to the affected area 1-2 times a day.
Side effects: irritation.

Caution: patients allergic to aspirin may react to this product.
Not to be used for: areas near the eyes, broken or inflamed skin, or on membranes (such as the mouth).
Not to be used with:
Contains: glycol salicylate, menthol, camphor, squalane, benzyl nicotinate, methyl salicylate.

Salonpas Plasters
(Salonpas)

A plaster used as an analgesic treatment for joint and muscle pain, such as stiff shoulders, simple backache, lumbago, sprains, strains, and bruises.

Dose: apply the patch to the affected area up to 3 times a day for up to 7 days.
Side effects: redness, itchiness, irritation.
Caution: children under 12 years, pregnant women, nursing mothers, and patients who are allergic to aspirin or salicylates should consult a doctor before using this product. Avoid contact with the eyes, mucous membranes, rashes, wounds, or damaged skin.
Not to be used for:
Not to be used with: heating pads.
Contains: methyl salicylate, glycol salicylate, camphor, menthol, thymol, tocopherol acetate.

Sciargo
(Potters)

A tablet or herbal teabag used as herbal diuretic and anti-inflammatory remedy to relieve the symptoms of sciatica and lumbago.

Dose: 2 tablets 3 times a day, or 1 teabag infused 5 times a day.

Side effects:
Caution:
Not to be used for: children, pregnant women, nursing mothers, or patients with poor kidney function.
Not to be used with:
Contains: shepherd's purse, wild carrot, clivers, uva ursi, juniper berry.

Seatone*
(Ferrosan Healthcare)

A capsule, available with or without added cod liver oil, used as a food supplement, and thought to assist in the mobility of joints, as in arthritis.

Dose: up to 5 capsules (standard product) each day, or up to 3 capsules (product with cod liver oil) each day, with meals.
Side effects: allergy, stomach upset.
Caution: patients with high blood pressure are advised to consult a doctor before using this product.
Not to be used for: patients with allergy to shellfish.
Not to be used with: other products containing vitamins A or D (product with cod liver oil only).
Contains: extract of green-lipped mussel. (Capsules with cod liver oil also contain cod liver oil and vitamins A, D, and E.)

---

starflower oil* see entry in 'Skin disorders' section

Tabritis
(Potters)

A tablet used as a herbal anti-inflammatory and analgesic remedy to relieve the symptoms of rheumatic pain and stiffness.

Dose: 2 tablets 3 times a day. (For best results take for at least 6 weeks.)

Side effects:
Caution:
Not to be used for: children or pregnant women.
Not to be used with:
Contains: elder flowers, prickly ash bark, yarrow, burdock, clivers, poplar bark, uva ursi.

Tiger Balm
(LRC Products)

An ointment (available in two strengths) used as a rubefacient to give temporary relief from minor muscular aches and pains.

Dose: rub on to affected area 2-3 times a day and cover.
Side effects: irritation.
Caution: avoid contact with eyes and mucous membranes. Pregnant women and nursing mothers should avoid using this product.
Not to be used for: children under 2 years, or on broken or irritated skin. Not to be used for inhalation.
Not to be used with: homeopathic remedies.
Contains: cajuput oil, peppermint oil. (The extra-strength product also contains menthol, clove oil, camphor, and cinnamon oil.)

Transvasin Heat Rub
(Seton Healthcare)

A cream used as a rubefacient for the relief of rheumatic and muscular pain.

Dose: use up to 3 times a day.
Side effects:
Caution:
Not to be used for: broken or sensitive skin, or for children under 6 years.

Not to be used with:
Contains: ethyl nicotinate, hexylnicotinate, tetrahydrofurfuryl salicylate.

Transvasin Heat Spray
(Seton Healthcare)

A spray used as an analgesic and rubefacient to treat muscular and rheumatic pain.

Dose: spray on affected area.
Side effects:
Caution: avoid inhalation, and contact with eyes, nose, and sensitive areas. Patients who are allergic to aspirin may react to this product.
Not to be used for: children under 5 years.
Not to be used with:
Contains: 2-hydroxyethyl salicylate, diethylamine salicylate, methyl nicotinate.

Vegetex
(Lane)

A tablet used as a herbal remedy to relieve the symptoms of rheumatic pain, fibrositis, and lumbago.

Dose: 3 tablets 3 times a day with meals.
Side effects: skin irritation, stomach upset, nausea, vomiting.
Caution:
Not to be used for: children under 12 years, pregnant women, nursing mothers.
Not to be used with:
Contains: celery, buckbean, black cohosh.

Weleda Massage Balm with Arnica
(Weleda)

A balm used as a herbal remedy to relieve muscular and rheumatic pain (including sporting use).

Dose: apply to damp skin after a warm bath or shower.
Side effects:
Caution:
Not to be used for: broken skin.
Not to be used with:
Contains: arnica flower, birch leaves, lavender, rosemary oil.

Simple pain killers

Drugs, such as aspirin, paracetamol, or codeine, form the basis of this section of over-the-counter preparations. Other items listed include ibuprofen products and migraine treatments. Many pain killers are combined with caffeine, which functions as a stimulant.

Analgesics should be taken only for short treatment courses for conditions such as headache, backache, period pain, and simple rheumatic conditions. They are also useful for treatment of fevers. The total daily dose should be monitored carefully, and manufacturers' recommendations should be followed.

Aspirin should not be given to children under 12 years, except on the advice of a doctor, or to anyone suffering from stomach disorders or bleeding problems (such as haemophilia), or patients taking anticoagulants. Asthmatics should also avoid aspirin, because asthma attacks may result.

Paracetamol should not be used by anyone with liver problems, but is suitable for children and babies over 3 months. (Children should not be treated for more than 3 days before consulting a doctor, however.) Babies aged 2 months may be given some of the paracetamol products for post-vaccination fever and discomfort.

Ibuprofen is a non-steroidal anti-inflammatory drug, but this product should be used with caution in elderly patients, who may need reduced doses. It may also inflame the stomach, so it should be avoided in patients with ulcers or other stomach disorders. It is closely related to aspirin, and should not be taken by patients who are allergic to aspirin or to other anti-inflammatory products. Patients with heart disease should also avoid this type of medication. Ibuprofen can interfere with many other drugs, (especially medicines used to treat high blood pressure, and some antibiotics), so anyone taking other medication should check with a pharmacist before taking ibuprofen as well. It can also precipitate asthmatic attacks in susceptible patients, so asthmatics should also avoid using this drug.

Actron
(Warner Wellcome Consumer Healthcare)

An effervescent tablet used as an analgesic and stimulant to relieve pain.

Dose: 2 tablets dissolved in water every 4 hours. (Maximum of 8 in 24 hours.)
Side effects: irritation of stomach and intestines.
Caution: in pregnant women and in patients with asthma or indigestion.
Not to be used for: children under 12 years, nursing mothers, or patients with stomach ulcers, haemophilia, or allergy to aspirin.
Not to be used with: anti-coagulants, some anti-epileptic drugs, other preparations containing paracetamol, some antibiotics, tablets coated to protect the stomach, excess tea or coffee.
Contains: aspirin, paracetamol, caffeine, sodium bicarbonate, citric acid.

Alka-Seltzer see entry in 'Stomach preparations' section
(Warner Wellcome Consumer Healthcare)

Alvedon
(Novex)

A suppository supplied at a strength of 125 mg and used to treat pain and fever in children.

Dose: 1-2 suppositories (according to age) inserted into the rectum up to 4 times a day.
Side effects: rash, itching, or soreness around the anus.
Caution: children suffering from epilepsy should see a doctor before using this product. The suppositories are not to be swallowed.

Not to be used for: children under 1 year.
Not to be used with: other medicines containing paracetamol.
Contains: paracetamol.

Ana-sed see entry in 'Sleeping problems and stress' section
(Potters)

Anadin
(Whitehall Laboratories)

A caplet used as an analgesic and stimulant to relieve pain.

Dose: 2 caplets every 4 hours. (Maximum of 12 in 24 hours.)
Side effects: irritation of stomach and intestines.
Caution: pregnant women and patients with asthma or
indigestion should consult a doctor before using this product.
Not to be used for: children under 12 years, nursing mothers,
or for patients with stomach ulcers, blood-clotting disorder, or
allergy to aspirin.
Not to be used with: anticoagulants, some anti-epileptic drugs,
excess tea or coffee.
Contains: aspirin, caffeine, quinine sulphate.

Anadin All Night
(Whitehall Laboratories)

A controlled-release tablet used as an analgesic for relief of
overnight pain.

Dose: 2 tablets 1-2 hours before bedtime.
Side effects: irritation of stomach and intestines, skin rash,
allergy, asthma.
Caution: patients with asthma or indigestion should consult a
doctor before using this product.
Not to be used for: pregnant women, children under 12 years,
nursing mothers, or patients with stomach ulcers, haemophilia,

or allergy to aspirin.

Not to be used with: anti-coagulants, some anti-epileptic drugs, any other painkillers.

Contains: aspirin.

Anadin Extra
(Whitehall Laboratories)

A tablet or soluble tablet used as an analgesic and stimulant to relieve pain.

Dose: 1-2 tablets every 4 hours. (Maximum 6 tablets in 24 hours.)

Side effects: irritation of stomach and intestines.

Caution: pregnant women and patients with asthma or indigestion should consult a doctor before using this product.

Not to be used for: children under 12 years, nursing mothers, or patients with stomach ulcers, blood-clotting disorder, or allergy to aspirin.

Not to be used with: anticoagulants, some anti-epileptic drugs, other medicines containing paracetamol, excess tea or coffee.

Contains: aspirin, paracetamol, caffeine.

Anadin Maximum Strength
(Whitehall Laboratories)

A capsule used as an analgesic and stimulant to relieve pain.

Dose: 1-2 capsules every 4 hours. (Maximum 8 in 24 hours.)

Side effects: irritation of stomach and intestines.

Caution: pregnant women and patients with asthma or indigestion should consult a doctor before using this product.

Not to be used for: children under 12 years, nursing mothers, or patients with stomach ulcers, haemophilia, or allergy to aspirin.

Not to be used with: anti-coagulants, some anti-epileptic

drugs, excess tea or coffee.
Contains: aspirin, caffeine.

Anadin Paracetamol see **paracetamol tablets**
(Whitehall Laboratories)

Ashton and Parsons Infants' Powders
(SmithKline Beecham Consumer Healthcare)

A herbal powder used to relieve pain and stomach upset associated with teething in infants.

Dose: infants under 6 months ½ powder, infants over 6 months 1 powder (taken dry on the tongue). Use twice a day or every 1, 2, or 3 hours if necessary.
Side effects:
Caution:
Not to be used for: more than 5 days.
Not to be used with:
Contains: tincture of matricaria.

Askit
(Askit Laboratories)

A powder or capsule used as an analgesic and stimulant to treat pain, especially when associated with periods or headaches.

Dose: 1 powder (in water) or 2 capsules every 4 hours.
Side effects: irritation of stomach and intestines, constipation.
Caution: in pregnant women and patients with asthma or indigestion.
Not to be used for: children under 12 years, nursing mothers, or for patients with stomach ulcers, haemophilia, or allergy to aspirin.
Not to be used with: anti-coagulants, some anti-epileptic

drugs, excess tea or coffee.
Contains: aspirin, aloxiprin, caffeine.

---

aspirin 300 mg tablets

A tablet or soluble tablet used as an analgesic to relieve pain and reduce fever.

Dose: 1-3 tablets every 4-6 hours as needed. (Maximum of 12 tablets in 24 hours.)
Side effects: irritation of stomach and intestines, allergy.
Caution: pregnant women and patients with asthma or indigestion should consult a doctor before using this product.
Not to be used for: children under 12 years, nursing mothers, or for patients with stomach ulcers, blood-clotting disorder, or allergy to aspirin.
Not to be used with: anticoagulants, some anti-epileptic drugs.
Contains: aspirin.

Aspro
(Roche Consumer Health)

A tablet used as an analgesic to relieve pain and reduce fever.

Dose: 2-3 tablets every 4 hours as needed. (Maximum of 12 tablets in 24 hours.)
Side effects: irritation of stomach and intestines, allergy.
Caution: pregnant women and patients with asthma or indigestion should consult a doctor before using this product.
Not to be used for: children under 12 years, nursing mothers, or for patients with stomach ulcers, blood-clotting disorder, or allergy to aspirin.
Not to be used with: anticoagulants, some anti-epileptic drugs.
Contains: aspirin.

Aspro Clear
(Roche Consumer Health)

A clear-dissolving tablet, available as normal and maximum strengths, used as an analgesic to relieve pain.

Dose: 2-3 normal-strength tablets or 1-2 maximum-strength tablets every 4 hours. (Maximum 13 normal strength or 8 maximum strength in 24 hours.)
Side effects: irritation of stomach and intestines.
Caution: pregnant women and patients with asthma, indigestion, or stomach disorder should consult a doctor before using this product.
Not to be used for: children under 12 years, nursing mothers, or patients with stomach ulcers, blood-clotting disorder, or allergy to aspirin.
Not to be used with: anticoagulants, some anti-epileptic drugs.
Contains: aspirin.

Barum Aspirin
(Wrafton Laboratories)

A tablet or soluble tablet used as an analgesic to relieve pain and reduce fever.

Dose: 1-3 tablets every 4 hours as needed. (Maximum of 12 tablets in 24 hours.)
Side effects: irritation of stomach and intestines, allergy.
Caution: pregnant women and patients with asthma or indigestion should consult a doctor before using this product.
Not to be used for: children under 12 years, nursing mothers, or patients with stomach ulcers, blood-clotting disorder, or allergy to aspirin.
Not to be used with: anticoagulants, some anti-epileptic drugs.
Contains: aspirin.

Barum Extra Power see **Anadin Extra**
(Wrafton Laboratories)

Barum Paracetamol see **paracetamol**
(Wrafton Laboratories)

Barum Paracetamol Plus see **Panadol Extra**
(Wrafton Laboratories)

Bayer Aspirin see **aspirin 300 mg tablets**
(Bayer)

Beechams Aspirin Tablets 75 mg
(SmithKline Beecham Consumer)

A tablet which disperses on the tongue without water, and used to relieve pain.

Dose: 4 tablets every 4 hours if required. (Maximum of 24 in 24 hours.)
Side effects: irritation of stomach and intestines.
Caution: pregnant women and patients receiving medical treatment, or with asthma or indigestion should consult a doctor before using this product.
Not to be used for: children under 12 years, nursing mothers, or patients with stomach ulcers, blood-clotting disorder, or allergy to aspirin.
Not to be used with: anticoagulants, some anti-epileptic drugs.
Contains: aspirin.

Beechams Lemon Tablets
(SmithKline Beecham Consumer)

A tablet (to dissolve in the mouth or swallow with water), used to relieve pain, fever, and cold symptoms.

Dose: 1-2 tablets every 3-4 hours. (Maximum of 12 in 24 hours.)
Side effects: irritation of stomach and intestines.
Caution: pregnant women and patients receiving medical treatment, or with asthma or indigestion should consult a doctor before using this product.
Not to be used for: children under 12 years, nursing mothers, or patients with stomach ulcers, blood-clotting disorder, or allergy to aspirin.
Not to be used with: anticoagulants, some anti-epileptic drugs.
Contains: aspirin, glycine.

Beechams Powders
(SmithKline Beecham Consumer Healthcare)

A powder or tablet used as an analgesic and stimulant to relieve pain and the symptoms of colds and influenza.

Dose: 1 powder in water or 2 tablets every 3-4 hours when required. (Maximum of 6 powders in 24 hours.)
Side effects: irritation of stomach and intestines.
Caution: pregnant women and patients with asthma or indigestion should consult a doctor before using this product.
Not to be used for: children under 12 years, nursing mothers, or patients with stomach ulcers, blood-clotting disorder, or allergy to aspirin.
Not to be used with: anticoagulants, some anti-epileptic drugs, excess tea or coffee.
Contains: aspirin, caffeine.

Boots Children's Pain Relief Syrup
(Boots)

A sugar-free syrup used as an analgesic to treat pain and fever in children.

Dose: children aged 3-12 months 2.5-5 ml (aged 1-6 years 5-10 ml) up to 4 times a day.
Side effects: occasionally allergy.
Caution: patients taking other medicines, pregnant women, and nursing mothers should consult a doctor before using this medicines. Do not use for more than 3 days without consulting a doctor.
Not to be used for: infants under 3 months.
Not to be used with: other medicines containing paracetamol.
Contains: paracetamol.

Boots Children's Soluble Paracetamol Tablets see **Disprol Junior**
(Boots)

Boots Herbal Menstrual Comfort Tablets see entry in 'Women's disorders' section
(Boots)

Boots Pain Relief Tablets
(Boots)

A tablet or clear-dissolving tablet used as an analgesic and stimulant to treat pain and fever.

Dose: adults 1-2 tablets up to four times a day, children aged 5-12 years half the adult dose.
Side effects:
Caution:
Not to be used for: children under 5 years.
Not to be used with: other medicines containing paracetamol, excess tea or coffee.
Contains: paracetamol, caffeine.

Boots Pain Relief Plus Capsules see **Paracodol**
(Boots)

Boots Pain Relief Plus Clear Dissolving Tablets see **Solpadeine**
(Boots)

Buscopan
(Windsor Healthcare)

For use in treating period pain see entry in 'Stomach preparations' section

---

Calpol Extra see **paracetamol tablets**
(Warner Wellcome Consumer Healthcare)

Calpol Infant
(Warner Wellcome Consumer Healthcare)

A syrup available in normal or sugar-free varieties, used as an analgesic to relieve pain and fever in children.

Dose: for post-vaccination fever at 2 months, 2.5 ml. For general use, children aged 3-12 months 2.5-5 ml (aged 1-6 years 5-10 ml) up to 4 times a day.
Side effects:
Caution: infants under 3 months should be seen by a doctor before using this product. Do not use for more than 3 days without consulting a doctor.
Not to be used for: infants under 2 months.
Not to be used with: other medicines containing paracetamol.
Contains: paracetamol.

Calpol Six Plus
(Warner Wellcome Consumer Healthcare)

A suspension available in normal or sugar-free varieties, used as an analgesic to treat pain and fever in children over 6 years old.

Dose: children aged 6-12 years 5-10 ml (adults 10-20 ml) 4 times a day.
Side effects:
Caution: Do not use for more than 3 days without consulting a doctor.
Not to be used for: children under 6 years.
Not to be used with: other medicines containing paracetamol.
Contains: paracetamol.

---

co-codamol

A tablet or effervescent/dispersible tablet used as an opiate analgesic to relieve pain.

Dose: adults 1-2 tablets every 4-6 hours to a maximum of 8 tablets a day; children 6-12 years half adult dose.
Side effects: constipation, dependence.
Caution: asthmatics should consult a doctor before using this product.
Not to be used for: children under 6 years.
Not to be used with: MAOIs, other medicines containing paracetamol.
Contains: codeine phosphate, paracetamol.

---

co-codaprin

A tablet or dispersible tablet used as an opiate analgesic to relieve pain.
Dose: 1-2 tablets every 4-6 hours as needed.

Side effects: irritation of stomach and intestines, constipation, dependence.
Caution: pregnant women, the elderly, and patients with asthma, impaired kidney or indigestion should consult a doctor before using this product.
Not to be used for: children under 12 years, nursing mothers, or for patients with stomach ulcers, blood-clotting disorder, or allergy to aspirin.
Not to be used with: anticoagulants, some anti-epileptic drugs, MAOIs.
Contains: aspirin, codeine phosphate.

Coda-Med
(Thompson Medical)

A tablet used as an opiate analgesic and stimulant to relieve tension headache.

Dose: adults 1-2 tablets every 4 hours (maximum of 8 in 24 hours); children aged 8-14 years 1 tablet every 4 hours (maximum of 4 in 24 hours).
Side effects: constipation, dependence.
Caution: asthmatics should consult a doctor or pharmacist before using this product.
Not to be used for: children under 8 years.
Not to be used with: MAOIs, other medicines containing paracetamol, excess tea or coffee.
Contains: paracetamol, codeine phosphate, caffeine.

Codanin
(Whitehall Laboratories)

A tablet used as an opiate analgesic to relieve pain and reduce fever.

Dose: adults 2 tablets every 3-4 hours when required

(maximum of 8 in 24 hours); children aged 6-12 years ½ tablet every 3-4 hours (maximum of 4 in 24 hours).
Side effects: constipation, dependence.
Caution: asthmatics should consult a doctor or pharmacist before using this product.
Not to be used for: children under 6 years.
Not to be used with: MAOIs, other medicines containing paracetamol.
Contains: paracetamol, codeine.

Codis 500 see **co-codaprin dispersible**
(Reckitt & Colman)

Cojene
(Roche Consumer Health)

A tablet used as an opiate analgesic and stimulant to relieve pain and symptoms of colds and influenza.

Dose: 1-2 tablets every 4 hours if needed. (Maximum of 6 in 24 hours.)
Side effects: irritation of stomach and intestines, constipation, dependence.
Caution: pregnant women and patients with asthma or indigestion should consult a doctor before using this product.
Not to be used for: children under 12 years, nursing mothers, or for patients with stomach ulcers, blood-clotting disorder, or allergy to aspirin.
Not to be used with: anticoagulants, some anti-epileptic drugs, MAOIs, excess tea or coffee.
Contains: aspirin, codeine phosphate, caffeine.

Cullens Headache Powders
(Cullen and Davison)

A powder supplied in a sachet and used as an analgesic and

536

stimulant to relieve headache.

Dose: 1 powder every 3-4 hours as needed. (Maximum of 6 in 24 hours.)
Side effects: irritation of stomach and intestines.
Caution: pregnant women and patients with asthma or indigestion should consult a doctor before using this product.
Not to be used for: children under 12 years, nursing mothers, or patients with stomach ulcers, blood-clotting disorder, or allergy to aspirin.
Not to be used with: anticoagulants, some anti-epileptic drugs, excess tea or coffee.
Contains: aspirin, caffeine, calcium phosphate.

Cuprofen
(Seton Healthcare)

A tablet supplied at a strength of 200 mg (Cuprofen) or 400 mg (Cuprofen Maximum Strength) and used as a non-steroidal anti-inflammatory treatment for pain and fever.

Dose: 1-2 Cuprofen tablets or 1 Cuprofen Maximum Strength tablet every 4 hours if required. (Maximum 6 Cuprofen or 3 Cuprofen Maximum Strength in 24 hours.)
Side effects: stomach discomfort, nausea, diarrhoea, stomach ulcers, rash, rarely blood disorders.
Caution: elderly patients may need lower doses.
Not to be used for: children under 12 years, pregnant women, patients with stomach ulcers, heart disease, asthma, allergy to aspirin or anti-inflammatory drugs.
Not to be used with: antihypertensives, some antibiotics, other non-steroidal anti-inflammatory products (purchased or prescribed).
Contains: ibuprofen.

De Witt's Analgesic Pills
(E. C. De Witt)

A pill used as an analgesic and stimulant to treat pain and fever.

Dose: 2-3 tablets every 4 hours. (Maximum of 12 in 24 hours.)
Side effects:
Caution:
Not to be used for: children under 12 years.
Not to be used with: other medicines containing paracetamol, excess tea and coffee.
Contains: paracetamol, caffeine.

Disprin see aspirin soluble tablets
(Reckitt & Colman)

Disprin Direct
(Reckitt & Colman)

A tablet which disperses on the tongue without water, used to treat pain and fever.

Dose: 2-3 tablets every 4 hours. (Maximum of 13 in 24 hours.)
Side effects: irritation of stomach and intestines.
Caution: pregnant women and patients receiving medical treatment, or with asthma or indigestion should consult a doctor before using this product.
Not to be used for: children under 12 years, nursing mothers, or for patients with stomach ulcers, blood-clotting disorder, or allergy to aspirin.
Not to be used with: anticoagulants, some anti-epileptic drugs.
Contains: aspirin.

Disprin Extra
(Reckitt & Colman)

A soluble tablet used to treat pain and fever.

Dose: 1-2 tablets in water every 4 hours. (Maximum of 6 in 24 hours.)
Side effects: irritation of stomach and intestines.
Caution: pregnant women and patients with asthma or indigestion should consult a doctor before using this product.
Not to be used for: children under 12 years, nursing mothers, or for patients with stomach ulcers, blood-clotting disorder, or allergy to aspirin.
Not to be used with: anticoagulants, some anti-epileptic drugs, other medicines containing paracetamol.
Contains: aspirin, paracetamol.

Disprol see **paracetamol tablets**
(Reckitt & Colman)

Disprol Infant see **Calpol Infant (sugar-free)**
(Reckitt & Colman)

Disprol Junior
(Reckitt & Colman)

A soluble sugar-free tablet used to treat pain and fever in children.

Dose: ½-4 tablets (according to age) every 4 hours, up to four times a day.
Side effects:
Caution: children under 3 months and those taking any other medicines should be treated only on the advice of a doctor. Do not use for more than 3 days without consulting a doctor.
Not to be used for:

Not to be used with: other medicines containing paracetamol.
Contains: paracetamol.

Doan's Backache Pills
(Zyma Healthcare)

A tablet used as an analgesic to relieve rheumatic pain,
including backache.

Dose: 2-3 tablets every 4 hours. (Maximum of 16 in 24 hours.)
Side effects: irritation of stomach and intestines.
Caution: pregnant women and patients with asthma or
indigestion should consult a doctor before using this product.
Not to be used for: children under 12 years, nursing mothers,
or patients with stomach ulcers, blood-clotting disorder, gout
or allergy to aspirin.
Not to be used with: anticoagulants, some anti-epileptic drugs,
other medicines containing paracetamol.
Contains: paracetamol, sodium salicylate.

E. P.
(Pharmax)

A tablet used as an opiate analgesic and stimulant to treat
period pain.

Dose: 2 tablets every 4 hours when needed. (Maximum of 8 in
24 hours.)
Side effects: constipation, dependence.
Caution: asthmatics should consult a doctor or pharmacist
before using this product.
Not to be used for: children under 12 years.
Not to be used with: MAOIs, other medicines containing
paracetamol, excess tea or coffee.
Contains: paracetamol, caffeine, codeine phosphate.

Fanalgic see **paracetamol**
(Mitchell International Pharmaceuticals)

Femigraine
(Roche Consumer Health)

An effervescent tablet used as an antihistamine and analgesic treatment for headache and nausea associated with migraine.

Dose: 2 tablets every 4 hours. (Maximum 8 in 24 hours.)
Side effects: drowsiness, irritation of stomach and intestines. (Rarely, rash and jaundice.)
Caution: pregnant women and patients with asthma or indigestion, or receiving medical treatment should consult a doctor before using this product.
Not to be used for: children under 12 years, nursing mothers, or for patients with stomach ulcers, other stomach disorders, blood-clotting disorder, or allergy to aspirin.
Not to be used with: anticoagulants, some anti-epileptic drugs, alcohol.
Contains: aspirin, cyclizine.

Feminax
(Roche Consumer Health)

A tablet used as an anti-spasm, stimulant, and analgesic treatment for period pain.

Dose: 2 tablets up to 3 times a day.
Side effects: constipation, dependence, drowsiness.
Caution: asthmatics should consult a doctor or pharmacist before using this product. Pregnant women should consult a doctor if this product is required.
Not to be used for: children under 12 years, or for patients suffering from glaucoma.
Not to be used with: MAOIs, other medicines containing

paracetamol, excess tea or coffee, other sedating medicines.
Contains: paracetamol, codeine phosphate, caffeine monohydrate, hyoscine hydrobromide.

Fenning's Children's Cooling Powders
(Waterhouse)

A powder used as an analgesic to treat pain and fever in children.

Dose: 1-4 powders (according to age) up to 4 times a day.
Side effects:
Caution: children under 3 months should be seen by a doctor before using this product.
Not to be used for:
Not to be used with: other medicines containing paracetamol.
Contains: paracetamol.

Fynnon Calcium Aspirin
(Seton Healthcare)

A tablet used as an analgesic to relieve pain (including rheumatic pain and stiffness), and symptoms of colds and influenza.

Dose: 1-2 tablets every 4 hours. (Maximum of 8 in 24 hours.)
Side effects: irritation of stomach and intestines.
Caution: pregnant women and patients with asthma or indigestion should consult a doctor before using this product.
Not to be used for: children under 12 years, nursing mothers, or for patients with stomach ulcers, blood-clotting disorder, or allergy to aspirin.
Not to be used with: anticoagulants, some anti-epileptic drugs.
Contains: aspirin, calcium carbonate.

Hedex see **paracetamol tablets**
(Sterling Health)

Hedex Extra see **Panadol Extra**
(Sterling Health)

---

ibuprofen tablets

A tablet available at a strength of 200 mg or 400 mg and used as a non-steroidal anti-inflammatory treatment for pain (including headache, muscular pain, period pain, and dental pain) and fever.

Dose: 400 mg initially, then 200-400 mg every 4 hours. (Maximum of 1200 mg in 24 hours.)
Side effects: stomach discomfort, nausea, diarrhoea, stomach ulcers, rash, rarely blood disorders.
Caution: elderly patients may need lower doses.
Not to be used for: children under 12 years, pregnant women, patients with stomach ulcers or other stomach disorder, heart disease, asthma, allergy to aspirin or anti-inflammatory drugs.
Not to be used with: antihypertensives, some antibiotics, other non-steroidal anti-inflammatory products (purchased or prescribed).
Contains: ibuprofen.

Infadrops
(Goldshield)

A sugar-free solution supplied with a measuring dropper, and used as an analgesic and antipyretic to reduce pain and fever (including post-vaccination fever) in babies and young children.

Dose: 0.6 ml-1.6 ml up to 4 times a day, according to age.
Side effects:
Caution: babies under 3 months should be seen by a doctor

before using this product. Do not use for more than 3 days without consulting a doctor.
Not to be used for: babies under 2 months.
Not to be used with: other medicines containing paracetamol.
Contains: paracetamol.

Inoven see **Nurofen**
(Janssen)

Jackson's Febrifuge see entry in 'Respiratory conditions – cough and cold remedies' section
(Waterhouse)

Junifen
(Crookes Healthcare)

A sugar-free liquid used as a non-steroidal anti-inflammatory treatment for pain and fever in children.

Dose: 2.5 ml-10 ml (according to age) 3 or 4 times a day.
Side effects: stomach discomfort, nausea, diarrhoea, stomach ulcers, rash, rarely blood disorders.
Caution: pregnant women, asthmatics, and patients who are taking other medication should see a doctor before using this product.
Not to be used for: children under 1 year, or for those weighing less than 7 kg or with stomach ulcers, other stomach disorder, heart disease, asthma, allergy to aspirin or anti-inflammatory drugs.
Not to be used with: antihypertensives, some antibiotics, other non-steroidal anti-inflammatory products (purchased or prescribed).
Contains: ibuprofen.

Librofem
(Zyma Healthcare)

A tablet used to treat period pain, muscular pain, and menstrual headache.

Dose: 2 tablets initially, then 1-2 tablets every 4 hours. (Maximum of 6 in 24 hours.)
Side effects: stomach discomfort, nausea, diarrhoea, stomach ulcers, rash, rarely blood disorders.
Caution: pregnant women, and patients with asthma, allergy to aspirin, or who receive regular medical treatment should see a doctor before using this product.
Not to be used for: children under 12 years, elderly patients, patients with stomach ulcers or other stomach disorders, heart disease, allergy to anti-inflammatory drugs.
Not to be used with: antihypertensives, some antibiotics, other non-steroidal anti-inflammatory products (purchased or prescribed).
Contains: ibuprofen.

Medinol Over 6 see **Calpol Six Plus**
(Seton Healthcare)

Medinol Under 6 (Paediatric) see **Calpol Infant**
(Seton Healthcare)

Medised
(Seton Healthcare)

A liquid used as an antihistamine and analgesic to treat pain and fever, and relieve the symptoms of chickenpox, influenza, and colds.

Dose: children aged 1-6 years 10 ml (aged 6-12 years 20 ml) up to 4 times a day, for a maximum of 3 days.

Side effects: drowsiness, sensitivity to light, disorientation, shaking, excitability, nightmares.
Caution: children under 1 year, or suffering from asthma, heart disease, bronchitis or epilepsy should be seen by a doctor before using this product.
Not to be used for:
Not to be used with: other sedating medicines, alcohol, other medicines containing paracetamol.
Contains: paracetamol, promethazine hydrochloride.

Midrid
(Rhone Poulenc Rorer)

A capsule used as a sympathomimetic and analgesic to treat migraine.

Dose: 2 capsules at the beginning of the migraine attack, then 1 capsule every hour to a maximum of 5 capsules in 12 hours.
Side effects: dizziness.
Caution: pregnant women and nursing mothers should consult a doctor before using this product.
Not to be used for: children, or for patients suffering from heart disease, gastritis, severe high blood pressure, or glaucoma.
Not to be used with: MAOIs, other medicines containing paracetamol.
Contains: isometheptene mucate, paracetamol.

Migrafen see **ibuprofen tablets**
(Chatfield)

Migraleve
(Charwell Healthcare)

A pink tablet and a yellow tablet used as an opiate analgesic, antihistamine treatment for migraine headache and associated nausea and vomiting.

Dose: adults and children over 14 years 2 pink tablets at the beginning of the attack and then 2 yellow tablets every 4 hours if needed to a maximum of 2 pink tablets and 6 yellow tablets in 24 hours. (Children aged 10-14 years, half the adult dose.)
Side effects: drowsiness, constipation, dependence.
Caution: asthmatics should consult a doctor before using this product.
Not to be used for: children under 10 years.
Not to be used with: other medicines containing paracetamol, other sedating medicines, alcohol, MAOIs.
Contains: paracetamol, codeine phosphate. (Pink tablets also contain buclizine hydrochloride.)

Nu-Seals 300 mg
(Lilly)

A tablet, coated to protect the stomach, supplied at a strength of 300 mg and used as an analgesic to treat pain and fever.

Dose: up to 3 tablets 3 times a day.
Side effects: irritation of stomach and intestines.
Caution: pregnant women, diabetics, and patients with asthma or indigestion should consult a doctor before using this preparation.
Not to be used for: children under 12 years, nursing mothers, or patients with stomach ulcers, blood-clotting disorder, or allergy to aspirin.
Not to be used with: anticoagulants, some anti-epileptic drugs, antacids.
Contains: aspirin.

Nurofen
(Crookes Healthcare)

A tablet available at a strength of 200 mg or 400 mg, and a sachet of microgranules (at a strength of 400 mg to add to water) used as a non-steroidal anti-inflammatory treatment for pain (including headache, muscular pain, period pain, and dental pain) and fever.

Dose: 400 mg initially, then 200 mg-400 mg every 4 hours. (Maximum of 1200 mg in 24 hours.)
Side effects: stomach discomfort, nausea, diarrhoea, stomach ulcers, rash, rarely blood disorders.
Caution: elderly patients may need lower doses.
Not to be used for: children under 12 years, pregnant women, patients with stomach ulcers or other stomach disorder, heart disease, asthma, allergy to aspirin or anti-inflammatory drugs.
Not to be used with: antihypertensives, some antibiotics, other non-steroidal anti-inflammatory products (purchased or prescribed).
Contains: ibuprofen.

Nurofen Plus
(Crookes Healthcare)

A tablet used as a non-steroidal anti-inflammatory and opiate analgesic treatment for pain.

Dose: 2 tablets initially, then 1-2 tablets every 4 hours. (Maximum of 6 in 24 hours.)
Side effects: stomach discomfort, nausea, diarrhoea, stomach ulcers, rash, rarely blood disorders, constipation, dependence.
Caution: elderly patients may need lower doses.
Not to be used for: children under 12 years, pregnant women, patients with stomach ulcers or other stomach disorder, heart disease, asthma, allergy to aspirin or anti-inflammatory drugs.
Not to be used with: antihypertensives, some antibiotics, MAOIs, other non-steroidal anti-inflammatory products (purchased or prescribed).

Contains: ibuprofen, codeine phosphate.

Nurse Sykes' Powders
(Waterhouse)

A powder used as an analgesic and stimulant to treat pain and fever.

Dose: 1 powder (in water) every 4 hours.
Side effects: irritation of stomach and intestines.
Caution: pregnant women and patients with asthma or indigestion should consult a doctor before using this product.
Not to be used for: children under 12 years, nursing mothers, or patients with stomach ulcers, blood-clotting disorder, or allergy to aspirin.
Not to be used with: anticoagulants, some anti-epileptic drugs, other medicines containing paracetamol, excess tea or coffee.
Contains: aspirin, caffeine, paracetamol.

Pacifene see **ibuprofen 200 mg tablets**
(Sussex)

Pacifene Maximum Strength see **ibuprofen 400 mg tablets**
(Sussex)

Pameton
(Sterling Health)

A tablet used as an analgesic (with antidote), to treat pain and fever, particularly when there is a possibility of misuse or overdose.

Dose: adults 2 tablets (children aged 6-12 years ½-1 tablet) every 4 hours if required. (Maximum of 8 in 24 hours for adults, 4 in 24 hours for children.)
Side effects:

Caution: pregnant women should consult a doctor before taking this product.
Not to be used for: children under 6 years.
Not to be used with: other medicines containing paracetamol, some anti-parkinson drugs.
Contains: paracetamol, methionine.

Panadeine see **co-codamol**
(Sterling Health)

Panadol Baby and Infant
(Sterling Health)

A suspension used as an analgesic to treat pain and fever.

Dose: babies aged 2-3 months 2.5 ml, babies aged 3-12 months 2.5-5 ml, children aged 1-6 years 5-10 ml, children aged 6-12 years 10-20 ml up to 4 times a day.
Side effects:
Caution: babies under 2 months, or premature babies under 3 months should be seen by a doctor before using this product. Do not use for more than 3 days without consulting a doctor.
Not to be used for:
Not to be used with: other medicines containing paracetamol.
Contains: paracetamol.

Panadol Extra
(Sterling Health)

A tablet or soluble tablet used as an analgesic and stimulant to treat pain and fever.

Dose: 2 tablets up to 4 times a day.
Side effects:
Caution:
Not to be used for: children under 12 years.

Not to be used with: other medicines containing paracetamol, excess tea and coffee.
Contains: paracetamol, caffeine.

Panadol Junior
(Sterling Health)

A powder supplied in sachets and used as an analgesic to treat pain and fever in children.

Dose: 1-2 sachets (according to age) up to 4 times a day.
Side effects:
Caution: do not use for more than 3 days without consulting a doctor.
Not to be used for: children under 3 years.
Not to be used with: other medicines containing paracetamol.
Contains: paracetamol.

Panadol Tablets/Capsules see **paracetamol tablets/capsules**
(Sterling Health)

Panadol Ultra
(Sterling Health)

A tablet used as an opiate analgesic for strong pain relief.

Dose: 2 tablets every 4 hours. (maximum 8 in 24 hours).
Side effects: constipation, dependence, drowsiness.
Caution: asthmatics should consult a doctor or pharmacist before using this product.
Not to be used for: children under 12 years.
Not to be used with: MAOIs, other medicines containing paracetamol, other sedating medicines.
Contains: paracetamol, codeine phosphate hemihydrate.

Panaleve Junior see **Calpol Infant**
(Pinewood Healthcare)

Panaleve 6+ see **Calpol Six Plus**
(Pinewood Healthcare)

Panerel
(Cox)

A tablet used as an opiate analgesic to treat pain.

Dose: adults 1-2 tablets up to 4 times a day; children aged 8-14 years 1 tablet up to 3 times a day.
Side effects: constipation, dependence.
Caution: asthmatics should consult a doctor or pharmacist before using this product.
Not to be used for: children under 8 years.
Not to be used with: MAOIs, other medicines containing paracetamol.
Contains: paracetamol, codeine phosphate.

---

paracetamol tablets/capsules

A tablet, soluble tablet, or capsule used as an analgesic to relieve pain and reduce fever.

Dose: adults 1-2 tablets or capsules 4 times a day; children 6-12 years ½-1 tablet 4 times a day.
Side effects:
Caution:
Not to be used for: children under 6 years (tablets), children under 12 years (capsules).
Not to be used with: other medicines containing paracetamol.
Contains: paracetamol.

Paracets see **paracetamol**
(Sussex)

Paraclear
(Roche Consumer Health)

A clear-dissolving tablet available as normal strength, and a plain tablet available as extra strength, used as an analgesic to treat pain.

Dose: 1-2 tablets up to 4 times a day. (Children over 6 years may take the normal strength tablets at half the adult dose.)
Side effects:
Caution: pregnant women or patients already receiving medical treatment should consult a doctor before using this product.
Not to be used for: children under 6 years (normal strength) or children under 12 years (extra strength).
Not to be used with: other medicines containing paracetamol. Avoid excessive intake of coffee and tea with extra-strength tablets.
Contains: paracetamol. (Extra-strength tablets also contain caffeine.)

Paracodol
(Roche Consumer Health)

A capsule or effervescent tablet used as an opiate analgesic to relieve pain.

Dose: adults 1-2 capsules or tablets every 4-6 hours to a maximum of 8 tablets in 24 hours; children 6-12 years may use tablets at half adult dose.
Side effects: constipation, dependence.
Caution: asthmatics should consult a doctor before using this product. Patients who need to restrict their intake of salt will also need medical advice if using the effervescent tablets.

Not to be used for: children under 6 years (tablets), or under 12 years (capsules).
Not to be used with: MAOIs, other medicines containing paracetamol.
Contains: paracetamol, codeine phosphate.

Paramin Junior Paracetamol Capsules
(Wallis)

A capsule used as an analgesic to treat pain and fever.

Dose: 1-4 capsules (according to age) up to 4 times a day.
Side effects:
Caution: do not use for more than 3 days without consulting a doctor.
Not to be used for: children under 3 years.
Not to be used with: other medicines containing paracetamol.
Contains: paracetamol.

Paramol
(Napp Consumer Products)

White tablets used as an opiate analgesic to treat pain and feverish conditions.

Dose: 1 or 2 tablets every 4 to 6 hours after meals. (Maximum of 8 in 24 hours.)
Side effects: constipation, dependence.
Caution: pregnant women, nursing mothers, and patients with asthma, breathing difficulty, or allergic disorder should consult a doctor before using this product.
Not to be used for: children under 12 years, patients with obstructed airways.
Not to be used with: other medicines containing paracetamol, MAOIs.
Contains: dihydrocodeine tartrate, paracetamol.

Phensic
(SmithKline Beecham Consumer)

A tablet used as an analgesic and stimulant to relieve pain.

Dose: 2 tablets every 3-4 hours when required. (Maximum of 12 in 24 hours.)
Side effects: irritation of stomach and intestines.
Caution: pregnant women and patients with asthma or indigestion should consult a doctor before using this product.
Not to be used for: children under 12 years, nursing mothers, or patients with stomach ulcers, blood-clotting disorder, or allergy to aspirin.
Not to be used with: anticoagulants, some anti-epileptic drugs.
Contains: aspirin, caffeine.

Phor Pain see **ibuprofen 200 mg tablets**
(Goldshield Healthcare)

Phor Pain Double Strength see **ibuprofen 400 mg tablets**
(Goldshield Healthcare)

Placidex
(E. C. De Witt)

A syrup used as an analgesic to treat pain and fever in children.

Dose: children aged 3-12 months 2.5-5 ml (aged 1-6 years 5-10 ml, aged 6-12 years 10-20 ml) up to 4 times a day.
Side effects:
Caution: infants under 3 months should be seen by a doctor before using this product. Do not use for more than 3 days without consulting a doctor.
Not to be used for:
Not to be used with: other medicines containing paracetamol.

Contains: paracetamol.

Powerin see **Anadin Extra**
(Whitehall Laboratories)

Proflex
(Zyma Healthcare)

A tablet or long-acting capsule used as a non-steroidal anti-inflammatory treatment for muscular aches and pains.

Dose: 1-2 tablets 3 times a day or 1-2 capsules twice a day.
Side effects: stomach discomfort, nausea, diarrhoea, stomach ulcers, rash, rarely blood disorders.
Caution: elderly patients may need reduced doses. Patients already taking medication should consult their doctor before using this product. Do not suck or chew the capsules.
Not to be used for: pregnant women, or for patients with stomach ulcers, heart disease, asthma, allergy to aspirin or anti-inflammatory drugs.
Not to be used with: antihypertensives, some antibiotics, other non-steroidal anti-inflammatory products (purchased or prescribed).
Contains: ibuprofen.

Propain
(Panpharma)

A tablet used as an opiate analgesic, antihistamine and stimulant treatment for headache, migraine, muscle pain, period pain, and fever.

Dose: 1-2 tablets every 4 hours to a maximum of 10 tablets in 24 hours.
Side effects: drowsiness, constipation, dependence.
Caution: asthmatics should consult a doctor before using this

product.

Not to be used for: children, pregnant women, or nursing mothers.

Not to be used with: alcohol, other sedating medicines, other medicines containing paracetamol, MAOIs, alcohol.

Contains: codeine phosphate, diphenhydramine hydrochloride, paracetamol, caffeine.

Relcofen see **ibuprofen tablets**
(Cox)

Resolve see entry in 'Stomach preparations' section
(SmithKline Beecham Consumer)

Safeway Paracetamol Plus Tablets see **Panadol Extra**
(Safeway)

Sea-band Head Band*
(Sea-band)

A head band with two rubber pressure pads, which are applied to the affected area during a headache, to relieve pain.

Solpadeine
(Sterling Health)

A tablet, effervescent tablet, or capsule used as an opiate analgesic and stimulant to relieve pain and fever.

Dose: adults 2 tablets or capsules 3-4 times a day.
Side effects: constipation, dependence.
Caution: asthmatics should consult a doctor before using this product. Patients who need to restrict their salt intake will also need medical advice if using the effervescent tablets.
Not to be used for: children under 12 years.

Not to be used with: other medicines containing paracetamol, excess tea or coffee, MAOIs
Contains: paracetamol, codeine phosphate, caffeine.

Syndol
(Marion Merrell Dow)

A tablet used as an opiate analgesic, antihistamine, and stimulant treatment for headache (including tension headache) and other pain, such as toothache, period pains, and post-operative pains.
Dose: 1-2 tablets every 4-6 hours up to a maximum of 8 tablets in 24 hours.
Side effects: drowsiness, constipation, dependence, dizziness, rarely blood disorders.
Caution: asthmatics should consult a doctor before using this product.
Not to be used for: children under 12 years and pregnant women.
Not to be used with: alcohol, MAOIs, other sedating medicines, other medicines containing paracetamol, excess tea or coffee.
Contains: paracetamol, codeine phosphate, doxylamine succinate, caffeine.

Tramil see **paracetamol capsules**
(Whitehall Laboratories)

Unichem Junior Paracetamol Capsules see **Paramin Junior Paracetamol Capsules**
(Unichem)

Unichem Pain Relief Syrup for Children
(Unichem)

A syrup used as an analgesic to treat pain and fever in children.

Dose: children aged 3-12 months 2.5-5 ml (aged 1-6 years 5-10 ml) up to 4 times a day.
Side effects:
Caution: infants under 3 months should be seen by a doctor before using this product. Do not use for more than 3 days without consulting a doctor.
Not to be used for:
Not to be used with: other medicines containing paracetamol.
Contains: paracetamol.

Unichem Paracetamol Seltzer see Paracetamol Soluble Tablets
(Unichem)

Veganin
(Warner Wellcome Consumer Healthcare)

A tablet used as an opiate analgesic to treat pain, fever, and symptoms of influenza and colds.

Dose: 1-2 tablets every 3-4 hours. (Maximum of 8 in 24 hours.)
Side effects: irritation of stomach and intestines, constipation, dependence.
Caution: pregnant women and patients with asthma or indigestion should consult a doctor before using this product.
Not to be used for: children under 12 years, nursing mothers, or patients with stomach ulcers, blood-clotting disorder, or allergy to aspirin.
Not to be used with: anticoagulants, some anti-epileptic drugs, MAOIs, other medicines containing paracetamol.
Contains: aspirin, paracetamol, codeine phosphate.

Sleeping problems and stress

The few products that have been licensed for use as aids to sleeping are intended only for occasional, short-term use. They should not be used for more than a few days, or repeatedly, because dependence on a drug to produce sleep may result. For persistent sleep problems, consult a doctor.

There are many herbal remedies available that can be used to relieve symptoms of stress-related disorders and insomnia. These are not a substitute for medical attention, however, and persistent or severe problems of this nature should be referred to a doctor.

Ana-sed
(Potters)

A tablet used as a sedative and mildly analgesic herbal remedy to treat symptoms of minor aches, irritability, and tension.

Dose: 1-2 tablets 3 times a day and 2 at bedtime.
Side effects:
Caution:
Not to be used for: children, women in the early stages of pregnancy, or nursing mothers.
Not to be used with:
Contains: hops, Jamaica dogwood, wild lettuce, passionflower, pulsatilla.

Avena Sativa Comp.
(Weleda)

A liquid used as a herbal sedative to aid relaxation at the end of the day.

Dose: adults 10-20 drops (children aged 2-12 years 5-10 drops) in water half an hour before retiring.
Side effects: drowsiness.
Caution: children under 2 years should be seen by a doctor before using this medicine.
Not to be used for: pregnant women or nursing mothers.
Not to be used with: other sedating medicines, alcohol.
Contains: oats, passionflower, valerian, coffea.

Bio-Strath Valerian Formula
(Cedar Health)

A liquid used as a herbal sedative to relieve the symptoms of tension, irritability, restlessness, stress, and strain, and to encourage natural sleep.

Dose: 20 drops (0.6 ml) in a little water 3 times a day before meals, or as directed by a doctor.
Side effects:
Caution:
Not to be used for: children, pregnant women, or nursing mothers.
Not to be used with: homeopathic remedies.
Contains: yeast, valerian, passionflower, peppermint.

___

Biophyllin
(Gerard House)

A tablet used as a herbal sedative to treat tension, restlessness, and nervous irritability.

Dose: 2 tablets after meals 3 times a day.
Side effects:
Caution: nursing mothers and patients taking other medication should consult a doctor before using this product.
Not to be used for: children under 12 years, or for pregnant women.
Not to be used with:
Contains: valerian, scullcap, Jamaican dogwood, black cohosh.

Boots Herbal Restful Night Tablets
(Boots)

A tablet used as a herbal remedy to promote natural sleep.

Dose: 2 tablets taken with the evening meal and 2 tablets before bedtime.
Side effects:
Caution: pregnant women and nursing mothers should consult a doctor before using this product.
Not to be used for: children under 12 years, or in early pregnancy.

Not to be used with:
Contains: passionflower.

Boots Herbal Stress Tablets
(Boots)

A tablet used as a herbal remedy to relieve the symptoms of stress, strain, and irritability.

Dose: 2 tablets 3 times a day after food and 2 tablets at bedtime.
Side effects:
Caution:
Not to be used for: children under 14 years, pregnant women, and nursing mothers.
Not to be used with:
Contains: passionflower, motherwort, dry extract of vervain and valerian.

Fragador
(Weleda)

A tablet used as a natural remedy to relieve occasional nerviness and edginess brought on by everyday stress and strain.

Dose: 2 tablets 3 times a day.
Side effects:
Caution:
Not to be used for: pregnant women and nursing mothers.
Not to be used with:
Contains: scurvy grass, conchae, wild strawberry, glycogen 10x, lovage, radix mel 1x, natrum carbonicum 1x, aniseed, sage, wheatgerm, stinging nettle, ferrum phosphoricum 4x.

Gerard 99
(Gerard House)

A tablet used as a herbal sedative to relieve symptoms of tension, irritability, and stress.

Dose: 2 tablets after meals 3 times a day.
Side effects:
Caution: patients using other medication should consult a doctor before using this product.
Not to be used for: children under 12 years or pregnant women.
Not to be used with:
Contains: hops, passionflower, valerian.

Heath & Heather Becalm
(Ferrosan Healthcare)

A tablet used as a herbal sedative to aid relaxation from stress.

Dose: 1 tablet 3 times a day.
Side effects: drowsiness.
Caution:
Not to be used for: children, pregnant women, or nursing mothers.
Not to be used with: other sedating medicines, alcohol.
Contains: valerian, hops, passionflower.

Heath & Heather Quiet Night Tablets
(Ferrosan Healthcare)

A tablet used as a herbal sedative to aid sleep.

Dose: 2 tablets 1 hour before bedtime.
Side effects: drowsiness, which may persist the next day.
Caution: pregnant women should consult a doctor before using this product.

Not to be used for: children.
Not to be used with: other sedating medicines, alcohol.
Contains: valerian, hops, passionflower.

___

Isocones*
(Sea-band)

Soft rubber buttons worn on the wrists (attached by plasters) at night to treat insomnia. (Not suitable for children under 5 years.)

___

Kalms
(Lane)

A tablet used as a herbal sedative used to relieve the symptoms of anxiety, irritability and stress, and to encourage natural sleep.

Dose: 2 tablets 3 times a day after meals.
Side effects:
Caution: patients taking other medication should consult a doctor before using this product. Not to be taken in large doses for extended periods of time.
Not to be used for: children, pregnant women, nursing mothers, or for patients suffering from clinical depression.
Not to be used with: (see above.)
Contains: hops, valerian, gentian.

___

Medinex
(Whitehall)

A liquid used as an antihistamine treatment for temporary sleep disturbance.

Dose: 10-25 ml at night.
Side effects: drowsiness.
Caution: pregnant women, nursing mothers, and patients

suffering from glaucoma, asthma or other lung disease, prostate or bladder problems, gastro-intestinal obstruction, or those taking other medicines should consult a doctor before using this product. Not for prolonged use.
Not to be used for: children under 16 years.
Not to be used with: other sedating drugs, alcohol, MAOIs.
Contains: diphenhydramine hydrochloride.

Motherwort Compound
(Gerard House)

A tablet used as a herbal sedative and anti-spasm remedy to treat the symptoms of stress and strain.

Dose: 2 tablets 3 times a day after meals.
Side effects:
Caution: pregnant women and patients with serious symptoms should consult a doctor before using this product.
Not to be used for: children.
Not to be used with:
Contains: passionflower, motherwort, lime flower.

Natracalm
(English Grains Healthcare)

A tablet used as a herbal remedy to relieve symptoms of stress, strain, and nervous tension.

Dose: 1 tablet 3 times a day.
Side effects:
Caution: pregnant women and patients taking prescribed tranquillizers should consult a doctor before using this product. (Do not discontinue treatment with prescribed medication until a doctor has agreed.)
Not to be used for: children.
Not to be used with: tranquillizers (see above).

Contains: passionflower.

Natrasleep
(English Grains Healthcare)

A tablet used as a herbal remedy to encourage natural sleep.

Dose: 1-3 tablets taken 30 minutes before bedtime.
Side effects:
Caution: pregnant women, nursing mothers, and patients taking other medication should consult a doctor before using this product.
Not to be used for: children.
Not to be used with: (see above.)
Contains: hops, valerian.

Naturest
(Lane)

A tablet used as a herbal sedative to treat temporary or occasional sleeplessness due to everyday problems.

Dose: 2 tablets 3 times a day and up to 3 more at bedtime.
Side effects:
Caution:
Not to be used for: children under 12 years, pregnant women, or nursing mothers.
Not to be used with:
Contains: passionflower.

Newrelax
(Potters)

A tablet used as a herbal sedative, analgesic, and anti-spasm remedy to relieve the symptoms of tension, irritability, stress, and strain.

Dose: 2 tablets 3 times a day. (Best results obtained if taken as a continuous course for a few weeks.)
Side effects:
Caution: patients taking other medications should consult a doctor before using this product.
Not to be used for: children, pregnant women, or nursing mothers.
Not to be used with:
Contains: hops, scullcap, valerian, vervain.

Nodoff
(Potters)

A liquid and tablet used as a herbal remedy to assist natural sleep.

Dose: 5 ml liquid (or 2 tablets) with the last meal, then 10 ml liquid (or 2-4 tablets) at bedtime.
Side effects: (liquid may cause drowsiness if taken in excess.)
Caution: pregnant women and nursing mothers should consult a doctor before using this product.
Not to be used for: children, or for women in early pregnancy.
Not to be used with: (liquid not to be used with alcohol or other sedating medicines.)
Contains: passionflower. (Liquid also contains scullcap, hops, valerian, Jamaica dogwood.)

Nytol
(Stafford-Miller)

A tablet available in two strengths, and used as an antihistamine treatment for relief of temporary sleep disturbance.

Dose: 2 regular tablets or 1 'one-a-night' tablet 20 minutes before bedtime.
Side effects: drowsiness, dizziness, dry mouth, nausea,

nervousness, reduced effect with continuous use, and rarely blood disorders.

Caution: patients with myaesthenia gravis, asthma, glaucoma, prostate or other bladder disorder, or stomach ulcer should consult a doctor before using this product. Patients using other medication should also seek advice. Not to be used for more than 2 weeks.

Not to be used for: children under 16 years, pregnant women, nursing mothers.

Not to be used with: other sedating drugs, MAOIs, alcohol.

Contains: diphenhydramine hydrochloride.

---

passiflora tablets
(Licensed preparations available from Gerard House, Potters)

A tablet used as a herbal remedy to promote natural sleep and assist relaxation. It also has mild pain-killing and anti-spasm properties.

Dose: as specified for the individual products.

Side effects:

Caution: pregnant women and nursing mothers should consult a doctor before using this product.

Not to be used for:

Not to be used with:

Contains: passionflower.

Phenergan Nightime
(Rhone-Poulenc Rorer)

A tablet used as a short-term antihistamine treatment for insomnia.

Dose: 1-2 tablets at night.

Side effects: drowsiness, nausea, reduced reactions, dizziness, disorientation, sensitivity to light, shaking, rigidity, dry mouth, difficulty passing water, headache, confusion, restlessness.

Caution: pregnant women, nursing mothers, and patients with asthma, bronchitis, glaucoma, epilepsy or coronary heart disease, or who take other medicines should consult a doctor before using this product. Do not use for more than 7 days, except on the advice of a doctor.

Not to be used for: children under 16 years.

Not to be used with: other sedating drugs, antidepressants, MAOIs, alcohol, pregnancy tests, allergy tests.

Contains: promethazine.

Quiet Life
(Lane)

A tablet used as a herbal sedative remedy to treat the symptoms of irritability, nervousness, tension, and sleeplessness, and to aid relaxation.

Dose: 2 tablets twice a day and 2-3 at bedtime.
Side effects: high doses may cause headaches or sickness.
Caution: patients taking other medication should consult a doctor before using this product.
Not to be used for: children, pregnant women, nursing mothers, or patients suffering from clinical depression.
Not to be used with:
Contains: hops, wild lettuce, valerian, motherwort, passionflower, vitamins B_1, B_2, B_3.

---

royal jelly* see entry in 'Vitamins and minerals' section

Serenity
(Gerard House)

A tablet used as a herbal remedy to relieve symptoms of stress, strain, and irritability.

Dose: 2 tablets 3 times a day after food.
Side effects:
Caution: pregnant women and nursing mothers should consult a doctor before using this product.
Not to be used for: children.
Not to be used with:
Contains: hops, valerian, passionflower.

Sominex
(SmithKline Beecham Consumer)

A tablet used to correct the sleep pattern during temporary sleep disturbance.

Dose: 1 tablet at bedtime.
Side effects: drowsiness.
Caution: not for prolonged use. (Patients suffering from prolonged sleep disturbance must consult a doctor.)
Not to be used for: children under 16 years.
Not to be used with: other sedating drugs, alcohol.
Contains: promethazine hydrochloride.

Somnus
(Gerard House)

A tablet used as a herbal remedy to relieve symptoms of restlessness and encourage relaxation and natural sleep.

Dose: 2 tablets 1 hour before bedtime.
Side effects:
Caution: pregnant women and nursing mothers should consult a doctor before using this product.
Not to be used for: children.
Not to be used with:
Contains: valerian, wild lettuce, hops.

Sunerven
(Lane)

A tablet used as a sedative herbal remedy to relieve symptoms of anxiety, stress, tension, irritability, fatigue, and sleeplessness, and to encourage natural sleep.

Dose: 2 tablets 3 times a day after meals and 2 tablets before bedtime.
Side effects:
Caution: pregnant women and nursing mothers should consult a doctor before using this product. Not to be taken in high doses for prolonged periods of time.
Not to be used for: children under 14 years.
Not to be used with:
Contains: valerian, passionflower, motherwort, vervain.

---

valerian

A herb used in various remedies as a sedative.

Dose: according to individual product instructions.
Side effects: possible drowsiness with high doses.
Caution: pregnant women and nursing mothers should consult a doctor before using this herb.
Not to be used for: children.
Not to be used with: avoid alcohol and sedating medicines with high doses.
Contains: valerian.

Valerian Compound
(Gerard House)

A tablet used as a herbal sedative to relieve the symptoms of restlessness and aid natural sleep.

Dose: 2 tablets in the early evening and 2 immediately before bedtime.
Side effects:

Caution: pregnant women and nursing mothers should consult a doctor before using this product.
Not to be used for: children under 12 years.
Not to be used with:
Contains: hops, passionflower, valerian, Jamaican dogwood, wild lettuce.

Valerina Day Tablets
(Kallo Foods)

A tablet used as a herbal remedy for stress, strain, tension, and irritability.

Dose: 2 tablets 3 times a day.
Side effects: possible drowsiness if taken in excess.
Caution:
Not to be used for: children under 16 years, pregnant women, or nursing mothers.
Not to be used with: avoid alcohol and sedating medicines with high doses.
Contains: valerian, lemon balm extract.

Valerina Night Tablets
(Kallo Foods)

A tablet used as a herbal remedy to relieve tension and irritability, and to help to promote natural sleep.

Dose: 2-4 tablets at bedtime.
Side effects: prolonged drowsiness with high doses.
Caution:
Not to be used for: children under 16 years, pregnant women, or nursing mothers.
Not to be used with: avoid alcohol and sedating medicines with high doses.
Contains: valerian, lemon balm, hops.

Tonics

(See also 'Vitamin and mineral preparations' section as well as 'Homeopathic remedies' sections.)

Tonics are generally given to improve appetite. Those listed here contain a variety of minerals and other preparations which are claimed to improve the desire to eat and produce a feeling of well-being. Stimulants are also included in this section, but repeated or prolonged use of such products is not recommended.

Eating disorders, such as anorexia nervosa or bulimia, require professional care.

Appetiser Mixture
(Potters)

A sugar-free liquid used as a herbal tonic to promote appetite and relieve wind.

Dose: 5 ml 3 times a day in water, before meals.
Side effects:
Caution:
Not to be used for: children, pregnant women, or nursing mothers.
Not to be used with:
Contains: camomile, calumba root, gentian.

Bio-Strath Elixir
(Cedar Health)

An elixir used as a herbal yeast formula to aid convalescence, improve appetite, and help symptoms of fatigue and tiredness.

Dose: 5 ml 3 times a day before meals.
Side effects:
Caution:
Not to be used for: children.
Not to be used with:
Contains: yeast.

Chlorophyll
(Potters)

A tablet used as a herbal stimulant remedy to relieve temporary tiredness.

Dose: 1-2 tablets 3 times a day.
Side effects: sleeplessness.
Caution: not for prolonged use.

Not to be used for: children.
Not to be used with: excess tea or coffee.
Contains: kola nut, chlorophyll.

Curzon
(Gerard House)

A tablet used as a herbal remedy to relieve temporary tiredness.

Dose: 2 tablets at night and 2 in the morning.
Side effects:
Caution: pregnant women and nursing mothers should consult a doctor before using this product.
Not to be used for: children.
Not to be used with:
Contains: damiana.

---

damiana*
(Licensed remedy available from Gerard House – see Curzon)

A herbal remedy thought to be useful for nerve strain by stimulating the nervous system. It is also traditionally reputed to be aphrodisiac.

Dose: as specified for each individual product.
Side effects:
Caution: pregnant women and nursing mothers should consult a doctor before using this product.
Not to be used for: children.
Not to be used with:
Contains: damiana.

Effico
(Pharmax Healthcare)

A liquid used as a stimulant and source of B vitamins for patients who are tired or run down after illness.

Dose: adults 10 ml (children 2.5-5 ml) 3 times a day after food.
Side effects:
Caution:
Not to be used for:
Not to be used with: excess tea or coffee.
Contains: vitamins B_1 and B_3, caffeine.

Elixir of Damiana and Saw Palmetto
(Potters)

An elixir used as a herbal restorative.

Dose: 10 ml 3 times a day for the first week, then 5 ml 3 times a day.
Side effects: mildly irritant to the lining of the genital and urinary tracts.
Caution: pregnant women and nursing mothers should consult a doctor before using this product.
Not to be used for: children.
Not to be used with:
Contains: damiana, cornsilk, saw palmetto.

---

ginseng* see entry in 'Miscellaneous' section

---

guarana*

A herbal remedy, available as a capsule or chewing gum, used for its natural stimulant effects. It is thought to revitalize the mind and body, fighting fatigue and maintaining alertness. It is used by people with demanding work periods, sportsmen and women, and those recovering from illness.

Dose: as specified for each individual product.
Side effects:

Caution:
Not to be used for:
Not to be used with: excess tea or coffee.
Contains: guarana.

Labiton
(LAB)

A liquid used as a tonic to relieve mental and physical fatigue.

Dose: 10-20 ml twice a day.
Side effects: drowsiness.
Caution:
Not to be used for: children.
Not to be used with: alcohol, other sedating medicines, excess tea or coffee.
Contains: kola nut dried extract, alcohol, caffeine, vitamin B$_1$.

Malted Kelp see entry in 'Miscellaneous' section
(Potters)

Metatone
(Warner-Lambert Healthcare)

A liquid used as a source of vitamin B$_1$ and minerals and used as a tonic, particularly after illness, when there is tiredness and loss of appetite.

Dose: 5-10 ml 2-3 times a day.
Side effects:
Caution:
Not to be used for: children under 12 years.
Not to be used with:
Contains: calcium glycerophosphate, manganese, potassium, sodium, vitamin B$_1$.

Metatone Junior Tonic
(Warner Wellcome Consumer Healthcare)

A liquid used as a vitamin B and mineral supplement, where appetite is poor, or when a tonic is needed after illness or trauma.

Dose: children over 6 years 5 ml 2-3 times a day before meals. (Dilute if required.)
Side effects:
Caution:
Not to be used for: children under 6 years.
Not to be used with: some anti-parkinson drugs.
Contains: vitamins B_1, B_2, B_3, B_6, calcium glycerophosphate, manganese glycerophosphate.

Minadex Tonic
(Seven Seas)

A liquid used as a vitamin and mineral supplement, particularly during and after illness, and if there is loss of appetite.

Dose: children aged 6 months-3 years 5 ml twice a day; children aged 3-12 years and pregnant women or nursing mothers 5 ml 3 times a day; adults 10 ml 3 times a day.
Side effects: nausea, stomach pain, altered bowel habit.
Caution:
Not to be used for: children under 6 months or for patients with a history of stomach ulcers.
Not to be used with: antacids, some antibiotics, some anti-parkinson drugs, other preparations containing vitamins A or D, some diuretics.
Contains: vitamins A and D_3, iron, potassium, calcium, potassium, manganese, copper.

Pro-Plus
(Roche Consumer Health)

A tablet used as a stimulant to relieve the symptoms of temporary tiredness.

Dose: 1-2 tablets when required. (Maximum 12 in 24 hours.)
Side effects: sleeplessness.
Caution: avoid taking a dose too close to bedtime. Not for prolonged or repeated use.
Not to be used for: children under 12 years.
Not to be used with: other stimulant medicines, excess tea or coffee.
Contains: caffeine.

Seven Seas Vitamin and Mineral Tonic
(Seven Seas)

A liquid used as a vitamin and mineral supplement, particularly during and after illness.

Dose: adults 10 ml (pregnant women or nursing mothers 5 ml) 3 times a day after meals.
Side effects: nausea, stomach pain, altered bowel habit.
Caution:
Not to be used for: patients with a history of stomach ulcers.
Not to be used with: antacids, some antibiotics, some anti-parkinson drugs, some diuretics, other preparations containing vitamins A or D.
Contains: vitamins A and D_3, iron, potassium, calcium, manganese, copper.

Strength Tablets
(Potters)

A tablet used as a stimulant herbal tonic after illness.

Dose: 2 tablets 3 times a day.
Side effects:
Caution:
Not to be used for: children.
Not to be used with: excess tea or coffee.
Contains: kola, damiana, saw palmetto.

Vitamin and mineral preparations

Many vitamin and mineral preparations are available over the counter. Some are combined (with vitamins and minerals in one product), and many appear as homeopathic remedies (see 'Homeopathic remedies' sections). Many products are not licensed as medicines, but are marketed purely as dietary supplements. (Such products are marked with * in the entries below to denote their unlicensed status.) Overdoses of vitamins and minerals can occur (see individual vitamin entries below), and this is particularly easy if taking more than one preparation, especially when they are of the combined type. (Always check ingredients carefully to ensure that accidental overdose does not occur.) The recommended daily amounts (RDAs) quoted for the various vitamins and minerals are based on EC regulations (March 1995), but RDAs are not quoted for children, and youngsters should be supplemented with caution.

It is uncertain whether healthy people benefit from supplements. Many claims are made about the effects of various dietary supplements, but often the evidence to support such claims is scant. (One controversial suggestion is that children do better academically when taking vitamin supplements.) Only products with a full medicinal product licence carry the reassurance of efficacy for the conditions stated. Provided certain warnings are heeded, however, (see individual product entries), supplements may be used safely, and many people will find them beneficial.

True deficiency states of vitamins are rare, but are seen occasionally nowadays, particularly B_{12} deficiency in vegetarians and those with pernicious anaemia, scurvy in elderly people who also do not eat enough fruit, and variations of rickets (vitamin D deficiency). B_6 deficiency is said to occur in premenstrual syndrome. Iron deficiency occurs in pregnant and nursing women, the elderly, and vegetarians. Calcium deficiency may occur in the elderly and in some bone conditions, sodium may be depleted in hot weather, and potassium levels can be reduced by overuse of diuretic tablets. High-dose supplementation with calcium, potassium, and sodium should always be monitored by a doctor, however, because of the possibility of adverse effects. Pregnant women (and those trying to become pregnant) are now routinely recommended to take folic acid until the twelfth week of pregnancy.

Also included in this section are products such as co-enzyme Q10 which is not a vitamin or mineral but which is usually to be found displayed with vitamin products in the stores, and which is used as a dietary supplement to improve health. Oral rehydration products, which contain minerals and which are used to treat fluid loss due to diarrhoea and sickness, are listed in the 'Bowel disorders' section.

Abidec
(Warner Wellcome Consumer Healthcare)

Drops used as a multivitamin preparation to treat vitamin deficiencies.

Dose: children over 1 year 0.6 ml once a day; infants under 1 year 0.3 ml once a day.
Side effects:
Caution:
Not to be used for: adults.
Not to be used with: some diuretics, some anti-parkinson drugs..
Contains: vitamins A, B_1, B_2, B_3, B_6, C, D_2.

---

antioxidant*

Various vitamins and minerals (such as vitamins A, D, E, selenium, and beta-carotene) function as 'antioxidants' in the body, mopping up free radicals that can cause tissue damage. (The free radicals are by-products in the body, and are increased on exposure to pollutants.) Antioxidants are also thought to prevent the changes in blood fats which scar and thicken the walls of blood vessels. These effects may help to protect the body against heart disease and cancer. The various antioxidants are available alone or in combination products, mostly as unlicensed food supplement tablets, capsules, or pastilles.

Dose: as specified for each individual product.
Side effects:
Caution:
Not to be used for:
Not to be used with:
Contains: varies according to product.

---

ascorbic acid* see **vitamin C***

BC 500
(Whitehall)

A tablet used as a source of vitamins B and C.

Dose: 1 tablet a day.
Side effects:
Caution:
Not to be used for: children.
Not to be used with: some anti-parkinson drugs.
Contains: vitamins B_1, B_2, B_3, B_6, B_{12}, C, calcium pantothenate, sodium ascorbate.

Becosym
(Roche Consumer Health)

A tablet used as a source of B vitamins to treat vitamin B deficiencies.

Dose: 1-3 tablets a day.
Side effects:
Caution:
Not to be used for: children.
Not to be used with: some anti-parkinson drugs.
Contains: vitamins B_1, B_2, B_3, B_6.

Becosym Forte
(Roche Consumer Health)

A stronger form of **vitamin B compound strong tablets**.

Benadon
(Roche Consumer Health)

A tablet available in two strengths, used as a source of vitamin B_6 to treat B_6 deficiency conditions.

Dose: 20 mg or 50 mg each day.
Side effects:
Caution:
Not to be used for:
Not to be used with: some anti-parkinson drugs.
Contains: vitamin B_6.

Benerva
(Roche Consumer Health)

A tablet available in various strengths used as a source of vitamin B_1.

Dose: 25-50 mg a day.
Side effects:
Caution:
Not to be used for: children.
Not to be used with:
Contains: vitamin B_1.

Benerva Compound see **vitamin B compound tablets**
(Roche Consumer Health)

---

beta-carotene*

An antioxidant (see separate entry) which is converted to vitamin A in the body. It is a safer means of taking vitamin A supplements because it does not have the same toxic effects in the body as vitamin A. Available as food-supplement tablets or capsules, either alone or in combination with other vitamins (especially with other antioxidants).

Dose: as specified for each individual product.
Side effects: excessive intake may cause the skin to become yellow.
Caution:

Not to be used for:
Not to be used with: vitamin A supplements.
Contains: beta-carotene.

___

bioflavonoids*

Compounds that assist in the absorption of vitamin C. They are found in food supplements either alone or in combination with vitamin C. Some bioflavonoids are also antioxidants (see separate entry).

Dose: as specified for each individual product.
Side effects:
Caution:
Not to be used for:
Not to be used with:
Contains: bioflavonoids.

___

biotin*

A vitamin in the B group, needed for digestion and the production of energy from food. It is also used to maintain the health of the hair, skin, bone marrow, nerves, heart, and circulation. Deficiency causes dermatitis and fatigue. Supplements may be useful to people taking antibiotics. (Available as food supplement capsules or tablets.)

Dose: recommended total daily intake (including dietary sources) for adults is 150µg (150 mcg), although supplements up to 200µg (200 mcg) per day are thought to be safe.
Side effects:
Caution:
Not to be used for:
Not to be used with:
Contains: biotin (also known as vitamin H).

___

Biovital
(Rhone-Poulenc Rorer Family Health)

A tablet or tonic liquid used as a multivitamin and iron supplement to prevent deficiency.

Dose: adults and children over 14 years 1 tablet or 20 ml liquid 3 times a day. (Children aged 5-14 years 1 tablet daily.)
Side effects: nausea, stomach pain, altered bowel habit.
Caution:
Not to be used for: children under 14 years (liquid), children under 5 years (tablets), or for patients with a history of stomach ulcers.
Not to be used with: antacids, some antibiotics, some anti-parkinson drugs.
Contains: vitamins B_1, B_2, B_6, B_{12} and C, nicotinamide, iron, manganese.

---

calciferol* see **vitamin D***

---

calcium*
(Licensed products available for use on recommendation of a doctor.)

A mineral required to build and maintain strong teeth and bones. (Deficiency will cause rickets.) Pregnant women, nursing mothers, and older people with osteoporosis may benefit from supplements, but a doctor should be consulted before taking high-dose supplements. (Available as licensed medicinal products, for use on the advice of a doctor. Unlicensed food supplements are also available, alone or in combination with other minerals or vitamins.)

Dose: recommended total daily intake (including dietary sources) for adults is 800 mg.
Side effects: excessive intake may cause stomach upset,

kidney disorders, disturbance of heart rhythm.
Caution: children and patients with kidney or heart disorders,
or sarcoidosis should consult a doctor before using calcium
supplements.
Not to be used for:
Not to be used with: some antibiotics, some diuretics, digoxin.
Contains: calcium.

---

calcium ascorbate* see **ascorbic acid***

---

calcium pantothenate* see **pantothenic acid***

---

cholecalciferol* see **vitamin D***

---

co-enzyme Q10*

A food-supplement tablet or capsule used because of its role
in the body of metabolizing fats and releasing energy. It is
believed to be essential for the health of all tissues and organs,
and may help to maintain a healthy heart and circulation. It is
also thought to be of help in maintaining healthy gums. It
functions as an antioxidant (see 'antioxidant' entry in this
section), and is normally made in the body, but the ability to
produce it decreases with age. It is taken particularly by athletes,
who require strength and stamina, and slimmers.

Dose: as specified for each individual product.
Side effects:
Caution:
Not to be used for: pregnant women or nursing mothers.
Not to be used with:
Contains: co-enzyme Q10.

---

cod liver oil*
(Some licensed liquid and capsule forms available see Seven Seas products)

A fish oil used as a source of omega-3 fatty acids, and vitamins A and D. Products available include the pure oil (with or without malt extract or orange syrup added), capsules of various strengths, and combination products with other minerals, vitamins, or food supplements. The licensed products are recommended for relief of joint pain and stiffness (as in arthritis or rheumatic conditions), but the products may be taken for the omega-3 fatty acids or vitamins content. (See individual entries for these components.)

Dose: as specified for each individual product.
Side effects:
Caution: pregnant women should consult a doctor before taking these products.
Not to be used for:
Not to be used with: other products containing vitamins A or D, some diuretics.
Contains: omega-3 fatty acids, vitamins A and D.

Comploment Continus
(Seton Healthcare)

A long-acting tablet used as a source of vitamin B_6 to treat vitamin B_6 deficiency including that developed by the contraceptive pill.

Dose: 1 tablet a day.
Side effects:
Caution: pregnant women should consult a doctor before using this product.
Not to be used for: children.
Not to be used with: some anti-parkinson drugs.
Contains: vitamin B_6.

Concavit
(Wallace)

A capsule, syrup, or drops used as a multivitamin treatment for vitamin deficiencies.

Dose: 1 capsule, 5 ml syrup, or 0.5 ml drops daily.
Side effects:
Caution: pregnant women should consult a doctor before using this product.
Not to be used for:
Not to be used with: other products containing vitamins A or D, some anti-parkinson drugs, some diuretics.
Contains: vitamins A, B_1, B_2, B_3, B_6, B_{12}, C, D. (Capsules also contain vitamin E and calcium pantothenate. Liquid and drops also contain dexpantherol.)

Cytacon
(Goldshield Healthcare)

A tablet or liquid used as a source of vitamin B_{12} for vegetarians, vegans, and the elderly.

Dose: adults 1-3 tablets a day or 5-10 ml liquid 2-3 times a day; children 1 tablet twice a day or 5 ml liquid 2-3 times a day.
Side effects: rarely allergy
Caution:
Not to be used for:
Not to be used with: vitamin B_{12}.
Contains: vitamin B_{12}.

Dalivit Drops
(Eastern)

Drops used as a multivitamin preparation in the prevention and treatment of vitamin deficiency in children.

Dose: 0-1 year 7 drops a day, over 1 year 14 drops a day.
Side effects:
Caution: pregnant women should consult a doctor before using this product.
Not to be used for:
Not to be used with: some anti-parkinson drugs, some diuretics, other products containing vitamins A and D.
Contains: vitamins A, B_1, B_2, B_3, B_6, C, D_2.

Ephynal
(Roche Consumer Health)

A tablet available in various strengths and used as a source of vitamin E.

Dose: adults 10-15 mg a day; children 1-10 mg per kg body weight a day.
Side effects:
Caution:
Not to be used for:
Not to be used with:
Contains: vitamin E.

---

ergocalciferol* see **vitamin D***

Feospan Spansule
(Evans Medical)

A long-acting capsule used as an iron supplement to treat iron deficiency (anaemia).

Dose: adults 1-2 capsules a day.
Side effects: mild stomach upset, diarrhoea, constipation, dark stools, loss of appetite.
Caution: children, pregnant women and patients receiving medication or medical treatment should consult a doctor before

using this product. Do not chew the capsule.
Not to be used for: infants under 1 year.
Not to be used with: some antibiotics, antacids, penicillamine.
Contains: ferrous sulphate.

Fergon
(Sanofi Winthrop)

A tablet used as an iron supplement to treat and prevent iron deficiency.

Dose: adults treatment 4-6 tablets a day in divided doses (prevention 2 tablets a day); children 6-12 years 1-3 tablets a day.
Side effects: nausea, stomach pain, altered bowel habit.
Caution:
Not to be used for: children under 6 years, or for patients with a history of stomach ulcers.
Not to be used with: some antibiotics, antacids, some anti-parkinson drugs.
Contains: ferrous gluconate.

Ferrocap-F
(Consolidated Chemicals)

A capsule used as an iron and folic acid supplement to treat anaemia in pregnancy.

Dose: 1 daily.
Side effects: nausea, stomach pain, altered bowel habit.
Caution:
Not to be used for: children, or for patients with a history of stomach ulcers.
Not to be used with: antacids, some antibiotics, some anti-epileptic drugs, some anti-parkinson drugs.
Contains: ferrous fumarate, folic acid.

Ferrocontin Continus
(ASTA Medica)

A long-acting tablet used as an iron supplement to treat iron deficiency.

Dose: 1 tablet a day.
Side effects: nausea, stomach pain, altered bowel habit.
Caution:
Not to be used for: children, or for patients with a history of stomach ulcers.
Not to be used with: some antibiotics, antacids, some anti-parkinson drugs.
Contains: ferrous glycine sulphate.

Ferrocontin Folic Continus
(ASTA Medica)

A long-acting tablet used as an iron and folic acid supplement to treat and prevent anaemia in pregnancy.

Dose: 1 tablet each day.
Side effects: nausea, stomach pain, altered bowel habit.
Caution:
Not to be used for: children, or for patients with a history of stomach ulcers.
Not to be used with: antacids, some antibiotics, some anti-parkinson drugs, some anti-epileptic drugs.
Contains: ferrous glycine sulphate, folic acid.

Ferrograd
(Abbott)

A long-acting tablet used as an iron supplement to treat iron deficiency.

Dose: 1 tablet a day before food.
Side effects: nausea, stomach pain, altered bowel habit.
Caution: in patients suffering from slow bowel actions.
Not to be used for: children, or for patients suffering from diverticular disease, blocked intestine, or with a history of stomach ulcers.
Not to be used with: antibiotics, antacids, some anti-parkinson drugs.
Contains: ferrous sulphate.

Ferrograd C
(Abbott)

A long-acting tablet used as an iron supplement to treat iron deficiency, especially where absorption is difficult.

Dose: 1 tablet a day.
Side effects: nausea, stomach pain, altered bowel habit.
Caution: in patients suffering from slow bowel action.
Not to be used for: children, or for patients suffering from diverticular disease, blocked intestine, or with a history of stomach ulcers.
Not to be used with: some antibiotics, antacids, some anti-parkinson drugs, some urine tests for glucose.
Contains: ferrous sulphate, vitamin C.

Ferrograd Folic
(Abbott)

A long-acting tablet used as an iron and folic acid supplement to treat anaemia in pregnancy.

Dose: 1 tablet a day.
Side effects: nausea, stomach pain, altered bowel habit.
Caution: in patients suffering from slow bowel movments.
Not to be used for: children, or for patients suffering from

diverticular disease, intestinal blockage, vitamin B_{12} deficiency, or with a history of stomach ulcers.

Not to be used with: some antibiotics, antacids, some anti-parkinson drugs, some anti-epileptic medications.

Contains: ferrous sulphate, folic acid.

---

ferrous gluconate tablets see Fergon

---

ferrous sulphate tablets

A tablet used as an iron supplement to treat or prevent iron deficiency.

Dose: to prevent deficiency, 1 tablet daily. (Patients who are definitely anaemic should consult a doctor for advice on treatment.)

Side effects: nausea, stomach pain, altered bowel habit.

Caution: pregnant women should consult a doctor before taking iron supplements.

Not to be used for: children, or patients with a history of stomach ulcers.

Not to be used with: antacids, some antibiotics, some anti-parkinson drugs.

Contains: ferrous sulphate.

Fersaday
(Goldshield Healthcare)

A tablet used as an iron supplement to treat iron deficiency.

Dose: 1 tablet a day.

Side effects: nausea, stomach pain, altered bowel habit.

Caution:

Not to be used for: children, or for patients with a history of stomach ulcers.

Not to be used with: antacids, some antibiotics, some anti-parkinson drugs.
Contains: ferrous fumarate.

Fersamal
(Forley)

A tablet or syrup used as an iron supplement to treat iron deficiency.

Dose: adults 1 tablet 3 times a day or 10 ml syrup twice a day; children 2.5–5 ml syrup twice a day.
Side effects: nausea, stomach pain, altered bowel habit.
Caution: children should be seen by a doctor before using this product.
Not to be used for: patients with a history of stomach ulcer.
Not to be used with: antacids, some anti-parkinson drugs, some antibiotics.
Contains: ferrous fumarate.

Folex-350
(Shire)

A tablet used as an iron and folic acid supplement to prevent anaemia in pregnancy.

Dose: 1 tablet a day.
Side effects: nausea, stomach pain, altered bowel habit.
Caution:
Not to be used for: children, or for patients suffering from vitamin B_{12} deficiency, or with a history of stomach ulcers.
Not to be used with: some antibiotics, some anti-parkinson drugs, antacids, some anti-epileptic medications.
Contains: ferrous fumarate, folic acid.

---

folic acid*
(Some licensed products available see Preconceive)

Necessary for healthy cell division, and for the formation of red blood cells. Supplements containing 400µg (400 mcg) are now being licensed for use in pregnant women to prevent neural tube defects (such as spina bifida) in the foetus. (Higher-strength products are available on prescription to treat women who have previously had this problem in pregnancy, and other serious blood disorders.) Deficiency causes diarrhoea and anaemia. Folic acid is also found in low doses in food supplements, both alone and in combination with other vitamins and minerals.

Dose: recommended total daily intake (including dietary sources) is normally 200µg (200 mcg) per day for adults. Women wishing to become pregnant should take 400µg (400 mcg) per day while trying to conceive and continue until the twelfth week of pregnancy.
Side effects: excessive intake will reduce zinc absorption.
Caution:
Not to be used for:
Not to be used with: some anti-epileptic medications.
Contains: folic acid.

Forceval
(Unigreg)

A capsule available in normal and junior strengths, and used as a source of multivitamins and minerals to treat vitamin and mineral deficiencies.

Dose: adults 1 normal-strength capsule a day; children over 5 years 2 junior-strength capsules a day.
Side effects:
Caution:
Not to be used for: children under 5 years.
Not to be used with: some anti-parkinson drugs, other products containing vitamins A and D. Normal-strength product should not be used with antacids or some antibiotics.

Contains: vitamins A, B$_1$, B$_2$, B$_3$, B$_6$, B$_{12}$, C, D$_2$, E, and K, folic acid, biotin, selenium, zinc, molybdenum, manganese, magnesium, iodine, copper, chromium. (Normal-strength product also contains calcium, iron, phosphorus, potassium.)

Galfer
(Galen)

A capsule and sugar-free syrup used as an iron supplement to treat iron-deficiency anaemia.

Dose: adults 1 capsule or 10 ml syrup once or twice a day; children 2.5-5 ml once or twice a day, according to age, or as directed by a doctor.
Side effects: nausea, stomach pain, altered bowel habit.
Caution:
Not to be used for: patients with a history of stomach ulcers.
Not to be used with: antacids, some antibiotics, some anti-parkinson drugs.
Contains: ferrous fumarate.

Gevral
(Lederle)

A capsule used as a source of multivitamins and minerals to treat vitamin and mineral deficiencies.

Dose: 1 capsule a day.
Side effects:
Caution: pregnant women should consult a doctor before using this product.
Not to be used for: children under 12 years.
Not to be used with: some anti-parkinson drugs, other products containing vitamin A, some anti-epileptic medications, antacids, some antibiotics.
Contains: vitamins A, B$_1$, B$_2$, B$_3$, B$_6$, B$_{12}$, C, and E, folic acid, iron, calcium, iodine.

---

halibut liver oil*

A capsule used as a source of vitamins A and D.

Dose: as specified for each individual product.
Side effects:
Caution: pregnant women should consult a doctor before using this product.
Not to be used for:
Not to be used with: other products containing vitamins A and D, some diuretics.
Contains: vitamins A and D.

Halycitrol
(LAB)

An emulsion used as a source of vitamins A and D.

Dose: adults and children over 6 months 5 ml teaspoonful a day; infants under 6 months 2.5 ml a day.
Side effects:
Caution: pregnant women and patients suffering from sarcoidosis (a chest disease that affects calcium levels) should consult a doctor before using this product.
Not to be used for:
Not to be used with: other products containing vitamins A or D, some diuretics.
Contains: vitamins A and D.

---

iodine*

A mineral required in the body to regulate metabolism by involvement with the thyroid gland. (Not available alone as a supplement, except for use by doctors for treating thyroid disease, but often included in multivitamin and multimineral supplements.)

Dose: recommended total daily intake for adults (including dietary sources) is 150 µg (150 mcg). [Toxic effects may appear if intake exceeds 1000 µg (1000 mcg) per day.]

Side effects: allergy. Excessive intake may cause headache, eye disorders, cold-like symptoms.

Caution: children, pregnant women, and patients suffering from thyroid disorders should consult a doctor before taking high doses of iodine supplements.

Not to be used for: nursing mothers.

Not to be used with:

Contains: iodine.

---

iron*

(Some licensed brands available see **Fefol**, **Feospan**, **Fergon**, **Ferrocontin**, **Ferrograd**, **ferrous sulphate tablets**, **Fersaday**, **Fersamal**, **Galfer**, **Niferex**, **Plesmet**, **Slow-Fe**, **Sytron**.)

A mineral required for the healthy formation of red blood cells, and transportation of oxygen around the body. Supplements may be required by women with heavy periods, or by pregnant women. (Available as single mineral supplements – licensed medicinal products or unlicensed food supplements – and in combination with minerals and vitamins.) Iron content may be expressed as the amount of salt or the amount of iron in the salt. Equivalent values are as follows:

200 mg ferrous fumarate	=	65 mg iron
300 mg ferrous gluconate	=	35 mg iron
100 mg ferrous succinate	=	35 mg iron
300 mg ferrous sulphate	=	60 mg iron
200 mg dried ferrous sulphate	=	65 mg iron

Dose: recommended total daily intake for adults (including dietary sources) is 14 mg iron. Do not exceed the doses recommended for individual products, because excessive intake is harmful.

Side effects: nausea, stomach pain, altered bowel habit.

Caution: children and pregnant women should consult a doctor before taking iron supplements. Patients with diagnosed anaemia should be treated by a doctor.
Not to be used for: patients with a history of stomach ulcers.
Not to be used with: antacids, some antibiotics, some anti-parkinson drugs.
Contains: iron.

---

magnesium*

A mineral needed for correct functioning of nerves and muscles, and the formation of protein in the body. It is also involved in the absorption of calcium and in various body enzyme systems. (It needs to be in balance with calcium in the body.) Deficiency causes tiredness, depression, and lack of co-ordination. It is thought that it may be helpful in treating premenstrual syndrome and asthma. Available as food-supplement tablets, powder, or capsules, alone or in combination with other minerals or vitamins.

Dose: recommended total daily intake for adults (including dietary sources) is 300 mg.
Side effects: excessive intake may cause diarrhoea.
Caution:
Not to be used for:
Not to be used with:
Contains: magnesium.

---

manganese*

A mineral required to maintain blood sugar levels and nerve function. It also activates certain vitamins in the body, and is needed for the development of bones and normal growth. Available as food supplements, alone or in combination with other minerals or vitamins.

Dose: as specified for each individual product.

Side effects: excessive intake may cause muscle disorders or tiredness.
Caution:
Not to be used for:
Not to be used with:
Contains: manganese.

Minadex Chewable Children's Vitamins*
(Seven Seas)

A chewable tablet used as a source of vitamins for children.

Dose: 1 tablet each day.
Side effects:
Caution:
Not to be used for: children under 3 years.
Not to be used with: other products containing vitamins A or D, some diuretics.
Contains: vitamins A, C, D.

Minadex Multivitamin Syrup
(Seven Seas)

A liquid used as a vitamin supplement in patients whose vitamin intake is not sufficient from the diet (including convalescents and patients on restricted diets).

Dose: adults and children over 6 months 10 ml once a day. (Children fed on dried milk, nursing mothers, and women who are, or who may become, pregnant should take only 5 ml.)
Side effects:
Caution:
Not to be used for: children under 6 months.
Not to be used with: other products containing vitamins A or D, some anti-parkinson drugs, some diuretics.
Contains: vitamins A, B_1, B_2, B_3, B_6, C, D_3, E.

Minadex Vitamin Drops
(Seven Seas)

A sugar-free liquid (supplied with a measuring dropper) used as a source of vitamins for infants and children.

Dose: babies and children up to 5 years 0.28 ml (older children 0.14 ml) once a day.
Side effects:
Caution:
Not to be used for:
Not to be used with: other products containing vitamins A or D, some diuretics.
Contains: vitamins A, C, D.

Minalka
(Cedar Health)

A tablet used to relieve symptoms of muscular pain and stiffness, and give a dietary supplement of minerals.

Dose: adults 4 daily. (Children half adult dose.) Full benefit of the treatment may take six weeks to be seen.
Side effects: nausea, vomiting, stomach pain, altered bowel habit.
Caution: pregnant women, nursing mothers, and patients suffering from indigestion or heart disease (or taking other medicines) should consult a doctor before using this product.
Not to be used for: patients with a history of stomach ulcers, or with high blood levels of calcium or potassium, or high urine levels of calcium.
Not to be used with: antacids, some antibiotics, other medicines containing vitamin D, some diuretics, some anti-parkinson drugs.
Contains: calcium, potassium, sodium, magnesium, cobalt, copper, zinc, potassium, iron, manganese, vitamin D_3.

---

niacin* see **vitamin B₃***

---

nicotinamide see **vitamin B₃***

---

nicotinic acid see **vitamin B₃***

Niferex
(Tillomed)

An elixir or capsule used as an iron supplement to treat iron deficiency anaemia.

Dose: adults treatment 5 ml or 1 capsule once or twice a day, (prevention 2.5 ml a day); children 0-2 years 1 drop per 0.45 kg body weight 3 times a day, older children 2.5-5 ml daily according to age.
Side effects: nausea, stomach pain, altered bowel habit.
Caution: children should be seen by a doctor before using this product.
Not to be used for: patients with a history of stomach ulcers.
Not to be used with: some antibiotics, some anti-parkinson drugs, antacids.
Contains: polysaccharide-iron complex.

Octovit
(Goldshield)

A tablet used as a multivitamin and mineral supplement.

Dose: 1 tablet a day.
Side effects:
Caution:
Not to be used for: children
Not to be used with: some antibiotics, some diuretics, some anti-parkinson drugs, antacids.

Contains: vitamins A, B$_1$, B$_2$, B$_3$, B$_6$, B$_{12}$, C, D$_3$, and E, iron, magnesium, zinc.

---

omega-3 fish oils* see entry in 'Miscellaneous' section

Orovite
(SmithKline Beecham Consumer)

A tablet used as a source of vitamins B and C to aid convalescence.

Dose: adults 1 tablet 3 times a day for up to 1 month.
Side effects:
Caution:
Not to be used for: children.
Not to be used with: some anti-parkinson drugs.
Contains: vitamins B$_1$, B$_2$, B$_3$, B$_6$, and C.

Orovite 7
(SmithKline Beecham Consumer)

Granules in a sachet used as a multivitamin treatment for vitamin deficiencies (particularly for patients on restricted diets or who miss meals, or who use a lot of physical energy).

Dose: 1 sachet in water once a day.
Side effects:
Caution:
Not to be used for: children under 5 years.
Not to be used with: some anti-parkinson drugs, some diuretics, other products containing vitamins A and D.
Contains: vitamins A, B$_1$, B$_2$, B$_3$, B$_6$, B$_{12}$, C, D$_3$.

---

pantothenic acid*

Needed for the release of energy from food, the production of hormones, tissue growth, and healthy hair and skin. It is also useful in improving resistance to infections. Supplements may be useful to people with a high alcohol intake or demanding lifestyle. Available in food supplements either alone or in combination with other vitamins and minerals.

Dose: recommended total daily intake for adults (including dietary sources) is 6 mg.
Side effects: excessive intake may cause stomach upset.
Caution:
Not to be used for:
Not to be used with:
Contains: pantothenic acid (also known as vitamin B_5).

Pharmaton
(Windsor Healthcare)

A sugar-free capsule containing minerals and vitamins, used to prevent deficiency.

Dose: 1 capsule daily.
Side effects: nausea, stomach pain, altered bowel habit.
Caution: pregnant women (or those trying to become pregnant) should consult a doctor before using this product.
Not to be used for: children, or for patients suffering from excess iron or calcium in the blood, or with a history of stomach ulcers.
Not to be used with: other vitamin preparations (unless allowances made), some anti-parkinson drugs, some diuretics, antacids, some antibiotics.
Contains: ginseng, dimethylaminoethanol hydrogen tartrate, vitamins A, B_1, B_2, B_3, B_6, B_{12}, C, D_2, and E, calcium, rutin, iron, calcium, copper, potassium, manganese, magnesium, zinc, lecithin.

---

phosphorus*

A mineral required to activate the B vitamins in the body. It is also used to maintain the health of teeth and bones, and for energy production. Deficiency may arise due to alcoholism or antacid abuse, (particularly overuse of aluminium antacids). Available as food supplements in combination with other minerals and vitamins.

Dose: recommended total daily intake for adults (including dietary sources) is 800 mg.
Side effects: excessive intake will interfere with iron absorption.
Caution:
Not to be used for:
Not to be used with:
Contains: phosphorus.

Phyllosan
(Seton Healthcare)

A tablet used as an iron and vitamin supplement for those with deficiencies, particularly after illness or when overworking or dieting.

Dose: 2 tablets 3 times a day after meals.
Side effects: nausea, stomach pain, altered bowel habit.
Caution:
Not to be used for: children under 12 years or patients with a history of stomach ulcers.
Not to be used with: antacids, some antibiotics, some anti-parkinson drugs.
Contains: iron, vitamins B_1, B_2, B_3, and C.

---

phytomenadione* see vitamin K*

Plesmet
(Link)

A syrup used as an iron supplement to treat iron-deficiency anaemia.

Dose: adults 5-10 ml 3 times a day; children 2.5-5 ml 2-3 times a day according to weight.
Side effects: nausea, stomach pain, altered bowel habit.
Caution: children should be seen by a doctor before using this product.
Not to be used for: patients with a history of stomach ulcers.
Not to be used with: some antibiotics, antacids, some anti-parkinson drugs.
Contains: ferrous glycine sulphate.

---

potassium*
(Licensed supplements available for use on a doctor's advice.)

A mineral needed for efficient functioning of the heart, nerves, and muscles. Along with sodium, it regulates the fluid balance in the body. High-dose supplements should be taken only on a doctor's advice. Available as food supplements, alone or in combination with other minerals and vitamins.

Dose: as specified for each individual product.
Side effects: excessive intake may cause irregular heart rhythm, muscle disorders, stomach upset, or stomach ulcers.
Caution: take after food. Patients with heart or kidney disorders, hiatus hernia, or a history of stomach ulcers should consult a doctor before using potassium supplements.
Not to be used for:
Not to be used with: some diuretics, some antihypertensives.
Contains: potassium.

Preconceive
(Lane)

A tablet used as a folic acid supplement, taken before and during pregnancy to help prevent spina bifida and other neural tube defects in the developing foetus.

Dose: 1 tablet each day until the end of the third month of pregnancy.
Side effects:
Caution: patients with epilepsy or anaemia should consult a doctor before using this medication.
Not to be used for:
Not to be used with: some anti-epileptic medications.
Contains: folic acid 400µg (400 mcg).

Pregaday
(Evans Medical)

A tablet used as a source of iron and folic acid, and used to prevent anaemia in pregnant women.

Dose: 1 tablet a day from the thirteenth week of pregnancy.
Side effects: nausea, stomach pain, altered bowel habit.
Caution: women in the first 3 months of pregnancy should not take this product unless a doctor advises.
Not to be used for: patients with a history of stomach ulcers, or with vitamin B_{12} deficiency.
Not to be used with: antacids, some antibiotics, some anti-parkinson drugs, some anti-epileptic medications.
Contains: ferrous fumarate, folic acid.

Pregnacare*
(Robinson Healthcare)

A capsule used as a folic acid, mineral, and vitamin supplement for women before conception and during pregnancy.

Dose: 1 each day.
Side effects: nausea, stomach pain, altered bowel habit.
Caution: patients with epilepsy or anaemia should consult a doctor before using this medication.
Not to be used for: children or patients with a history of stomach ulcers.
Not to be used with: antacids, some antibiotics, some anti-epileptic medications, some anti-parkinson drugs.
Contains: folic acid, beta-carotene, vitamin B_{12}, zinc, iron.

---

propolis*

A food supplement tablet or lozenge, used as an anti-oxidant and thought to increase physical fitness and stamina.

Dose: as specified for each individual product.
Side effects:
Caution:
Not to be used for:
Not to be used with:
Contains: propolis.

---

pyridoxine* see vitamin B_6*

Redoxon*
(Roche Consumer Health)

A range of products (tablets, chewable tablets, and effervescent tablets), available in various strengths and used as a source of vitamin C.

Dose: as specified for each individual product.
Side effects: diarrhoea.
Caution:
Not to be used for:
Not to be used with:

Contains: vitamin C.

---

retinol* see **vitamin A***

---

royal jelly*

A food supplement capsule used as a rich source of nutrients (vitamins and iron), and thought to give a general health boost, which is useful for people with busy lives. It may also be useful for increasing resistance to disease, and relieving symptoms of psoriasis, arthritis, and insomnia.

Dose: as specified for each individual product.
Side effects:
Caution:
Not to be used for:
Not to be used with:
Contains: royal jelly.

Scott's Emulsion
(SmithKline Beecham Healthcare)

An emulsion used as a source of vitamins A and D.

Dose: adults and children over 6 years 10 ml twice a day. (Children aged 1-6 years, half adult dose.)
Side effects:
Caution:
Not to be used for:
Not to be used with: other products containing vitamin A or D, some diuretics.
Contains: cod liver oil (vitamins A and D).

---

selenium*

A mineral that functions as an antioxidant (see separate entry in this section). It is thought to be of help in maintaining healthy blood vessels, immune system, and tissue repair. Available as food supplements, alone or in combination with other minerals and vitamins.

Dose: as specified for each individual product.
Side effects:
Caution:
Not to be used for:
Not to be used with:
Contains: selenium.

Seven Seas Cod Liver Oil Capsules
(Seven Seas)

A capsule used as a source of vitamins and as a traditional remedy for the symptoms of joint pains and stiffness.

Dose: adults and children over 6 years 2 capsules 3 times a day. (Pregnant women/nursing mothers should use only half the recommended dose.)
Side effects:
Caution:
Not to be used for: children under 6 years.
Not to be used with: other products containing vitamins A or D, some diuretics.
Contains: vitamins A, D_3, and E, cod liver oil.

Seven Seas Cod Liver Oil and Orange Syrup
(Seven Seas)

A liquid used as a source of vitamins and as a traditional remedy for the symptoms of joint pains and stiffness.

Dose: adults and children over 1 year 10 ml (children under 1 year 2.5-5 ml according to age) once a day. (Babies fed on dried milk and pregnant women/nursing mothers should use only half the recommended dose.)
Side effects:
Caution:
Not to be used for:
Not to be used with: other products containing vitamins A or D, some anti-parkinson drugs, some diuretics.
Contains: vitamins A, B_6, C, D_3, and E, cod liver oil.

Seven Seas Pure Cod Liver Oil
(Seven Seas)

A liquid used as a source of vitamins and as a traditional remedy for the symptoms of joint pains and stiffness.

Dose: adults and children over 1 year 10 ml (children under 1 year 2.5-5 ml according to age) once a day. (Babies fed on dried milk and pregnant women/nursing mothers should use only half the recommended dose.)
Side effects:
Caution:
Not to be used for:
Not to be used with: other products containing vitamins A or D, some diuretics.
Contains: vitamins A, D_3, and E, cod liver oil.

Slow Sodium
(Ciba)

A tablet used as a salt supplement to treat and prevent sodium deficiency.

Dose: adults 4-8 tablets a day (in divided doses).
Side effects:
Caution: children and patients receiving medical treatment or

taking medicines should be seen by a doctor before using this product.
Not to be used for: patients suffering from fluid retention, heart disease, heart failure.
Not to be used with: diuretics, lithium.
Contains: sodium chloride.

Slow-Fe
(Ciba)

A long-acting tablet used as an iron supplement to treat iron-deficiency anaemia.

Dose: adults 1 tablet a day; children 6-12 years 1 tablet a day.
Side effects: nausea, stomach pain, altered bowel habit.
Caution:
Not to be used for: children under 6 years or patients with a history of stomach ulcers.
Not to be used with: some antibiotics, some anti-parkinson drugs, antacids.
Contains: ferrous sulphate.

---

sodium*
(Licensed supplements available see Slow Sodium)

A mineral needed for efficient functioning of the heart, nerves, and muscles. Along with potassium, it regulates the fluid balance in the body. Supplements may be needed by people who sweat excessively (for example, athletes, or people in tropical climates). High-dose supplements should be taken only on a doctor's advice.

Dose: as specified for each individual product.
Side effects: excessive intake may cause fluid retention.
Caution: take after food. Pregnant women and patients with high blood pressure, or heart or kidney disorders, should consult

a doctor before using sodium supplements.
Not to be used for: patients with fluid retention.
Not to be used with:
Contains: sodium.

Solvazinc
(Thames)

An effervescent tablet used as a zinc supplement to treat zinc deficiency.

Dose: adults 1 tablet 1-3 times a day after meals.
Side effects: stomach upset.
Caution: children should be seen by a doctor before using this product.
Not to be used for:
Not to be used with: some antibiotics, iron preparations.
Contains: zinc sulphate.

Super Plenamins
(3M Health Care)

A tablet used as a source of multivitamins and minerals.

Dose: 1 tablet each day.
Side effects: nausea, stomach pain, altered bowel habit.
Caution:
Not to be used for: children under 10 years, or for patients with a history of stomach ulcers.
Not to be used with: other products containing vitamins A or D, antacids, some antibiotics, some anti-parkinson drugs, some diuretics.
Contains: vitamins A, B_1, B_2, B_3, B_6, B_{12}, C, D, and E, calcium, copper, iodine, iron, magnesium, manganese, phosphorus, potassium, zinc.

Super Wate-On
(Dendron)

An emulsion used to treat weight loss and debility due to poor appetite and dietary deficiency.

Dose: 30 ml 3 times a day between meals.
Side effects:
Caution:
Not to be used for: children.
Not to be used with: some diuretics, some anti-parkinson drugs, other products containing vitamin D.
Contains: vitamins B_1, B_2, B_3, B_6, and D_2, calcium pantothenate, lysine.

Sytron
(Link)

An elixir used as an iron supplement to treat iron-deficiency anaemia.

Dose: adults 5-10 ml 3 times a day; children 2.5-5 ml 2-3 times a day according to age.
Side effects: nausea, stomach pain, altered bowel habit.
Caution: children should be seen by a doctor before using this product.
Not to be used for: patients with a history of stomach ulcers.
Not to be used with: some antibiotics, antacids, some anti-parkinson drugs.
Contains: sodium iron edetate.

---

thiamine* see **vitamin B_1***

---

tocopheryl acetate* see **vitamin E***

---

vitamin A*

Necessary for healthy skin, bones, teeth, mucous membranes, and general growth. Also used to maintain vision in dim light. It functions as an antioxidant (see 'antioxidant' entry in this section), and is needed particularly by those with a high alcohol intake. Deficiency causes night-blindness and dry eyes. 1 i.u. is equivalent to 0.3 µg (0.3 mcg) for vitamin A. Available alone in tablet or capsule form as food supplements, but also in combination with other vitamins and minerals.

Dose: recommended total daily intake for adults (including dietary sources) is 800µg [800 mcg (2664 i.u.)] – 6 mg or more may produce toxic effects.
Side effects: excessive intake may cause headache, nausea, vomiting, drowsiness, irritability, muscle and bone pain, loss of hair, skin problems, and liver damage. The developing foetus can be damaged in a pregnant woman.
Caution: pregnant women should consult a doctor before taking vitamin A supplements.
Not to be used for:
Not to be used with:
Contains: vitamin A (also known as retinol).

---

vitamin B₁*
(Licensed tablet form available see Benerva)

Necessary for the production of energy from food, and the correct functioning of the nervous system. Supplements may be needed by smokers and people with a high alcohol intake or a physically demanding lifestyle. Deficiency causes beri-beri and anaemia. Available alone or in combination with other vitamins and minerals.

Dose: recommended total daily intake for adults (including dietary sources) is 1.4 mg, but excessive intake is unlikely to cause toxic effects.

Side effects:
Caution:
Not to be used for:
Not to be used with:
Contains: vitamin B_1 (also known as thiamine).

---

vitamin B_2*

Necessary for the production of energy from food and correct liver function. It also helps to maintain healthy skin, nails, hair, and mucous membranes, and the correct sensitivity of eyes to light. Supplements may be needed by smokers, the elderly, and those with a high intake of alcohol. Deficiency causes skin problems, sensitivity to light, cracked lips, and nervous disorders. (Available in capsule form as food supplements, and in combination with other vitamins and minerals.)

Dose: recommended total daily intake for adults (including dietary sources) is 1.6 mg, but excessive intake is unlikely to cause toxic effects.
Side effects: may darken the urine.
Caution:
Not to be used for:
Not to be used with:
Contains: vitamin B_2 (also known as riboflavine).

---

vitamin B_3*
(Licensed generic products of nicotinic acid and nicotinamide tablets available)

Necessary for the release of energy from food, and the maintenance of healthy skin, muscles, and nerves, and the correct sensitivity of eyes to light. It is involved in the production of various enzymes, antibodies, and blood components, and is therefore needed for general health, and to maintain the appetite. Uses such as relief of migraine, stress, and sleeplessness have been suggested, but the effects on these disorders have not been proved. Supplements may be needed by those with a high alcohol intake. Available both as licensed medicinal products and as unlicensed food supplements, either alone or in combination with other vitamins and minerals.

Dose: recommended total daily intake for adults (including dietary sources) is 18 mg.

Side effects: excessive intake may cause reddening of the skin or other skin disorders, expanded blood vessels, and liver disorders.

Caution: diabetics and patients with glaucoma or stomach ulcers should consult a doctor before using vitamin B_3 supplements.

Not to be used for:

Not to be used with:

Contains: vitamin B_3 (also known as niacin, nicotinamide, nicotinic acid).

---

vitamin B5* see **pantothenic acid***

---

vitamin B_6*
(Licensed tablet forms available see Benadon, Comploment)

Necessary for energy production from food, and the correct functioning of the nervous system. Deficiency is rare, but there may be an increase in requirement by women taking the contraceptive pill. Women with premenstrual irritability and tension may also find supplements useful. Available as licensed medicinal products and as unlicensed food supplements, either alone or in combination with other vitamins and minerals.

Dose: recommended total daily intake for adults (including dietary sources) is 2mg, but a supplement dose of 20 mg or 50 mg each day is usual. Women suffering from premenstrual symptoms may require 50 mg twice a day, but this should not be exceeded, because toxic effects may occur above 100 mg daily.

Side effects: excessive intake causes clumsiness, inability to co-ordinate muscles, numbness around the mouth, and permanent damage to sensory nerves.

Caution: children and pregnant women should consult a doctor before using vitamin B_6 supplements.

Not to be used for:

Not to be used with: some anti-parkinson drugs.

Contains: vitamin B_6 (also known as pyridoxine).

---

vitamin B_{12}*
(Licensed products available see Cytacon)

Necessary for healthy maintenance of the nervous system, normal growth, the production of energy from food, and the formation of blood cells. Deficiency causes damage to the spinal cord, anaemia and mental disturbances. Supplements are recommended for vegans (and may be useful for some vegetarians), because most dietary sources are of animal origin.

Dose: recommended total daily intake (including dietary sources) for adults is 1μg (1 mcg).

Side effects: allergy.

Caution: children, pregnant women, and nursing mothers should consult a doctor before using this product.

Not to be used for:

Not to be used with: some anti-diabetic drugs.

Contains: vitamin B_{12} (also known as cyanocobalamin).

---

vitamin B compound tablets

A tablet used as a source of B vitamins to prevent vitamin B deficiency.

Dose: adults 1-2 tablets a day.

Side effects:
Caution:
Not to be used for: children.
Not to be used with:
Contains: vitamins B_1, B_2, B_3.

---

vitamin B compound strong tablets

A tablet used as a source of B vitamins to treat vitamin B deficiency.

Dose: adults 1-2 tablets 3 times a day.
Side effects:
Caution:
Not to be used for: children.
Not to be used with: some anti-parkinson drugs.
Contains: vitamins B_1, B_2, B_3, B_6.

---

vitamin C*
(Some licensed generic tablet brands available)

Necessary for healthy bones, teeth, and gums, tissue repair, and iron absorption. It also functions as an antioxidant (see 'antioxidant' entry in this section). The use of vitamin C to treat or prevent colds is controversial, and there is little evidence as yet to suggest that it is effective. Deficiency causes scurvy, bleeding gums, and poor healing of body tissues. Supplements may be useful to smokers and physically injured people. (Available as licensed medicinal products, or as unlicensed food supplements of powder, tablets, or soluble tablets.)

Dose: recommended total daily intake (including dietary sources) for adults is 60 mg. Supplements of more than 1000 mg (1 g) per day may produce toxic effects.
Side effects: excessive intake causes diarrhoea, kidney damage, diarrhoea, and dependency. Sudden withdrawal of high-dose supplements can lead to deficiency symptoms.

Caution:
Not to be used for:
Not to be used with: high-dose supplements may affect the low-dose contraceptive pills.
Contains: vitamin C (also known as ascorbic acid, or as calcium ascorbate).

---

vitamin D*

Necessary for calcium and phosphorus absorption, and for healthy teeth and bones. Vitamin D is manufactured normally in the body by the effect of sunlight on the skin. Deficiency causes rickets. Supplements may be required by people who are not exposed to sunlight. 1µg (1 mcg) is equivalent to 40 i.u. for vitamin D. (Not generally available as the single vitamin – only in combination products.)

Dose: recommended total daily intake (including dietary sources) for adults is 5 µg (5 mcg) or 200 i.u., but this should be produced within the body from sunlight in normal circumstances. (Toxic effects are possible if intake exceeds 125 µg (125 mcg) or 5000 i.u..)
Side effects: excessive intake causes muscle weakness, nausea, vomiting, constipation, excessive urine output, itching, high calcium levels in the blood, kidney and bladder stones, and damage to the heart and circulation.
Caution: high doses should not be taken by nursing mothers.
Not to be used for:
Not to be used with: some diuretics.
Contains: vitamin D – may be expressed as vitamin D_2 (also known as ergocalciferol or calciferol) or vitamin D_3 (also known as cholecalciferol).

---

vitamin E*

There is little evidence for any real value from vitamin E supplements. It is thought to be involved in some rare medical disorders (such as bile disorders), but its actual function remains obscure. It may play a role in the body's use of oxygen, and in maintaining a healthy skin, immune system, and reproductive system. It functions as an antioxidant (see 'antioxidant' entry in this section). For synthetic vitamin E, 1 mg is equivalent to 1 i.u., but the unit equivalents may vary according to the source of the vitamin E. Available as food-supplement capsules and tablets, and in cosmetic creams, believed to be of use in healing tissue and scars.

Dose: recommended total daily intake (including dietary sources) for adults is 10 mg (10 i.u.). Supplements above 1000 mg (1000 i.u.) may cause toxic effects.

Side effects: excessive intake may cause headache, tiredness, raised blood pressure, blood clots, disturbance of vision, diarrhoea, and abdominal pain.

Caution: patients with high blood pressure, heart disease, or circulatory disorder should consult a doctor before taking vitamin E supplements.

Not to be used for:

Not to be used with:

Contains: vitamin E (also known as tocopheryl acetate).

---

vitamin H* see **biotin***

---

vitamin K*
(Licensed tablet form is available for use on advice of a doctor)

Necessary for correct functioning of the blood-clotting mechanism and normal bone calcification. Although included in many multivitamin preparations, there is no reason to self-medicate with a vitamin K supplement. (Deficiencies or suspected deficiencies should be treated by a doctor.) Supplements are sometimes given by doctors to newborn babies, because deficiency can cause bleeding.

Dose: only as directed by a doctor.

Side effects: excessive intake causes anaemia, liver disease, and itching.
Caution: not recommended for self-medication.
Not to be used for:
Not to be used with: anticoagulants.
Contains: vitamin K (also known as phytomenadione).

Yeast-Vite
(Seton Healthcare)

Tablets used as a vitamin supplement and stimulant to relieve tiredness.

Dose: 2 tablets every 3 to 4 hours if required. (Maximum of 12 in 24 hours).
Side effects:
Caution: children under 12 years should be seen by a doctor before using this product.
Not to be used for: nursing mothers.
Not to be used with: excess tea or coffee.
Contains: caffeine, vitamins B_1, B_2, B_3.

---

zinc*
(Some licensed brands available see Solvazinc, Z-Span)

A mineral required for maintenance of the nervous system and skin, and for normal development of the reproductive organs and bones. It may also be useful in maintaining an efficient immune system. It is often used to treat cold symptoms, but there is little evidence to suggest that this is effective. It is available as single supplements, but these should be taken only if there is proven deficiency. It is also included in many multivitamin and multimineral preparations.

Dose: recommended total daily intake (including dietary sources) for adults is 15 mg. (Toxic effects may be seen if intake exceeds 50 mg per day.)

Side effects: excessive intake may cause nausea, vomiting, abdominal pain, indigestion.
Caution:
Not to be used for:
Not to be used with: some antibiotics, iron supplements.
Contains: zinc.

Zincomed*
(Medo)

A capsule used as a zinc supplement to treat and prevent zinc deficiencies.

Dose: adults 1 capsule 3 times a day after food.
Side effects: stomach upset.
Caution:
Not to be used for:
Not to be used with: some antibiotics, iron supplements.
Contains: zinc sulphate.

Z Span Spansule
(Goldshield Healthcare)

A long-acting capsule used as a zinc supplement for the prevention and treatment of zinc deficiency.

Dose: adults and children over 1 year 1 capsule 1-3 times a day.
Side effects: stomach upset.
Caution: do not chew the capsule (contents can be sprinkled on to cool food if necessary).
Not to be used for: infants under 1 year.
Not to be used with: some antibiotics, iron.
Contains: zinc sulphate monohydrate.

Food products

The food supplements included here are those which may be required for patients suffering from common dietary intolerances, such as coeliac disease or milk intolerance. Patients requiring more complex food products should seek medical advice. The common branded infant milks are included, although own-brand varieties from various stores are also available. (It should be remembered, however, that in all cases breast-feeding is preferable where this is possible.) Soya formula milks are suitable for infants and for children allergic to cow's milk, but transfer from a standard infant feed to a soya-based feed should be attempted only after consultation with a doctor. Furthermore, soya-based formulas are not recommended for premature babies or for those with kidney problems.

Food supplements that are used to treat deficiencies or remedy ailments are listed in the 'Vitamin and mineral products' section.

Aglutella*
(Ultrapharm)

A low-protein rice, used for patients requiring a low-protein diet.

Aproten*
(Ultrapharm)

Low-protein, gluten-free preparations supplied as anellini, ditalini, rigatoni, tagliatelle, biscuits, crispbread, bread mix, and cake mix. It is used for patients suffering from phenylketonuria, kidney and liver failure, cirrhosis of the liver, and gastro-enteritic diseases where sensitivity to gluten is present. A gluten-free flour is also available.

Arnotts Rice Cookies*
(Ultrapharm)

Gluten-free cookies used for patients suffering from coeliac disease or other digestive disorders where sensitivity to gluten occurs.

Barkat*
(Gluten Free Foods)

Gluten-free bread mix used for patients suffering from coeliac disease or other digestive disorders where sensitivity to gluten occurs.

Bi-Aglut*
(Ultrapharm)

Gluten-free preparations supplied as a biscuit and cracker toast, used for patients suffering from coeliac disease or other digestive disorders where sensitivity to gluten is present.

Boots Vita* see Complan
(Boots)

Build-Up*
(Nestlé Health Care)

A gluten-free powder containing skimmed milk, glucose, sugar, minerals, and vitamins made into drinks or soups by mixing with milk, and used as a source of energy and protein for those in need of extra supplementation (e.g. convalescents, pregnant women, nursing mothers, and the elderly). Not suitable for children under 3 years except on medical advice. Diabetics should consult a dietician or doctor before using this product.

Complan*
(Heinz)

A powder containing skimmed milk, maltodextrin, sugar, vegetable oil, minerals, and vitamins made into drinks by mixing with water, and used as a source of energy and protein for those in need of extra supplementation (e.g. convalescents, pregnant women, nursing mothers, and the elderly). Not suitable for children under 1 year except on medical advice. Diabetics should consult a dietician or doctor before using this product.

Cow & Gate Infasoy*
(Cow & Gate Nutricia)

A complete milk-free, soya-based nutrition used as an infant formula feed for babies from birth onwards. (Consult a doctor before changing a baby's milk to a soya formula.)

Cow & Gate Plus*
(Cow & Gate Nutricia)

A nutritionally complete dried infant formula, suitable for hungrier babies from birth until 12 months.

Cow & Gate Premium*
(Cow & Gate Nutricia)

A nutritionally complete dried milk infant formula, close in composition to breast milk, suitable from birth until 12 months.

Cow & Gate Step-up*
(Cow & Gate Nutricia)

A follow-on dried milk formula, suitable for infants from 6 months of age as a complement to solid food.

Dextro Energy Tablets*
(CPC)

A tablet, available in various flavours, containing dextrose and vitamin C, and used as a source of energy. (Particularly useful to diabetics as a quick source of sugar when the blood sugar level is too low.)

---

dp*
(Nutricia Dietary Products)

Low-protein cookies used for patients suffering from phenylketonuria, liver and kidney disease.

Ener-G*
(General Dietary)

Gluten-free and wheat-free preparations supplied as brown or white rice bread, tapioca bread, pasta and brown rice pasta, used for patients suffering from disorders of the digestive system in which there is sensitivity to gluten. Gluten-free rice bran and gluten-free, low-protein egg replacer are also available.

Farley's First Milk*
(Heinz)

A nutritionally complete dried milk formula, suitable for babies from birth to 12 months when breastfeeding is not possible.

Farley's Follow-on Milk*
(Heinz)

A follow-on dried milk formula, suitable for babies from 6 months to 2 years as part of a mixed diet.

Farley's Second Milk*
(Heinz)

A nutritionally complete dried milk formula, suitable for hungrier babies from birth to 12 months, when breastfeeding is not possible.

Farley's Soya Formula*
(Heinz)

A complete milk-free, soya-based nutrition used as an infant formula feed for babies from birth onwards, children, and adults. (Consult a doctor before changing a baby's milk to a soya formula.)

GF Dietary*
(Nutricia Dietary Products)

Gluten-free products supplied as beta fibre, cooking crumbs, muesli, and thin wafers, used for patients suffering from coeliac disease or other digestive disorders where sensitivity to gluten occurs.

glucose powder*

A powder available in various brands, (with or without added vitamin C), which can be added to drinks or food and used as a source of energy (e.g. during illness or when exercising).

Glutafin*
(Nutricia Dietary Products)

Gluten-free preparations supplied as biscuits, crackers, pasta, loaves (fibre or white), baking mix (fibre or white), and white rolls used for patients suffering from coeliac disease or other digestive disorders where sensitivity to gluten occurs. (The white loaves and rolls are also wheat free.)

Glutano*
(Gluten Free Foods)

Gluten-free biscuits, crackers, pretzels, bread, flour mix, pasta, rolls, and bread with added soya bran, used for patients suffering from coeliac disease or other digestive disorders where sensitivity to gluten occurs.

Infasoy*
(Cow & Gate)

A nutritionally complete milk-free, soya-based formula for infants, children, and adults. (Consult a doctor before changing a baby's milk to a soya formula.)

Isomil*
(Abbott)

A nutritionally complete, milk-free, soya-based formula for infants. (Consult a doctor before changing a baby's milk to a soya formula.)

Juvela*
(Scientific Hospital Supplies)

Gluten-free products supplied as loaves and mixes (white or fibre), bread rolls, biscuits, crispbread, and mince pies, and used for patients suffering from coeliac disease or other digestive disorders where sensitivity to gluten occurs. Additionally available are gluten-free, low-protein products (loaves, rolls, cookies, and flour mix) used also for patients suffering from phenylketonuria, liver and kidney disease.

Lifestyle*
(Ultrapharm)

Gluten-free products supplied as bread (white, brown, or high fibre) and rolls, and used for patients suffering from coeliac disease or other digestive disorders where sensitivity to gluten occurs.

Liga*
(Jacobs Bakery)

Gluten-free, low-sugar rusks used for patients with coeliac disease and other digestive disorders where sensitivity to gluten occurs.

Loprofin*
(Nutricia Dietary Products)

Low-protein products supplied as loaves, biscuits, crackers, cookies, cream wafers, egg replacer, pasta, and a drink, and used for patients suffering from phenylketonuria, liver and kidney disease. (All products, except the PKU drink, are also gluten free and therefore suitable for use by patients suffering from coeliac disease or other digestive disorders where sensitivity to gluten occurs.)

Milumil*
(Milupa)

A nutritionally complete dried milk formula, suitable for hungrier babies from birth to 12 months, when breastfeeding is not possible.

Milupa Aptamil with Milupan*
(Milupa)

A nutritionally complete dried milk formula, closely matched to breast milk, suitable for babies from birth until 12 months.

Milupa Forward*
(Milupa)

A follow-on dried milk formula, suitable for babies from 6 months to 2 years as part of a mixed diet.

Orgran*
(Foodwatch Health Products)

Low-protein pasta used for patients suffering from phenylketonuria, liver and kidney disease.

Pastariso*
(General Designs)

Gluten-free and wheat-free brown rice pastas used for patients suffering from coeliac disease or other digestive disorders where sensitivity to gluten occurs.

Polial*
(Ultrapharm)

Gluten-free biscuit used for patients suffering from coeliac disease or other digestive disorders where sensitivity to gluten occurs.

PremCare*
(Farley's-Heinz)

A milk powder formula for infants of low birth weight (2 kg and over).

Prosobee*
(Mead Johnson Nutritionals)

A nutritionally complete milk-free, soya-based powder or liquid formula for infants, children, and adults. (Consult a doctor before changing a baby's milk to a soya formula.)

Rite-Diet gluten-free*
(Nutricia Dietary Products)

Gluten-free preparations supplied as cakes, cookies, biscuits, flour mix, white bread mix, brown bread mix, white and high-fibre loaf and rolls, baking powder, hot breakfast cereal, Christmas pudding, mince pies, and gravy mix, and used for patients suffering from coeliac disease or other digestive disorders where sensitivity to gluten occurs.

Caution: unsuitable for low-protein diets.

Rite-Diet low protein*
(Nutricia Dietary Products)

Low-protein preparations supplied as flour mix, baking mix, canned bread, and egg-white replacer, and used for patients suffering from phenylketonuria and kidney or liver disorders. (The flour mix and bread are also gluten-free and therefore additionally suitable for patients suffering from coeliac disease and other digestive disorders, where sensitivity to gluten occurs.)

Caution: biscuits and wafers are not suitable for gluten-sensitive digestive disorders.

Sanatogen Original Powder*
(Roche Consumer Health)

A powder mixed into water or a drink, and used as a source of protein to build up strength and help maintain the nervous system (e.g. after illness or injury, when pregnant or breastfeeding), or to maximize muscle performance in athletes.

Schar*
(Ultrapharm)

Gluten-free products supplied as bread, bread mix, rolls, cake mix, crackers, crispbread, pasta, pizza bases, and Savoy biscuits, and used for patients suffering from coeliac disease or other digestive disorders where sensitivity to gluten occurs.

SMA Gold*
(SMA Nutrition)

An infant milk formula, available as powder or ready-to-feed milk, suitable from birth onwards.

SMA Progress*
(SMA Nutrition)

A follow-on dried milk formula, suitable for babies from 6 months to 2 years as part of a mixed diet. (Contains no animal fat.)

SMA White*
(SMA Nutrition)

An infant milk formula, available as powder or ready-to-feed milk, suitable for hungrier bottle fed babies.

Sunnyvale*
(Everfresh Natural Foods)

Gluten-free mixed grain bread used for patients suffering from coeliac disease or other digestive disorders where sensitivity to gluten occurs.

Thick & Easy*
(Fresenius)

A powder added to liquids to thicken them for patients who have difficulty swallowing.

Thompson's Slippery Elm Food*
(Lane)

A powder available in a malted or unmalted form, and added to milk to make it easier to digest (e.g. for invalids, convalescents, elderly patients, and those with digestive disorders).

Trufree*
(Larkhall)

Gluten-free flour products supplied as plain flour, flour with rice bran, flour for cantabread, white flour, brown flour, and self-raising flour used for patients suffering from coeliac disease or other digestive disorders where sensitivity to gluten occurs.

Ultra*
(Ultrapharm)

Gluten-free products supplied as crackerbread, high-fibre bread, and canned white or brown bread, and used for patients suffering from coeliac disease or other digestive disorders where sensitivity to gluten occurs. The canned breads are, additionally, low-protein products, and therefore suitable for patients suffering from phenylketonuria, liver and kidney disease.

Miscellaneous products

Aspirin is now widely used to prevent strokes and heart attacks in susceptible patients. Various 75 mg tablets are now available for this purpose, but it is recommended that anyone wishing to take this type of treatment consults a doctor first. (There may be reasons why long-term aspirin treatment is inadvisable, and prolonged treatment without a doctor's supervision may be harmful.) The products listed here are for prevention only. Anyone with a suspected heart attack or stroke must receive immediate medical attention.

Various unlicensed food supplement products, (such as ginseng* and ginkgo biloba*) are listed in this section, because the claims made for them are diverse and cover many disorders. Various claims are made about the effects of these dietary supplements, but often the evidence to support such claims is scant. (Only products with a full medicinal product licence carry the reassurance of efficacy for the conditions stated.) Provided certain warnings are heeded, however, (see individual product entries) supplements may be safely used, and many people will find them beneficial.

Various herbal products, such as slimming aids, feverfew, and garlic, are also included in this section. Slimming aids should be used with caution, and are not a substitute for a calorie-controlled diet.

acidophilus*

A food supplement capsule consisting of a live organism normally resident in the body. Antibiotics can kill this organism, as well as the ones causing ill-health, leaving the body deficient and causing gastro-intestinal disturbance. This supplement corrects the deficiency.

Dose: as specified for each individual product.
Side effects: bloating.
Caution:
Not to be used for: young children or pregnant women.
Not to be used with:
Contains: lactobacillus acidophilus bacteria.

Angettes
(Bristol-Myers)

A tablet used as an anti-platelet agent to help prevent strokes and heart attacks.

Dose: as advised by a doctor.
Side effects: irritation of stomach and intestines, noises in the ears, allergy, asthma.
Caution: all users (but especially pregnant women, diabetics, and patients with asthma or indigestion) are advised to consult a doctor before using this product. Dissolve the tablets in water before use.
Not to be used for: children under 12 years, nursing mothers, or for patients with stomach ulcers, blood-clotting disorder, or allergy to aspirin.
Not to be used with: anticoagulants, some anti-epileptic drugs, antacids.
Contains: aspirin.

---

aspirin 75 mg tablets

A soluble tablet, or tablet which disperses on the tongue without water, used as an anti-platelet agent to help prevent strokes and heart attacks.

Dose: as advised by a doctor.
Side effects: irritation of stomach and intestines, noises in the ears, allergy, asthma.
Caution: all users (but especially pregnant women, diabetics, and patients with asthma or indigestion) are advised to consult a doctor before using this product. Dissolve the tablets in water before use.
Not to be used for: children under 12 years, nursing mothers, or for patients with stomach ulcers, blood-clotting disorder, or allergy to aspirin.
Not to be used with: anticoagulants, some anti-epileptic drugs, antacids.
Contains: aspirin.

Boldo Herbal Aid to Slimming
(Potters)

A tablet used as a herbal diuretic and remedy to increase the activity of the digestive organs, to aid slimming in conjunction with a calorie-controlled diet.

Dose: 1-2 tablets 3 times a day. (Elderly patients should take only 1 tablet 3-4 times a day.)
Side effects:
Caution: do not exceed the recommended dose. Large doses cause vomiting.
Not to be used for: children.
Not to be used with:
Contains: dandelion root, butternut bark, boldo, bladderwrack.

Boots Herbal Diet-aid Tablets
(Boots)

A tablet used as a herbal remedy to aid slimming, as part of a calorie-controlled diet, by increasing the activity of the digestive organs.

Dose: 1-2 tablets 3 times a day. (Elderly patients use only 1 tablet 4 times a day.)
Side effects:
Caution:
Not to be used for: children under 12 years, pregnant women, and nursing mothers.
Not to be used with:
Contains: dandelion root, butternut bark, boldo extract, fucus extract.

---

feverfew*

Feverfew is available as food-supplement tablets, and is used to relieve symptoms of migraine. It is also thought to be helpful in controlling symptoms of arthritis, menstrual disorders, vertigo, fever, toothache, insect bites, and tinnitus.

Dose: as specified by individual product.
Side effects: contraction of smooth muscles (such as the uterus), mouth ulcers, sore mouth and tongue, allergy, abdominal pain, diarrhoea, and vomiting.
Caution: patients with arthritis and rheumatism should consult a doctor before using this product.
Not to be used for: pregnant women, nursing mothers, children.
Not to be used with:
Contains: feverfew.

---

garlic*

Opinions differ regarding the value of fresh garlic compared to that of supplements. (Fresh garlic is generally held to be the most therapeutic form, but supplements may be more convenient to take daily or to reduce odour.) Garlic is licensed as an over-the-counter medicine to treat the symptoms of colds and catarrh, but it is also thought to be useful in maintaining a healthy heart and circulation. (It can lower cholesterol levels in the blood, reducing the risk of blood clots that may lead to heart attacks or strokes, and may also function as a weak anti-platelet agent, and help to dissolve existing clots.) It may also help to protect against colds and infections of many types. Some studies suggest that it may protect against some kinds of tumour (particularly stomach cancer). For details of licensed products see 'Respiratory conditions – cough and cold remedies' section.

Dose: see manufacturer's instructions for individual product.
Side effects: there is some evidence to suggest that too much fresh garlic may irritate or damage the lining of the digestive tract, or cause anaemia.
Caution: Gerard House recommends that garlic supplements are not given to young children.
Not to be used for:
Not to be used with:
Contains: garlic (*Allium sativum*).

---

ginkgo biloba*

Ginkgo is available as a food-supplement tablet, and is thought to help maintain healthy circulation to all parts of the body (including the brain), and this has led to its use to help revitalize older people, in an attempt to improve thought processes and reaction time. It may also be of use in relieving asthma symptoms (although this should not replace prescribed medication).

Dose: as specified for each individual product.

Side effects: headache, mild stomach upset, allergy.
Caution: pregnant women and nursing mothers should consult a doctor before using this product.
Not to be used for:
Not to be used with:
Contains: Ginkgo biloba.

ginseng*

Ginseng is available as food-supplement tablets or capsules (often in combination with vitamins and minerals) and is thought to be of help in various ways in the body. Increased stamina and performance under stress, improved mood, regulation of blood pressure, and increased resistance to shock or fatigue have all been attributed to the use of ginseng. The main use, however, is as a tonic and to prevent fatigue and infection, especially in elderly or debilitated patients.

Dose: as specified for each individual product.
Side effects: high blood pressure, insomnia, swollen breasts, vaginal bleeding, diarrhoea, stimulation, and skin rashes have all been reported with overuse of this product.
Caution: normal doses may be taken for up to 4 weeks, then a gap of at least 4 weeks is recommended before resuming. Continuous use for more than 3 months is not recommended, although the elderly or chronically sick patients may take low doses on a regular basis. Not generally recommended for healthy adults under the age of 40 years.
Not to be used for: children, diabetics, or patients with high blood pressure.
Not to be used with: steroids, anti-diabetic drugs, anti-hypertensive drugs.
Contains: ginseng.

kelp*
(licensed product available from Gerard House)

Kelp products are licensed as medicines for use as a source of minerals (including iodine which is needed for healthy metabolism), and for the symptomatic relief of rheumatic pain. Some are also recommended in the treatment of obesity (when associated with low thyroid function) and as an aid to convalescence. They are also thought to be of help in maintaining a healthy scalp and hair, relieving symptoms of rheumatic pain, and to function as a mild diuretic.

Dose: see manufacturer's instructions for individual product.
Side effects:
Caution: pregnant women, nursing mothers, and patients with thyroid disorders (or taking thyroxine) should consult a doctor before using these products.
Not to be used for: children under 5 years
Not to be used with: thyroxine (see above).
Contains: kelp.

Lactaid*
(Myplan)

A tablet used to treat inability to digest milk or dairy foods.

Dose: 2-6 tablets with each meal of dairy food.
Side effects: stomach upset, allergy.
Caution:
Not to be used for:
Not to be used with:
Contains: lactase enzyme.

---

lecithin*

A food supplement, available as capsules or granules, and used as a source of choline, inositol, and fatty acids. These components are used by the body to mobilize fat and convert it to energy. It is thought to help maintain a healthy heart and circulation by reducing cholesterol levels, and may also be of

645

use in maintaining a healthy nervous system. It is also thought to be an aid to dietary pollution, by helping the liver to fight pollutants in food.

Dose: as specified for each individual product.
Side effects:
Caution:
Not to be used for:
Not to be used with:
Contains: choline, inositol, fatty acids.

Malted Kelp Tablets
(Potters)

A tablet used as a herbal supplementary source of minerals to aid convalescence, and to help manage the symptoms of rheumatic pain.

Dose: adults 1 tablet 3 times a day after food; children over 5 years 1 tablet twice a day after food.
Side effects:
Caution: pregnant women and patients with thyroid disorders (or taking thyroxine) should consult a doctor before using these products.
Not to be used for: children under 5 years.
Not to be used with: thyroxine (see above).
Contains: kelp, malt extract.

Nu-Seals 75 mg
(Lilly)

A tablet, coated to protect the stomach, used as an anti-platelet agent to help prevent heart attacks, angina, or mini-strokes.

Dose: 1 tablet daily, or as advised by a doctor.
Side effects: irritation of stomach and intestines, noises in the ears, allergy, asthma.

Caution: all users (but especially pregnant women, diabetics, and patients with asthma or indigestion) are advised to consult a doctor before using this product.

Not to be used for: children under 12 years, nursing mothers, or patients with stomach ulcers, blood-clotting disorder, or allergy to aspirin.

Not to be used with: anticoagulants, some anti-epileptic drugs, antacids.

Contains: aspirin.

---

omega-3 fish oils*

A food supplement (capsule or liquid) derived from selected species of oil-rich fishes, which provides extra EPA and DPA in the diet and is thought to help maintain a healthy heart and circulation, lowering cholesterol levels and decreasing the risk of heart disease, strokes, or high blood pressure. Some fish-oil products (especially cod liver oil – see entry in 'Vitamins and minerals' section) are used to relieve symptoms of arthritis and rheumatism. There is some suggestion that asthma and skin conditions, such as acne and psoriasis, may also benefit from fish-oil supplements.

Dose: as specified for each individual product.
Side effects:
Caution:
Not to be used for:
Not to be used with:
Contains: eicosapentanenoic acid (EPA), docosahexaenoic acid (DPA).

Homeopathic preparations

Homeopathic remedies are prepared from minute amounts of that same substance which would create the disease if taken in crude form. For example, Apis mel., which is made from the honey bee venom, is used to treat hot red swellings with burning, stinging pains.

Homeopathic products are now licensed under a Homeopathic Registration Scheme which ensures the safety and quality of the product. Hence, consumers can now be assured that all licensed remedies bearing an HR number on the label have been properly examined and are safe to use.

The remedies are prepared by a process of dilution and succussion (repeated hard shaking) until they reach the desired potency, as follows:

6x: dilution 1:9, succussion, process repeated 6 times;

6c: dilution 1:99, succussion, process repeated 6 times;

30c: dilution 1:99, succussion, process repeated 30 times.

Homeopathic remedies are made in a very wide range of potencies, but the 6x, 6c, and 30c are the ones available over the counter at health food shops and pharmacies. These potencies are all suitable for first-aid use and to treat everyday ailments. It is best to begin with 6x and 6c, however, until you get to know the action of the remedies. The 30c is stronger and will be used for more serious conditions such as severe burns or shock, and for those where emotional or mental phenomena play a part. Their repetition should vary according to the severity of the complaint but, as a general guide:

Acute conditions

6x: every 15-30 minutes

6c: every 15-60 minutes

30c: every 15 minutes to once a day.

Chronic conditions
6x: 3-4 times a day
6c: 2-3 times a day
30c: once a week or less.

The suggested dose is 2 tablets for adults and 1 for children for the 6c potency. (New Era recommends a dose of 4 tablets for adults, 2 for children, and 1 for infants with its 6X range.) The tablets should be taken on a clean tongue and not at the same time as food. (An interval of at least 20 minutes is suggested.) Handle the tablets as little as possible. It is important to stop the tablets when the symptoms start to improve or worsen. Then wait and restart the remedy only if the original symptoms return.

1 Classical remedies
The descriptions of the remedies that follow are confined to those ailments that you might reasonably try to treat at home. For any more serious complaints or if your condition does not improve, you should consult a professional homeopath or physician. Many times when homeopathy fails to work it is because the correct remedy has not bee selected – this requires perceiving the patient clearly so that it is best, wherever possible, to visit a qualified practitioner.

Because homeopathy is patient based rather than symptom based, some brief descriptions of the patient's disposition have been included. If you are dealing with an acute or first-aid situation, however, these will be less relevant than when taking a remedy for a long-term ailment. Note that the paragraph headed 'Low time' refers to the time of day when symptoms may worsen or when the patient feels a dip in energy.

Aconite
(Weleda 6c, 30c; Nelsons 6c; Boots 6c)

Prepared from entire plant *Aconitum napellus* (wolfbane).

Uses: emotional shock, panic attacks, intense fear, anxiety, restlessness; useful in the first stages of a cold or fever – up to 48 hours from onset, complaints come on suddenly and patient may have hot red cheeks and be thirsty for cold drinks although everything tastes bitter; sudden high fevers with intense thirst and dry skin, burning sore throat, intolerable pain, toothache or earache after exposure to cold dry wind; croup, dry suffocating barking cough, insomnia with anxious dreams.
Suited to: patients suffering from illness following fright or shock.
Symptoms better for: open air, reduced covering.
Symptoms worse for: fright, shock, bad news, warm room, heat of sun, cold dry winds, lying on affected side, tobacco smoke, music.
Low time: midnight.

Actaea racemosa (Actaea rac.)
(Weleda 6c, 30c; Nelsons 6c.)

Prepared from root of *Cimicifuga racemosa* plant (black cohosh).

Uses: depression, claustrophobia, irritability, headaches with severe pains which start at the back of the head and spread upwards and which are relieved by cool fresh air, neuralgia, stiff neck, tinnitus, painful muscles after exercise, rheumatic pains in back and neck, heavy exhausting menstruation, chilliness.
Suited to: patients who are sensitive, nervous, excitable, and talkative and who may also become despondent.
Symptoms better for: warmth, eating.
Symptoms worse for: cold, damp, motion, menstruation.
Low time: morning.

Allium cepa
(Weleda 6c)

Prepared from entire *Allium cepa* plant (red onion).

Uses: hayfever, catarrh, inflammation of mucous membranes, colds with profuse burning watery discharge, eyes watering, burning, and smarting, laryngitis.
Symptoms better for: cold room, open air.
Symptoms worse for: warm room.
Low time: evening.

Apis mellifica (Apis mel.)
(Weleda 6c, 30c; Nelsons 6c; Boots 6c)

Prepared from honey bee venom.

Uses: burning stinging pains, cystitis with constant desire to urinate, arthritis with red, swollen, shiny joints, hot red swelling anywhere in body, swollen ankles, swollen lower eyelids, bites and stings which become red and swollen, allergic reactions (if the reaction is severe or there is difficult breathing, seek medical help immediately), urticaria, symptoms tend to affect the right side of the body most, thirstlessness, burning sore throat.
Suited to: busy, restless people who may become ill after emotional upset.
Symptoms better for: cold bathing, open air.
Symptoms worse for: heat, touch, after sleep, fright, anger, grief, bad news.
Low time: mid-afternoon.

Argentum nitricum (Argent nit.)
(Weleda 6c, 30c; Nelsons 6c; Boots 6c)

Prepared from silver nitrate.

Uses: nervousness, anticipatory fear, heartburn, acidity,

flatulence, headache relieved by pressure, mental strain, vertigo with buzzing in the ears, tremor, agoraphobia, claustrophobia, nervous diarrhoea, hoarseness.
Suited to: hurried, fidgety, impulsive, nervous people who suffer from anticipatory fear.
Symptoms better for: open air, cold bathing.
Symptoms worse for: anticipatory fear, overwork, overstudy, sugar, ice-cream, warmth.
Low time: night.

Arnica
(Weleda 6x, 6c, 30c; Nelsons 6c; Boots 6c)

Prepared from entire *Arnica montana* plant (mountain tobacco).

Uses: after physical shock or injury; bruises, sprains, exhaustion, jet lag, aching muscles; body feeling sore and bruised all over, concussion, haemorrhages, compound fractures.
Symptoms better for: lying down with head low.
Symptoms worse for: touch, movement, cold, damp.
Low time:

Arsenicum album (Arsen. alb.)
(Weleda 6c, 30c; Nelsons 6c; Boots 6c)

Prepared from the white oxide of metallic arsenic.

Uses: food poisoning, holiday stomach upsets, sudden violent vomiting and diarrhoea, restlessness, icy chills, burning pains especially throat or stomach, anxiety, fear, insomnia with overactive mind and anxious dreams.
Suited to: patients who are tidy, fastidious, precise, and anxious.
Symptoms better for: heat, cool air around head.
Symptoms worse for: cold, cold food and drinks.
Low time: after midnight.

Belladonna
(Weleda 6c, 30c; Nelsons 6c; Boots 6c)

Prepared from entire *Atropa belladonna* (deadly nightshade) plant when beginning to flower.

Uses: severe throbbing headache, sudden fevers with flushed face and dilated pupils, excitability during fever, skin is dry hot and burning, sunstroke, throbbing earache, acne, acute local inflammations which are red and throbbing; symptoms tend to be on right side of body.
Suited to: lively, cheerful, excitable children or adults who become restless and agitated when ill.
Symptoms better for: warmth, sitting upright.
Symptoms worse for: touch, movement, noise, sun.
Low time: mid-afternoon.

Bryonia
(Weleda 6c, 30c; Nelsons 6c; Boots 6c)

Prepared from root of *Bryonia alba* plant (white bryony).

Uses: dry, painful, irritating cough, dry mucous membranes, dry lips, fevers which develop slowly over a few days, irritability, mastitis, arthritis, sharp stitching pains; headache accompanies many acute complaints and patient will often be very thirsty.
Suited to: lean, dark-haired people.
Symptoms better for: keeping absolutely still, lying on painful side, pressure, fresh air, cold, cold food and drinks.
Symptoms worse for: movement, touch, warmth.
Low time: mid-evening.

Calcarea carbonica (Calc. Carb.)
(Weleda 6c, 30c; Nelsons 6c; Boots 6c)

Prepared from calcium carbonate from middle layer of oyster shell.

Uses: obesity, cold extremities, cracked itching skin, profuse sour perspiration especially on head, vertigo, anxiety, indigestion, poor assimilation of nutrients, swollen glands, premenstrual tension, insomnia, menses early, profuse, painful, and protracted, constipation; children – difficult and delayed dentition, head sweats, slow closure of fontanelles, poor calcium absorption.

Suited to: fair-haired, timid patients who tend to put on weight easily.

Symptoms better for: dry weather, lying on painful side.

Symptoms worse for: cold, damp, draughts, teething, drinking milk, exertion, standing.

Low time:

Calcarea fluorica (Calc. fluor.)

(New Era 6x; Weleda 6c, 30c; Nelsons 6c)

Prepared from calcium fluoride.

Uses: promotes elasticity of tissues; varicose veins, stretch marks, arthritis, prevention of adhesions after surgery, haemorrhoids, croup, head colds with discharge, catarrh, deficient enamel of teeth.

Symptoms better for: movement, warmth.

Symptoms worse for: rest, damp.

Low time:

Calcarea phosphorica (Calc. phos.)

(New Era 6x; Weleda 6c, 30c; Nelsons 6c)

Prepared from tricalcic phosphate.

Uses: adolescents lacking energy and concentration, emaciation, cough with yellow mucus, stomach pains after eating, acne, enlarged adenoids, headache from overstudying, swollen glands, chronic catarrh, non-union of fractures, debility remaining after acute disease.

Suited to: general debility with discontent.
Symptoms better for: summer, lying down.
Symptoms worse for: cold, damp, draughts, wet weather, fresh air, mental exertion.
Low time:

Calcarea sulphurica (Calc. Sulph.)
(New Era 6x)

Prepared from calcium sulphate.

Uses: blood purifier, helps rid the body of toxins, aids healing of abcesses after they have begun to discharge, acne, catarrh, boils, wounds which won't heal.
Symptoms better for: open air, bathing, eating, heat to the affected part.
Symptoms worse for: hot stuffy rooms, touch, draughts.
Low time:

Cantharis
(Weleda 6c, 30c; Nelsons 6c; Boots 6c)

Prepared from the *Cantharis vesicatoria* beetle.

Uses: cystitis with burning pains before and after urination, constant urge to urinate, severe difficulty urinating and with scalding sensation, burning pains; second degree burns and scalds before blisters form or where blistering is present, sunburn.
Symptoms better for: warmth, rest; pain of burns is better for cold compresses.
Symptoms worse for: urination, touch, coffee, drinking cold water.
Low time:

Carbo vegetabilis (Carbo veg.)
(Weleda 6c, 30c; Nelsons 6c; Boots 6c)

Prepared from vegetable charcoal.

Uses: indigestion with excessive flatulence, bloated abdomen with rumbling, sluggish venous circulation, shivering but with a desire for open window, cold limbs at night, violent racking cough, hoarseness, loss of voice, tinnitus with nausea and vertigo.
Symptoms better for: eructations, being fanned.
Symptoms worse for: fatty foods, warm damp weather.
Low time: evening, night.

Causticum
(Weleda 6c)

Prepared from potassium hydrate.

Uses: sore throat with raw burning pain, hoarseness, hollow spasmodic cough which is constant and exhausting, chemical burns and third degree burns (seek medical help immediately), to relieve soreness in the site of old burns, constipation with ineffectual urging, cystitis with frequent urging but difficulty passing urine, retention of urine, incontinence of urine on coughing, raw sore pains.
Suited to: patients who are lean, dark haired, and sensitive.
Symptoms better for: mild wet weather, cold drinks.
Symptoms worse for: dry cold or raw air, winds, drafts, grief.
Low time: evening.

Chamomilla
(Weleda 3x, 30c; also available from Weleda in 3x drops and pillules – see 'Miscellaneous homeopathic' section; Boots 6c)

Prepared from entire plant *Chamomilla recutita* (German camomile – formerly known as *Matricaria chamomilla*).

Uses: severe pains, irritability, toothache which is worse for warm drinks, oversensitivity to unpleasant stimuli, period pains which worsen after anger, sleeplessness from pain, anger, or too much coffee; children – babies who cry constantly and are quiet only when carried, teething remedy, colic, green diarrhoea especially during teething, earache.
Suited to: children who are irritable and restless when ill and want to be carried all the time.
Symptoms better for: being carried.
Symptoms worse for: teething, anger, coffee.
Low time: morning, evening, night.

Cina
(Weleda 6c)

Prepared from the unexpanded flower heads of *Artemisia maritima* (sea wormwood).

Uses: children very irritable, petulant, capricious, want to be rocked but not touched or carried, digestive problems, extreme hunger, refuses mother's milk, grinding teeth or crying out during sleep, intestinal worms.
Symptoms better for: lying on abdomen, rocking, movement.
Symptoms worse for: touch, during sleep.
Low time: morning, night.

Cocculus
(Weleda 6c; Boots 6c)

Prepared from powdered seeds of *Cocculus indicus* plant.

Uses: travel sickness, loss of sleep, jet lag especially after long-haul flights, effects of crossing time zones, vertigo with sensation as if at sea, nausea, vomiting, weakness and great pain with menses which are early and profuse.
Suited to: patients who are fair haired and sensitive.
Symptoms better for: sitting, lying on side.

Symptoms worse for: motion of cars, boats; swimming, touch, emotion, open air, noise, eating, menses.
Low time:

Coffea
(Weleda 6c; Boots 6c)

Prepared from raw coffee berries.

Uses: sleeplessness from mental activity, excessive sensitivity to noise and pain, agitation, toothache with shooting pains which is better for holding ice-cold water in the mouth, one-sided nervous headache.
Suited to: patients who are tall, dark haired, and cheerful.
Symptoms better for: sleep, warmth, lying down.
Symptoms worse for: noise, touch, odours, open air, mental exertion, excitement, emotion, overeating, alcohol.
Low time: night.

Colocynthis (Colocynth.)
(Weleda 6c; Boots 6c)

Prepared from pulp of *Citrullus colocynth* fruit (bitter cucumber).

Uses: abdominal colic, cramps and spasms, diarrhoea, vomiting from pain, neuralgic pains, sciatica, trigeminal neuralgia, vertigo from turning the head quickly, cramp in calves.
Symptoms better for: heat, pressure, doubling up.
Symptoms worse for: anger, lying on painless side.
Low time:

Cuprum metallicum (Cuprum met.)
(Weleda 6c, 30c; Nelsons 6c)

Prepared from copper.

Uses: cramps and spasms, cramp in fingers, legs, or toes, nausea and vomiting with abdominal cramps, diarrhoea, metallic taste in mouth, spasmodic cough with shortness of breath and vomiting, cold hands and feet, bluish face and lips.
Symptoms better for: cold drinks.
Symptoms worse for: cold air, touch, before menstruation, coughing, after vomiting.
Low time: evening, night.

Drosera
(Weleda 6c, 30c; Nelsons 6c)

Prepared from *Drosera rotundifolia* (round-leaved sundew) plant.

Uses: constant tickling cough, violent attacks of coughing which may end in vomiting, deep, hoarse, barking cough with retching, sore throat which is worse for swallowing, laryngitis with a dry throat making speech difficult.
Symptoms better for: open air.
Symptoms worse for: talking, laughing, drinking, lying down, warmth.
Low time: after midnight.

Euphrasia
(Weleda 6c, 30c; Nelsons 6c; Boots 6c)

Prepared from entire plant *Euphrasia officinalis* (eyebright).

Uses: colds with watering eyes and streaming nose, hayfever, conjunctivitis with burning tears, photophobia, cough which comes only during the day and has copious mucus.
Symptoms better for: dim light, cold applications.
Symptoms worse for: sunlight, warmth, being indoors.
Low time: evening.

Ferrum Phosphoricum (Ferr. Phos.)
(Weleda 6c, 30c; New Era 6x; Nelsons 6c)

Prepared from white phosphate of iron.

Uses: early stages of colds (after Aconite), early stages of fever and inflammation before exudation begins, anaemia, sluggish venous circulation, hammering congestive headaches, nosebleeds, rheumatism.
Suited to: pale, delicate people who flush easily on exertion.
Symptoms better for: cold applications, summer.
Symptoms worse for: touch, noise, cold.
Low time: night.

Feverfew
(Weleda 6x)

Prepared from feverfew plant (*Chrysanthemum parthenium*).

Uses: to reduce frequency and severity of migraine attacks. The indications for homoeopathic feverfew are the same as for taking it as a herbal remedy. The potentized form has been prepared because some patients were complaining of mouth ulcers after taking the herbal form (which is not licensed as a medicine).

Gelsemium
(Weleda 6c, 30c; Nelsons 6c; Boots 6c)

Prepared from bark of the root of *Gelsemium sempervirens* (yellow jasmine).

Uses: Influenza and its after-effects, fatigue, aching, trembling, weakness, heaviness, sneezing, sore throat, difficulty swallowing, headache, chills up and down the spine, vertigo, drooping eyelids, anticipatory fear.

Suited to: excitable, sensitive people who suffer from anticipatory fear.
Symptoms better for: urination, sweating.
Symptoms worse for: humidity, heat of sun, receiving bad news, shocks, anticipation, tobacco.
Low time: mid-morning.

Graphites
(Weleda 6c, 30c; Nelsons 6c; Boots 6c)

Prepared from amorphous carbon.

Uses: eczema which cracks and weeps, thickening and hardening of skin, cracks and fissures, wounds which tend to suppurate, styes, overweight, constipation, anal fissures, tinnitus, hot flushes, dandruff.
Suited to: cautious, indecisive people who tend to put on weight.
Symptoms better for: touch, more clothing, eating.
Symptoms worse for: during and after menstruation, cold, light.
Low time: night.

Hamamelis
(Weleda 6c, 30c; Nelsons 6c)

Prepared from fresh bark of twigs and roots of *Hamamelis virginica* (witch hazel).

Uses: varicose veins, haemorrhoids, bruised soreness, chilblains with bluish colour, nosebleeds, venous congestion.
Symptoms better for:
Symptoms worse for: injuries, bruises, day, touch, pressure, humidity.
Low time: night.

Hepar Sulphuris (Hepar Sulph.)
(Weleda 6c, 30c; Nelsons 6c; Boots 6c)

Prepared from a sulphide of calcium made by burning the white interior of oyster shells and sulphur together.

Uses: hypersensitivity, irritability, intolerance of pain, skin highly sensitive to touch, eczema, acne, intense chilliness, croup, cough brought on by exposure to cold air, wheezing, sensation of splinter at back of throat, tonsillitis, earache; all wounds tend to suppurate; will hasten abcesses; establishes suppuration around and removes foreign body.
Symptoms better for: warmth, humidity.
Symptoms worse for: cold dry air, winter, drafts, touch, noise, exertion.
Low time: night.

Hypericum
(Weleda 6c, 30c; Nelsons 6c)

Prepared from entire plant *Hypericum perforatum* (perforate St John's wort).

Uses: painful injuries to parts rich in nerve endings especially fingers and toes, lacerated wounds involving nerve endings, violent shooting pains, falls injuring spine especially coccyx, blows or crush injuries to fingers or toes, headache after blow to the occiput.
Symptoms better for: bending backwards, rubbing.
Symptoms worse for: shock, touch, movement, cold damp.
Low time:

Ignatia
(Weleda 6c, 30c; Nelson 6c; Boots 6c)

Prepared from the seeds of the *Ignatia amara* tree.

Uses: grief, fright, bereavement, exhaustion from prolonged grief, sighing, spasms, sensation of lump in throat, sore throat which is better for swallowing, piercing headache, haemorrhoids which are better when walking, croup, irritating cough which worsens with coughing, constipation.

Suited to: sensitive, emotional people who prefer to be alone.

Symptoms better for: being alone, eating.

Symptoms worse for: emotion, worry, coffee, tobacco smoke.

Low time: morning.

Ipecacuanha (Ipecac.)
(Weleda 6c, 30c: Nelsons 6c)

Prepared from dried root of *Cephaelis ipecacuanha* plant.

Uses: nausea, vomiting, morning sickness, travel sickness, gastric upset with clean tongue, bronchitis, loose coarse rattle in chest without expectoration, nausea and shortness of breath accompany most complaints.

Symptoms better for: open air, rest, closing eyes, cold drinks, pressure.

Symptoms worse for: warmth, overeating, change of weather, vomiting, motion.

Low time:

Kalium Bichromicum (Kali. Bich.)
(Weleda 6c, 30c: Nelsons 6c; Boots 6c)

Prepared from potassium bichromate.

Uses: catarrh which is stringy and tenacious, hard cough with plugs of mucus, pain in small spots (can be covered with point of finger), sore throat, migraine with blurred vision preceding the attack.

Suited to: reserved, conscientious people with a tendency to put on weight.

Symptoms better for: movement, pressure.
Symptoms worse for: alcohol, hot weather.
Low time: morning, 2-3 am.

Kalium Muriaticum (Kali. Mur.)
(New Era 6x)

Prepared from potassium chloride.

Uses: a blood purifier and cleanser, may help prevent blood from clotting too easily; white or greyish-white coated tongue and throat, sore throat, swollen glands, tonsillitis, thick white sticky catarrh, deafness from catarrh and blocked eustachian tubes, indigestion from fatty food, rheumatic swellings.
Symptoms better for: cold drinks, rubbing.
Symptoms worse for: open air, menstruation, movement, dampness, rich food.
Low time:

Kalium Phosphoricum (Kali. Phos.)
(Weleda 6c, 30c; New Era 6x; Nelsons 6c; Boots 6c)

Prepared from potassium phosphate.

Uses: nervous exhaustion, nervousness, insomnia, depression, anxiety, vertigo, headache with humming in the ears, shingles, nervous asthma, hoarseness, dry tongue; night fears in children.
Symptoms better for: sleep, eating, gentle movement.
Symptoms worse for: worry, excitement, touch, pain, overwork.
Low time:

Kalium Sulphuricum (Kali. Sulph.)
(New Era 6x)

Prepared from potassium sulphate.

Uses: skin problems with scaling, psoriasis, athlete's foot, brittle nails, yellow slimy coating on the tongue, yellow catarrh, rheumatism which moves from joint to joint.
Symptoms better for: cool open air, walking.
Symptoms worse for: warmth of room, noise.
Low time: evening.

Lachesis
(Weleda 6c)

Prepared from venom of *Trigonocephalus lachesis* snake (surukuku).

Uses: throbbing headache with head feeling hot and heavy, hot flushes, hot perspiration, menopause, intolerance of touch, pressure of clothing aggravates, symptoms occur more on left side of body or travel from left to right, poor circulation with bluish mottled appearance, sore throat extending to ear — better for swallowing solids but worse for liquids, tonsillitis.
Suited to: talkative excitable people.
Symptoms better for: open air, cold drinks, menstruation.
Symptoms worse for: sleep, heat, spring, summer, sun, touch, pressure, alcohol, hot drinks.
Low time: morning.

Ledum
(Weleda 6c)

Prepared from entire plant *Ledum palustre*.

Uses: puncture wounds, insect bites, bee stings, bruised or bloodshot eyes, cold blue swellings, chilliness, rheumatic or arthritic conditions which start in the lower limbs and ascend, gout.
Symptoms better for: cold applications, resting.
Symptoms worse for: warmth, movement, alcohol.

Low time: night.

Lycopodium
(Weleda 6c, 30c; Nelsons 6c; Boots 6c)

Prepared from *Lycopodium clavatum* plant (common club moss).

Uses: abdominal bloating and flatulence, excessive hunger but a few mouthfuls satiate, loud rumbling especially in lower abdomen, craving sweets although they aggravate, symptoms are mainly on the right side of body or moving from right to left, ailments from anticipation, fear of failure, cystitis, gout.
Suited to: people who may appear proud or argumentative but are lacking in self-confidence.
Symptoms better for: warm drinks, movement, eructations.
Symptoms worse for: pressure of clothes, eating, sleep, bread, onions, cabbage, wine, coffee, smoking.
Low time: late afternoon to mid-evening.

Magnesia Phosphorica (Mag. Phos.)
(New Era 6x)

Prepared from magnesium phosphate.

Uses: colic, cramps, spasms, neuralgic pains, right-sided complaints, sharp lightning-like pains, writer's cramp, menstrual cramp, facial neuralgia, headache relieved by warmth, sciatica.
Suited to: dark-haired, thin, nervous people.
Symptoms better for: warmth, hot bathing, pressure, rubbing, doubling up.
Symptoms worse for: cold, being uncovered.
Low time: night.

Mercurius Solubilis (Merc. Sol.)
(Weleda 6c, 30c, Nelsons 6c; Boots 6c).

Prepared from dimercurous ammonium nitrate.

Uses: suppuration, abcesses, mouth ulcers, sore throat, tonsillitis, excessive saliva, metallic taste in mouth, bad breath, tongue swollen and flabby showing imprint of teeth, profuse sweats, feverish head cold with offensive green/yellow catarrh, earache, diarrhoea with straining, tremor.
Suited to: those who are hurried and impulsive.
Symptoms better for: even temperature, rest.
Symptoms worse for: temperature changes.
Low time: night.

Natrum Muriaticum (Nat. Mur.)
(Weleda 6c, 30c; New Era 6x; Nelsons 6c; Boots 6c)

Prepared from sodium chloride.

Uses: excessive moisture or dryness in any part of the system, profuse watery colds, hayfever, severe headache, migraine, vertigo, pain in eyes from reading, effects of longstanding grief, depression, dry skin, eczema, cold sores, warts, menstrual pain, constipation, incontinence.
Suited to: thin, pale, reserved people who, though emotionally sensitive, dislike consolation.
Symptoms better for: open air, cool bathing.
Symptoms worse for: sun, emotion, consolation, touch, noise, music, salt, seaside.
Low time: mid- to late morning

Natrum Phosphoricum (Nat. Phos.)
(New Era 6x)

Prepared from sodium phosphate.

Uses: an acid neutralizer; helps remove excesses of lactic and uric acid from the body and thus aids digestive and rheumatic disorders, sour vomiting, yellow creamy coating at base of

tongue, dyspepsia, tightness of muscles and tendons, gout.
Symptoms better for: cold.
Symptoms worse for: sugar, milk, fatty food.
Low time: evening.

Natrum Sulphuricum (Nat. Sulph.)
(New Era 6x)

Prepared from sodium sulphate.

Uses: regulates density of intercellular fluids by eliminating excess water; aids the healthy functioning of the liver, biliousness, bitter taste in mouth, brown tongue, yellow diarrhoea, painful flatulence, rumbling abdomen, photophobia, inflammation of nailbed.
Symptoms better for: open air, changing position.
Symptoms worse for: all forms of damp, night air, music.
Low time: morning.

Nux vomica (Nux vom.)
(Weleda 6c, 30c; Nelsons 6c; Boots 6c)

Prepared from seeds of *Strychnos nux-vomica* (strychnine) tree.

Uses: hypersensitivity to external stimuli, irritability, effects of overwork, effects of overeating, hangover, headache with nausea or dizziness, dyspepsia, nausea, vomiting, travel sickness, hiccough, raw sore throat, colds, hayfever, violent cough, spasms, menstrual cramps, colic, constipation with ineffectual urging, itching haemorrhoids.
Suited to: solid, compact, muscular people who are inclined to be impatient, irritable, and fastidious.
Symptoms better for: warmth, evening, resting.
Symptoms worse for: cold, alcohol, coffee, noise, light, odours, music, mental exertion, vexation.
Low time: early morning.

Phosphorus
(Weleda 6c, 30c; Nelsons 6c; Boots 6c)

Prepared from red amorphous phosphorus.

Uses: cough with difficult rapid breathing, bronchitis, painful hoarseness, laryngitis, vomiting, diarrhoea, heartburn, burning sensations in small areas, need to eat often, anxiety, oversensitivity, vertigo, exhaustion with weakness and trembling, tendency to bleed or bruise easily.
Suited to: tall, slender, fine-boned, sensitive people.
Symptoms better for: cold food, ices, sleep.
Symptoms worse for: cold, thunderstorms, emotional upset, warm food, mental fatigue, lying on left side.
Low time: evening.

Phytolacca
(Weleda 6c)

Prepared from roots, berries and leaves of *Phytolacca decandra* plant (Virginian pokeweed).

Uses: mastitis, breast abscess, sore throat with intense burning and dryness, tonsillitis, rheumatism, shooting pains like shocks through the body, teething pains which are better when infant bites on something.
Symptoms better for: lying on abdomen, rest.
Symptoms worse for: movement, menstruation, cold damp, swallowing hot drinks.
Low time:

Pulsatilla
(Weleda 6c, 30c; Nelsons 6c; Boots 6c)

Prepared from entire flowering *Pulsatilla nigricans* plant (wind anemone).

Uses: changeability of symptoms and of mood, pains which move and change, menstrual irregularities, menstrual pain, colds with thick bland yellow catarrh, thick coated white tongue, stomach upsets from rich fatty foods, thirstless even though mouth is dry, weepy, yielding, babies who are quiet only when carried, styes, arthritis, cystitis, poor circulation, varicose veins.
Suited to: affectionate, emotional people easily moved to laughter or tears, fair haired, tend to put on weight easily.
Symptoms better for: open air, slow movement, consolation.
Symptoms worse for: rich foods, stuffy rooms.
Low time: evening.

Rhus toxicodendron (Rhus tox.)
(Weleda 6c 30c; Nelsons, 6c; Boots 6c)

Prepared from leaves of *Rhus toxicodendron* plant (oakleaf poison ivy) gathered at sunset just before flowering.

Uses: strains, sprains, overexertion, strains of muscles and tendons, pain in ligaments, rheumatism, stiffness, arthritis, sciatica, shooting pains, cold sores, herpes, eczema, tickling cough, restlessness.
Symptoms better for: continued movement, heat, hot bathing, rubbing, stretching, warm dry weather.
Symptoms worse for: first movement, cold, wet, drafts, before storms.
Low time: after midnight.

Ruta graveolens (Ruta grav.)
(Weleda 6c, 30c; Nelson 6c)

Prepared from entire *Ruta graveolens* plant (rue).

Uses: bruised bones, injuries to periosteum (membrane covering the bone), strains and sprains where Rhus tox. is ineffective, bruised sore aching with restlessness, synovitis, rheumatism, tennis elbow, eye strain.

Symptoms better for: warmth, movement, rubbing.
Symptoms worse for: overexertion, cold, menstruation.
Low time: evening.

Sepia
(Weleda 6c, 30c; Nelsons 6c; Boots 6c)

Prepared from the ink of *Sepia officinalis* (common cuttlefish).

Uses: depression, indifference to loved ones, menopause, hot flushes, hot sweats, hair loss, irregular periods, premenstrual tension, uterine pain with bearing down sensation, loss of sex drive, headache comes in shocks, sluggish irregular circulation, sudden tiredness.
Suited to: those who become depressed easily and lose interest in work, pleasure, loved ones, and sex.
Symptoms better for: exercise, dancing, hot applications.
Symptoms worse for: cold air, rest.
Low time: afternoon, evening.

Silica/Silicea
(Weleda 6c, 30c; New Era 6x; Nelsons 6c; Boots 6c)

Prepared from flint.

Uses: abcesses, boils, expulsion of foreign bodies, acne, fungal infections, athlete's foot, tendency to suppurate, whitlow, offensive sweats particularly of the feet, persistent colds, hayfever, chilliness, swollen glands, migraine, poor assimilation of nutrients, brittle unhealthy nails, white spots on nails, constipation.
Suited to: delicate, pale, fair-haired people who are both timid and obstinate.
Symptoms better for: warmth, summer, humidity.
Symptoms worse for: cold, drafts, noise, touch, alcohol.
Low time: morning.

Sulphur

(New Era 6c, 30c; Nelsons 6c; Boots 6c)

Prepared from sublimated sulphur.

Uses: skin eruptions which are hot and burning, redness, eczema, acne, burning pains, excoriating discharges, itching, mid-morning hunger, early morning diarrhoea, unrefreshing sleep, flushes of heat, burning soles of feet, burning itching haemorrhoids, insomnia.
Suited to: intellectual, self-absorbed, and untidy people.
Symptoms better for: open air, walking, movement.
Symptoms worse for: bathing, becoming overheated, standing, eating sweets, atmospheric changes.
Low time: late morning

Symphytum

(Weleda 6c; Boots 6c)

Prepared from *Symphytum officinale* plant (comfrey).

Uses: facilitates union of fractured bones (do not take unless you know the bones are in good alignment), pricking stitching pains, cartilage injuries, painful old injuries, blows to the eye from blunt objects.
Symptoms worse for: touch.
Symptoms better for:
Low time:

Thuja

(Weleda 6c, 30c; Nelsons 6c; Boots 6c)

Prepared from fresh green twigs of *Thuja occidentalis* tree (American arbor vitae, northern white cedar).

Uses: warts, catarrh, stabbing headaches, migraine, vertigo

when closing the eyes, tooth decay at roots, ear inflammations, cystitis, insomnia, rumbling and flatulence in abdomen.
Suited to: dark-haired, dark-skinned, reserved and perhaps inflexible people.
Symptoms better for: warmth, movement, sneezing, rubbing.
Symptoms worse for: cold, damp, menstruation, tea, coffee, sweets, onions, bright light, sun.
Low time: mid-afternoon, night.

Urtica Urens
(Weleda 6c)

Prepared from the flowering *Urtica urens* plant
(nettle).

Uses: skin rashes and irritations especially from heat or allergy, stinging and burning pains, urticaria, itchy red raised blotches, minor burns which do not blister, sunburn, insufficient breast milk, gout.
Symptoms better for:
Symptoms worse for: cool bathing, cool moist air, touch.
Low time:

Homeopathic preparations

2 Formulated remedies

These remedies are formulated with ingredients specific for one ailment only, and they are marketed specifically for this purpose. Specific doses are recommended, and these are quoted for each product.

Bach Flower Remedies
(Bach Flower Remedies)

A series of liquid concentrates, prepared from various flower sources. 5x extract available from: agrimony, aspen, beech, centaury, cerato, cherry plum, chestnut bud, chicory, clematis, crab apple, elm, gentian, gorse, heather, holly, honeysuckle, hornbeam, impatiens, larch, mimulus, mustard, oak, olive, pine, red chestnut, rock rose, rock water, scleranthus, star of Bethlehem, sweet chestnut, vervain, vine, walnut, white chestnut, wild oat, wild rose, willow. Rescue Remedy contains 5x extracts of cherry plum, clematis, impatiens, rock rose, star of Bethlehem.

Uses: treatment of patients with various moods or states of mind that may hinder recovery from illness. The flower remedies do not work on the physical illness itself. (See manufacturer's literature to determine which remedy is suitable for specific symptoms.) The Rescue Remedy is intended to calm patients who have received bad news or had a startling experience.

Dose: the remedy is diluted before use, according to the manufacturer's instructions. More than one remedy can be taken at one time. The Rescue Remedy (liquid and cream*) can be applied directly to the skin.

Bryonia Cough Linctus
(Nelsons)

A linctus prepared with bryonia alba 6c.

Uses: coughs and chestiness.
Dose: 5 ml 3 times a day.

Candida
(Nelsons)

A tablet prepared with candida albicans 6c.

Uses: candida infections (thrush, athlete's foot).
Dose: adults 2 tablets every hour for 6 doses, then 2 tablets 3 times a day; children use half the adult dose. Stop the treatment when symptoms have gone.

Chamomilla Drops
(Weleda 3x)

A liquid prepared from the root of *Chamomilla recutita* (German camomile – formerly known as *Matricaria chamomilla*).

Uses: For the relief of colicky pain and teething troubles in infants.
Dose: 5-10 drops to be taken in a little water 3 times a day, or, if necessary, 5 drops can be taken every half-hour until the condition improves, for up to 4 hours.

Chamomilla Pillules
(Weleda 3x)

A pillule prepared from the root of *Chamomilla recutita* (German camomile – formerly known as *Matricaria chamomilla*).

Uses: For the relief of colicky pain and teething troubles in infants.
Dose: 1-5 pillules dissolved in the mouth every half-hour until the condition improves. For children under 6 months the pillules may be crushed.

Coldenza
(Nelsons)

A tablet prepared with gelsemium sempervirans 6c.

Uses: influenza and colds.
Dose: adults 2 tablets every hour for 6 doses, then take 2 tablets

3 times a day; children use half adult dose. Stop the treatment when symptoms have gone.

Combination A
(New Era)

Combination of Ferr. Phos. 6x, Kali. Phos. 6x, Mag. Phos. 6x.

Uses: sciatica, neuralgia, neuritis, (consultation with a doctor is also advised).

Combination B
(New Era)

Combination of Calc. Phos. 6x, Kali. Phos. 6x, Ferr. Phos 6x.

Uses: general debility, nervous exhaustion, (consultation with a doctor is also advised).

Combination C
(New Era)

Combination of Mag. Phos. 6x, Nat. Phos. 6x, Nat. Sulph. 6x, Silica 6x.

Uses: acidity, heartburn, indigestion.

Combination D
(New Era)

Combination of Kali. Mur. 6x, Kali. Sulph. 6x, Calc. Sulph. 6x, Silica 6x.

Uses: minor skin ailments.

Combination E
(New Era)

Combination of Calc. Phos. 6x, Mag. Phos. 6x, Nat. Phos. 6x, Nat Sulph. 6x.

Uses: wind, colic, indigestion.

Combination F
(New Era)

Combination of Kali. Phos. 6x, Mag. Phos. 6x, Nat. Mur. 6x, Silica 6x.

Uses: migraine, nervous headaches.

Combination G
(New Era)

Combination of Calc. Fluor. 6x, Calc. Phos. 6x, Kali. Phos. 6x, Nat. Mur. 6x.

Uses: backache, lumbar pain (consultation with a doctor is also advised).

Combination H
(New Era)

Combination of Mag. Phos. 6x, Nat. Mur. 6x, Silica 6x.

Uses: hayfever, allergic rhinitis.

Combination I
(New Era)

Combination of Ferr. Phos. 6x, Kali. Sulph. 6x, Mag. Phos. 6x.

Uses: fibrositis, muscular pain.

Combination J
(New Era)

Combination of Ferr. Phos. 6x, Kali. Mur. 6x, Nat. Mur. 6x.

Uses: coughs, colds, chestiness (consultation with a doctor is also advised, especially if other medications are being taken).

Combination K
(New Era)

Combination of Kali. Sulph. 6x, Nat. Mur. 6x, Silica 6x.

Uses: brittle nails, falling hair (consultation with a doctor is also advised, especially if other medications are being taken).

Combination L
(New Era)

Combination of Calc. Fluor. 6x, Ferr. Phos. 6x, Nat. Mur. 6x.

Uses: varicose veins, circulatory disorders.

Combination M
(New Era)

Combination of Nat. Phos. 6x, Nat. Sulph. 6x, Kali. Mur. 6x, Calc. Phos. 6x.

Uses: rheumatism (consultation with a doctor is also advised).

Combination N
(New Era)

Combination of Calc. Phos. 6x, Kali. Mur. 6x, Kali. Phos. 6x, Mag. Phos. 6x.

Uses: menstrual pain (for adult use only).

Combination P
(New Era)

Combination of Calc. Fluor. 6x, Calc. Phos. 6x, Kali. Phos. 6x, Mag. Phos. 6x.

Uses: aching legs and feet.

Combination Q
(New Era)

Combination of Ferr. Phos. 6x, Kali. Mur. 6x, Kali. Sulph. 6x, Nat. Mur. 6x.

Uses: catarrh, sinus disorders.

Combination R
(New Era)

Combination of Calc. Fluor. 6x, Calc. Phos. 6x, Ferr. Phos. 6x, Mag. Phos. 6x, Silica 6x.

Uses: infants' teething pains.

Dose: 2 tablets dissolved on the tongue 3 times a day at feeding time when teething. For acute pain give 2 tablets in water every 15 minutes.

Combination S
(New Era)

Combination of Kali. Mur. 6x, Nat. Phos. 6x, Nat. Sulph. 6x.

Uses: stomach upsets, sick headaches, biliousness.

Elasto
(New Era)

Combination of Calc. Fluor. 6x, Calc. Phos. 6x, Ferr. Phos. 6x, Mag. Phos. 6x.

Uses: promotes the formation of elastin which is responsible for the repair and maintenance of the elastic tissues in the body; for aching legs and allied conditions.
Dose: adults 2 tablets (children 1 tablet) 3 times a day, or every 30 minutes in acute conditions.

Graphites Cream
(Nelsons)

A cream prepared with graphites 6x.

Uses: dermatitis, to soothe and protect the skin from irritation.
Dose: apply when required.

Mixed Pollen
(Weleda 30c)

Prepared from the following pollens: grasses – bent, brome, cocksfoot, crested dogtail, false oat, fescue, meadowgrass, rye grass, timothy grass, vernal, Yorkshire fog; trees – alder, ash, beech, silver birch, elm, hazel, oak, plane, poplar, willow; flowering plants – heather, nettle, plantain, fat hen, mugwort, borage, rape.

Uses: the relief of hayfever resulting from the above pollens.

Nervone
(New Era)

Combination of Calc. Phos. 6x, Kali. Mur. 6x, Kali. Phos. 6x, Mag. Phos. 6x, Nat. Phos. 6x.

Uses: nerve pains and allied conditions.
Dose: adults 2 tablets (children 1 tablet) 3 times a day (or every 30 minutes in acute cases).

Noctura
(Nelsons)

A tablet prepared with a combination of kali brom 6c, coffea 6c, passiflora 6c, avena sativa 6c, alfalfa 6c, valeriana 6c.

Uses: insomnia.
Dose: 2 tablets 4 hours before bedtime, 2 tablets immediately before bedtime, and 2 more tablets during the night if needed.

Ointment for Chilblains
(Nelsons)

An ointment prepared with tamus communis 6X.

Uses: unbroken chilblains.
Dose: apply as often as needed.

Pollenna
(Nelsons)

A tablet prepared with a combination of allium cepa 6c, euphrasia officinalis 6c, sabadilla officinarum 6c.

Uses: hayfever.
Dose: adults 2 tablets every 2 hours for 6 doses, then 2 tablets 3 times a day; children use half the adult dose. Stop the treatment when symptoms have gone.

Rheumatica
(Nelsons)

A tablet prepared from rhus toxicodendron 6c.

Uses: rheumatic pain.
Dose: adults 2 tablets every hour for 6 doses, then 2 tablets 3 times a day; children use half the adult dose. Stop the treatment when symptoms have gone.

Teetha
(Nelsons)

A powder prepared with chamomilla 6c.

Uses: symptoms of teething.
Dose: the contents of one sachet placed into the child's mouth every 2 hours for up to 6 doses.

Travella
(Nelsons)

A tablet prepared with a combination of apomorph 6c, staphisagria 6c, cocculus 6c, theridion 6c, petroleum 6c, tabacum 6c, nux vomica 6c.

Uses: travel sickness.
Dose: adults 2 tablets every hour for 2 hours before journey, then 2 tablets every hour during journey; children should use half adult dose.

Glossary of medical terms

adrenal glands

the adrenal glands are organs situated above the kidneys which produce hormones, including steroids.

anaesthetic

a substance that induces a loss of sensation and decreases the sensitivity to pain. A local anaesthetic decreases sensation of a body surface, (for example, the skin or the mucous membranes of the throat); example, benzocaine.

analgesic

a substance that relieves pain; example, paracetamol.

antacid

a preparation that reduces the acid content of the stomach, used to relieve indigestion; example, magnesium trisilicate mixture.

anti-platelet

a drug (usually a low-dose aspirin product) used to reduce the risk of blood-clotting disorders, such as stroke or heart attack.

antibiotic

a drug used to destroy bacteria (or to reduce their growth), example penicillin. Most antibiotics are available only on prescription, although a few can be purchased in remedies for throat infections.

anticholinergic

a drug that blocks the action of acetyl choline, a nerve transmitter. Anticholinergics are used to reduce muscle spasm. The effects include dry mouth, difficulty passing urine, and possibly confusion. Example, hyoscine.

anticoagulant

a drug used to prevent blood from clotting, example warfarin. Anticoagulants are available only on prescription.

antihistamine

a preparation that blocks the histamine response in the body which occurs during an allergic reaction. Antihistamines are used to treat all types of allergy (skin rashes, hayfever, etc.). Example, chlorpheniramine.

antihypertensive
a preparation used to lower blood pressure; example, BETA-BLOCKERS. Antihypertensives are available only on prescription.

beta-blocker (ß-blocker)
a drug that blocks some of the effects of adrenaline in the body. Beta-blockers are used to treat angina, high blood pressure, and other conditions. Example, propranolol.

bronchodilator
a drug that relaxes the muscles controlling the bronchi in the chest, causing the tubes to widen, thus easing breathing difficulty; example, theophylline.

carminative
a medicine used to relieve wind.

corticosteroid see steroid

counter-irritant
a substance applied externally to relieve muscular or joint pain by irritating the overlying skin. Counter-irritants are usually found in the warming balms, ointments, and lotions used to treat rheumatic conditions.

diuretic
a drug that removes salt and water from the body, thus treating fluid retention; example, frusemide.

expectorant
a remedy that assists the removal of sputum from the chest by coughing; example, guaiphenesin.

histamine H_2-receptor antagonist
a drug that works on the stomach to reduce acid production, by blocking the histamine pathway; example, ranitidine.

MAOI (mono-amine oxidase inhibitor)
an antidepressant agent that may interact with some foods and other drugs. Example, tranylcypromine.

non-steroidal anti-inflammatory drug (NSAID)

an antirheumatic preparation that has pain-killing properties. An NSAID may cause stomach upsets. Example, ibuprofen.

opiate

a medicine containing an opium-like substance. It acts on the central nervous system to reduce pain and suppress coughs, but may be addictive or cause sedation in high doses. Example, codeine.

rubefacient

a substance applied externally to cause reddening and warming of the skin. Rubefacients are usually found in products used to treat muscle and joint disorders.

steroid

a preparation that supplements the hormones naturally produced by the adrenal gland. Corticosteroids (e.g. prednisolone) are used to suppress inflammatory or allergic disorders, such as asthma, rheumatic conditions, or eczema. Anabolic steroids (e.g. stanazolol) are used to treat vascular disorders, thinning of the bones, and some bone marrow disorders. The anabolic steroids may be abused by some athletes because of their body-building properties. All internal steroids are obtainable only on prescription, but steroids may be purchased for use on the skin or in the mouth (e.g. hydrocortisone creams, hydrocortisone lozenges).

sympathomimetic

a drug that functions like adrenaline and causes narrowing of the blood vessels, but which may open other organs, such as the bronchial tubes; example, pseudoephedrine.

Glossary of herbal names

Agrimony	*Agrimonia eupatoria*
Alder buckthorn	*Rhamnus frangula*
American blackberry	*Rubus villosus*
American ginseng	*Panax quinquefolium*
Angelica	*Archangelica*
Aniseed	*Pimpinella anisum*
Aqua cherry laurel	*Laurocerasus*
Arnica	*Arnica montana*
Artichoke	*Cynara scolymus*
Asafoetida	*Ferula foetida*
Balm of Gilead	*Populus candicans*
Bay	*Laurua nobilis*
Barberry	*Berberis*
Bayberry	*Myrica cerifera*
Birch	*Betula verrucosa*
Black cohosh	*Cimicifuga racemosa*
Blackthorn	*Prunus spinosa*
Bladderwrack	*Fucus vesiculosus*
Blue flag	*Iris versicolor*
Bogbean	*Menyanthes trifoliata*
Boldo	*Peumus boldo*
Boneset	*Eupatorium perfoliatum*
Buchu	*Agathosma betulina (Barosma betulina)*
Buckbean	*Menyanthes trifoliata*
Buckthorn	*Rhamnus catharticus*
Burdock	*Arctium lappa*
Butternut bark	*Juglans cinerea*
Calumba	*Jateorhiza palmata*
Camphor	*Cinnomomum camphora*
Caraway	*Carum carvi*
Cardamom	*Elattaria cardamom*
Cascara	*Rhamnus purshiana*
Cayenne	*Capsicum frutescens*
Celery	*Apium graveolens*
Centaury	*Centaurium erythraea*
Camomile	*Chamaemelium nobile*
Chickweed	*Stellaria media*

Chinese ginseng	*Panax ginseng*
Cinnamon	*Cinnamomum verum*
Clivers	*Galium aparine*
Clove	*Caryophyllin*
Coltsfoot	*Tussilago farfara*
Comfrey	*Symphytum officinale*
Coneflower	*Echinacea angustifolia*
Coriander	*Coriandrum sativum*
Cornsilk	*Zea mays*
Couchgrass	*Agropyron repens*
Cranesbill	*Geranium maculatum*
Damiana	*Turnera diffusa*
Dandelion	*Taraxacum officinale*
Dog's mercury	*Mercurialis perennis*
Elder leaves	*Folia sambuci*
Elderflowers	*Sambucus*
Elecampane	*Inula helenium*
Eucalpytus	*Eucalyptus globulus*
Evening primrose	*Oenothera biennis*
Fennel	*Foeniculum vulgare*
Fenugreek	*Trigonella foenum-graecum*
Feverfew	*Tenacetum parthenium*
Flag lily	*Iris versicolor*
Fumitory	*Fumaria officinalis*
Garlic	*Allium sativum*
Gentian	*Gentiana lutea*
German camomile	*Matricaria chamomilla*
Ginger	*Zingiber officinale*
Golden seal	*Hydrastis*
Gravel root	*Eupatorium purpureum*
Ground ivy	*Glechoma hederacea*
Guaiacum	*Guaiacum officinale*
Guarana	*Paullinia cupana*
Hemlock spruce	*Tsuga canadensis*
Holy thistle	*Cnicus benedictus*
Hops	*Humulus lupulus*
Horehound	*Marrubium vulgare*
Horse chestnut	*Aesculus hippocastanum*
Horseradish	*Amoracia rusticana*
Horsetail	*Equisetum*
Hydrangea	*Hydrangea arborescens*

Hyssop	*Hyssopus officinalis*
Iceland moss	*Cetraria islandica*
Ipecacuanha	*Cephaelis ipecacuanha*
Irish moss	*Chondrus crispus*
Jamaica dogwood	*Piscidia erythrina*
Juniper	*Juniperus communis*
Kava	*Piper methysticum*
Kelp	*Fucus vesiculosus*
Kola	*Cola acuminata*
Korean ginseng	*Panax ginseng*
Lavender	*Lavender angustifolia*
Lemon	*Citrus limon*
Lemon balm	*Melissa*
Lettuce	*Lactuca virosa*
Lime flower	*Tilia cordata/platyphylla*
Liquorice	*Glycyrrhiza glabra*
Lobelia	*Lobelia inflata*
Loosestrife	*Lysimachia nummularia*
Lovage	*Levisticum*
Lungwort	*Pulmonaria officinalis*
Mandrake	*Mandragora*
Marigold	*Calendula officinalis*
Marshmallow	*Althaea officinalis*
Mate	*Ilex paraguariensis*
Meadowsweet	*Filipendula ulmaria*
Motherwort	*Leonurus cardiaca*
Myrrh	*Commiphora molmol*
Nutmeg	*Myristica fragrans*
Oak	*Quercus robur*
Oats	*Avena sativa*
Parsley	*Petroselinum crispum*
Parsley piert	*Aphanes arvensis*
Passionflower	*Passiflora incarnata*
Peppermint	*Mentha piperita*
Pilewort	*Ranunculus ficaria*
Pleurisy root	*Asclepias tuberosa*
Prickly ash	*Zanthoxylum americanum*
Poison oak	*Rhus toxicodendron*
Pokeweed	*Phytolacca americana*
Primula	*Primula officinalis*
Psyllium	*Plantago ovata*

Purple coneflower	*Echinacea purpurea*
Pumilio pine	*Pinus mugo*
Quassia	*Picrasma excelsa*
Quince	*Cydonia oblonga*
Raspberry leaf	*Rubus idaeus*
Rhubarb	*Rheum officinale*
Rosemary	*Rosmarinus officinalis*
Rue	*Ruta graveolens*
Sage	*Salvia officinalis*
St John's Wort	*Hypericum perforatum*
Saw palmetto	*Serenoa repens*
Sarsaparilla	*Smilax ornata*
Scullcap	*Scutellaria lateriflora*
Scurvy grass	*Cochlearia officinalis*
Senega	*Polygala senega*
Senna	*Cassia angustifolia/senna*
Shepherd's purse	*Capsella bursa-pastoris*
Siberian ginseng	*Eleutherococcus senticosus*
Skunk cabbage	*Symplocarpus foetidus*
Slippery elm	*Ulmus rubra*
Small nettle	*Urtica urens*
Snake root	*Polygala senega*
Southernwood	*Artemisia abrotanum*
Spindle tree	*Euonymus*
Squill	*Drimia maritima*
Stinging nettle	*Urtica dioica*
Stone root	*Collinsonia*
Thistle seed	*Carduus marianus*
Thyme	*Thymus vulgaris*
Unicorn root	*Helonias*
Uva ursi	*Arctostaphylos uva-ursi*
Valerian	*Valeriana officinalis*
Vervain	*Verbena officinalis*
White horehound	*Marrubium vulgare*
White willow	*Salix alba*
Wild anemone	*Pulsatilla*
Wild carrot	*Daucus carota*
Wild cranesbill	*Geranium maculatum*
Wild lettuce	*Lactuca virosa*
Wild pansy	*Viola tricolor*
Wild strawberry	*Fragaria vesca*

Willow	*Salix purpurea*
Witch hazel	*Hamamelis*
Wolfbane	*Aconitum napellus*
Woody nightshade	*Solanum dulcamara*
Yarrow	*Achillea millefolium*
Yellow dock	*Rumex crispus*

Index